MW00845418

Musculoskeletal Ultrasound

Musculoskeletal Ultrasound

Anatomy and Technique

John O'Neill, MD
Editor

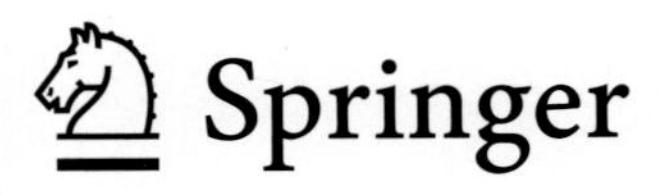

Editor
John M.D. O'Neill, MB, B.A.O, B.Ch, MRCPI, MSc, FRCR(UK)
Assistant Professor
McMaster University
Staff Radiologist, Musculoskeletal Imaging
Diagnostic Imaging Department
St. Joseph's Healthcare
Hamilton, Ontario
Canada

ISBN: 978-0-387-76609-6 e-ISBN: 978-0-387-76610-2
DOI: 10.1007/978-0-387-76610-2

Library of Congress Control Number: 2008924092

Printed on acid-free paper

9 8 7 6 5

springer.com

Dedicated to the memory of my father and
the love and strength of my mother.

Alva, Sam, and Sophie . . . Love . . .

. . . Always.

Preface

Ultrasound is an excellent imaging modality in the evaluation of the musculoskeletal system. It can, however, be intimidating due to the vast array of anatomy that is present and the different techniques and dynamic maneuvers required for a complete study. Many of the excellent musculoskeletal ultrasound texts have opening chapters on technique and anatomy, but the main aim of these texts is to describe the multitude of musculoskeletal pathology and its ultrasound appearance. Often it is necessary to use an anatomy reference text and atlas in addition to these texts. In this book we address the relevant anatomy of the musculoskeletal system by providing a detailed review of the anatomy relevant to that area followed by its normal ultrasound appearance. Anatomy is aided by multiple color illustrations, line drawings, magnetic resonance images, and anatomy review tables. Particular points of interest are highlighted in "Insider Information" boxes.

The normal ultrasound anatomy of structures is described in Section 1. The second half of each chapter details the ultrasound approach and the various techniques employed. This is supported by an extensive array of ultrasound images of the normal anatomy and the corresponding transducer positions. Ultrasound of the peripheral nervous system, including the brachial plexus, is gaining increasing interest, so we dedicated the third section of this text to the peripheral nervous system. Finally, the Appendix outlines the standard ultrasound imaging protocols for the major upper and lower limb joints, including dedicated protocols for assessment of mass lesions, synovitis, and assessment of the hands and feet.

The accompanying DVD, more than 2 hours in length, details the examination of the major joints of the upper and lower limbs. These examinations are presented by many of the individual chapter authors and follow the same imaging guidelines described in the text. All the authors use a structured approach to perform their examinations that is based on anatomy and anatomical landmarks. The evaluation of each joint is presented with a side-by-side arrangement of transducer position and the corresponding ultrasound image. Key anatomical structures and surface anatomy are highlighted throughout the demonstrations.

We hope that this book will encourage and stimulate all those interested in musculoskeletal ultrasound including radiologists, clinicians, sonographers, residents, and medical students.

ACKNOWLEDGMENTS

We would like to extend our gratitude to all who have supported and contributed to this endeavor: Mr. Michael Szabo, St Josephs Healthcare audiovisual department, has gone above the call of duty, devoting numerous hours to editing the DVD and images. Terry Popwich provided expertise and guidance in ultrasound technique. Mike Huska and Michael Lintack from GE Healthcare Canada provided the technical expertise and state-of-the art imaging equipment; Julie Turcotte modeled endlessly for both images and DVD. I thank Toni Cormier and Naveen Parasu for their help in the acquisition of the MRI images, Catriona Kerr and Simon Barrick from Primal Pictures, and Magda Dobranowski for her detailed illustrations. Thanks to my editors who have supported this endeavor, Merry Post and Sadie Forrester, and last, but not least, all my previous mentors for their outstanding teaching.

Contents

Contributors

Julian Dobranowski, MD, FRCPC
Associate Clinical Professor, McMaster University, Diagnostic Imaging Department, St. Joseph's Healthcare, Hamilton, Ontario, Canada

Karen Finlay, MD, FRCPC
Assistant Professor, McMaster University, Staff Radiologist, Diagnostic Imaging, Hamilton Health Sciences–Henderson Division, Hamilton, Ontario, Canada

Lawrence Friedman, MBBCh, FRCPC, FACR
Associate Professor, McMaster University, Radiology Department, Hamilton Health Sciences–Henderson Division, Hamilton, Ontario, Canada

Gandikota Girish, MD, MBBS, FRCS, FRCR
University of Michigan, Musculoskeletal Radiology, Ann Arbor, MI, USA

Aaron Glickman, MSc, MD, FRCPS
Musculoskeletal Radiologist, Toronto East General Hospital, Diagnostic Imaging Department, Toronto, Ontario, Canada

Srinivasan Harish, MD, FRCR, FRCPC
Assistant Professor, McMaster University, Department of Diagnostic Imaging, St. Joseph's Healthcare, Hamilton, Ontario, Canada

Jon A. Jacobson, MD
Associate Professor of Radiology, University of Michigan, Director, Division of Musculoskeletal Radiology, Ann Arbor, MI, U.S.A.

John M.D. O'Neill, Editor, MB, B.A.O, B.Ch, MRCPI, MSc, FRCR(UK)
Assistant Professor, McMaster University, Staff Radiologist, Musculoskeletal Imaging, Diagnostic Imaging Department, St. Joseph's Healthcare, Hamilton, Ontario, Canada

Section 1

Introduction

1

Introduction to Musculoskeletal Ultrasound

John O'Neill

Ultrasound is an effective and established technique in musculoskeletal imaging; its role in diagnostic imaging is continuing to expand with the development of further clinical applications and with the advancement of ultrasound technology. It is well established in Europe as a first line imaging modality in the investigation of musculoskeletal pathology and is rapidly gaining popularity in North America, as shown by the popularity of musculoskeletal ultrasound teaching courses. Ultrasound is, however, operator dependent and requires a detailed knowledge of the relevant anatomy, ultrasound artifacts, technique, and ultrasound appearance of both normal and abnormal structures for the conduction and interpretation of the study. This chapter will detail the anatomy and ultrasound appearance of the constituents of the musculoskeletal system. This is preceded by a brief overview of the history of musculoskeletal ultrasound.

Although musculoskeletal ultrasound may be considered as one of the later developments in ultrasound applications, it was first used, as far back as 1958, in the assessment of the acoustic attenuation of musculoskeletal tissues by K.T Dussik et al.[1,2] Dussik had also been the first to use ultrasound as a medical imaging modality in 1942.[1,3] Ultrasound developed slowly until 1960, when Donald and colleagues produced the first automatic scanner.[1] For the next decade ultrasound was predominantly limited to the evaluation of abdominal and pelvic diseases.

By 1972 the first B-scan image of a joint was reported in the differentiation of a Baker's cyst and thrombophlebitis.[4] Graf, in 1980, published his landmark paper on the use of ultrasound in the diagnosis of congenital hip-joint dislocation.[5] In 1988, L. De Flaviis described ultrasound of the hand in rheumatoid patients including erosions, 10 years after Cooperberg described features of synovial thickening and joint effusion in the rheumatoid knee.[6,7] Since this time, particularly in the past decade, there has not only been a rapid development in ultrasound technology, but also widespread use of ultrasound in the investigation of musculoskeletal disorders to the point where it is now firmly established as a key imaging modality. Ultrasound advances include high-resolution linear array transducers, extended field of view, tissue harmonics, compound imaging, and, recently, early forays into three- and four-dimensional (3-D and 4-D) imaging use in musculoskeletal imaging.

Muscle

There are three different varieties of muscle found in the human body: skeletal, smooth, and cardiac. This description will focus on the structure and ultrasound appearance of skeletal muscle. Muscle is composed of individual fibers, cylindrical or prismatic in shape.[8,9] Each fiber, in general, measures up to 1.5 inches in length and 0.02 inches in breadth. The length of individual fibers is, however, highly variable; those of the sartorius measure up to 2 feet. Individual fibers are surrounded by a sheath: the sarcolemma. A bundle of fibers is called a fasciculus. The fasciculi are prismatic in shape and align parallel to one another, oblique or parallel to the longitudinal axis of the muscle. The endomysium, composed of connective tissue, separates individual muscle fibers. It is derived from the perimysium, which envelops the fasciculus, whereas the epimysium invests the entire muscle (Figure 1.1). Nerves and blood vessels are supported within this connective tissue framework.[8]

Muscles have an origin, a belly, and an insertion. The origin and insertion attachment sites can be multiple, including bones, cartilage, ligaments, and skin. By definition, the insertion is the attachment that has the greatest movement on muscle contraction. There are multiple different arrangements of fiber orientation with respect to the tendon (Figure 1.2). In the quadrilateral type, the fibers are parallel and run in the same longitudinal axis as the tendon, e.g., quadratus femoris, pronator quadratus. The fusiform type, a variation of the quadrilateral, is as the name implies, a fusiform arrangement of the fibers in which the fibers are curved with proximal and distal tapering to the tendon, e.g., biceps (Figure 1.3a). Triangular muscles, such as the infraspinatus, have a wide origin with convergence of fibers into a narrow point of insertion (Figure 1.3b). Feather-like or pennate muscles have a fiber orientation oblique to the tendon. They can be unipennate, bipennate, or multipennate. In unipennate muscles, the tendon lies on one side of the muscle and the fibers insert into it through the length of the muscle, e.g., the extensor digitorum longus. Bipennate muscles have a central tendon with oblique insertion fibers on both sides, e.g., the rectus femoris (Figure 1.3c). Multipennate muscles can have a central tendon with circumferential fiber insertion, e.g., tibialis anterior, or be composed of two or more series in a bipennate arrangement.

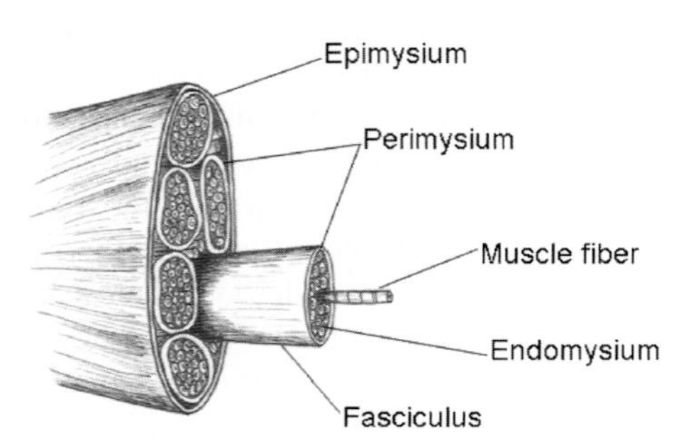

Figure 1.1. Muscle fiber: cross section.

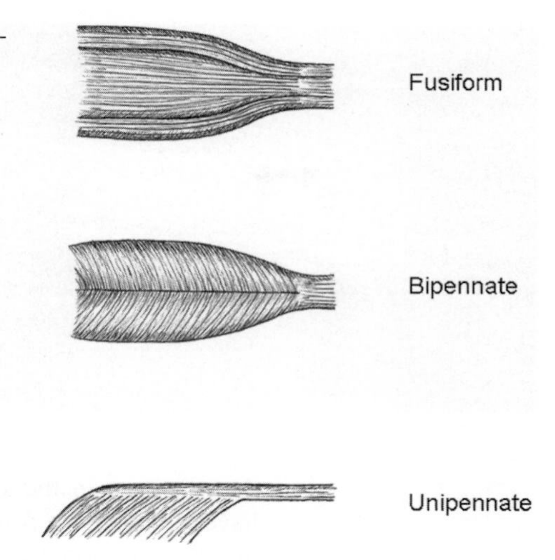

Figure 1.2. Muscle structure: some of the different arrangements of fiber orientation.

The fasciculi can be identified as separate structures on ultrasound.[10,11] They are best identified in the longitudinal plane as hypoechoic cylindrical structures, separated by the hyperechoic intervening connective tissue, the perimysium (Figure 1.4). Individual fibers and the endomysium are not individually discernible. The epimysium, fascia, and intermuscular fat are all thin, linear hyperechoic structures on ultrasound. Ultrasound can also differentiate the different arrangements of muscle fibers: quadrilateral, fusiform, triangular, unipennate, bipennate, or multipennate, as previously described.

During muscle contraction, there is a shortening of fibers and an apparent increase in muscle bulk (Figure 1.5). The hypoechoic fascicles appear thicker and give a more hypoechoic appearance to the muscle in the contracted state. When comparing the echotexture of the contralateral muscle, it is important

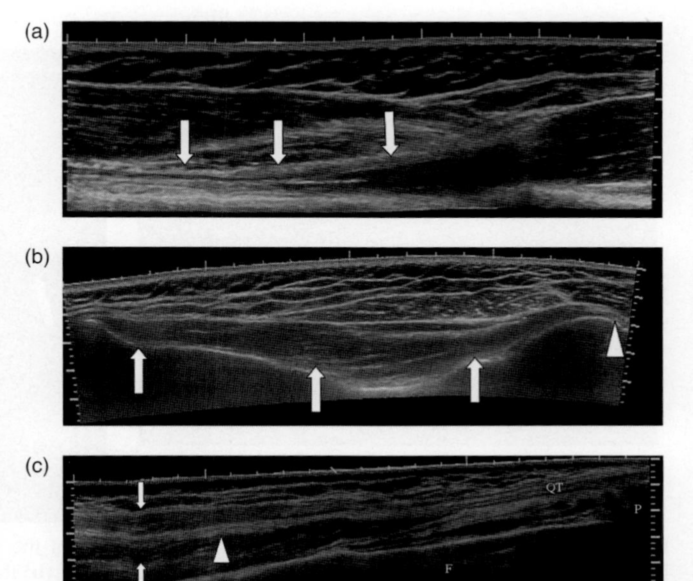

Figure 1.3. **(a)** Longitudinal ultrasound image of the long head biceps tendon at its musculotendinous junction (arrows) demonstrating the fusiform arrangement with proximal tapering of the muscle. **(b)** Extended field of view (EFOV) ultrasound image of the infraspinatus muscle (arrows); an example of the triangular configuration with a wide origin with convergence of fibers into a narrow point of insertion (arrowhead). **(c)** Bipennate: longitudinal EFOV ultrasound image of the distal anterior thigh demonstrating the rectus femoris muscle (arrows) as an example of a bipennate structure with a central tendon (arrowhead) and bilateral oblique insertion fibers. P, patella; F, femur; QT, quadriceps tendon.

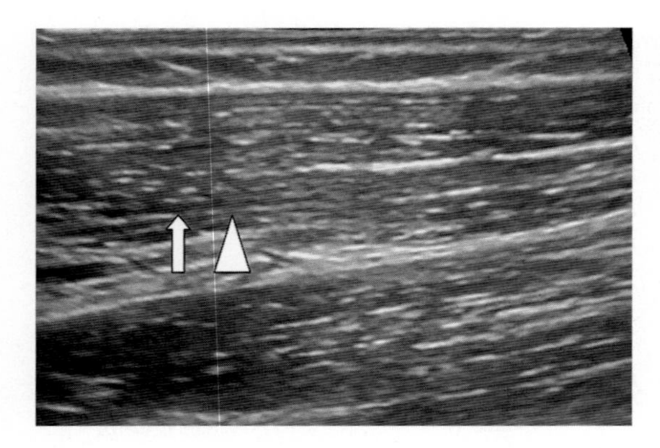

Figure 1.4. Longitudinal ultrasound image of the biceps muscle demonstrating multiple, linear, hypoechoic cylindrical structures: the fasciculi. A muscle fasciculus (arrow) is shown separated by the thin hyperechoic intervening connective tissue, the perimysium (arrowhead).

that they are in the same state of relaxation or contraction. Recent studies have assessed the role of dynamic evaluation in the contraction patterns of muscles in normal and abnormal states. Abnormal contraction patterns may explain different functional capabilities in patients with similar pathology.[12]

Insider Information 1.1
A bundle of muscle fibers, called a fasciculus, can be seen on ultrasound, in its longitudinal axis, as parallel hypoechoic cylindrical structures separated by the intervening hyperechoic connective tissue, the perimysium.

Individual chapters will outline the technical guidelines for specific regions, but, in general, linear array transducers are preferred with higher frequencies for superficial muscles.[10] Deeper muscles may require the use of a curvilinear probe with a frequency of 5 MHz to allow for deeper penetration. Extended field of view can allow for the full length of the muscle to be captured on

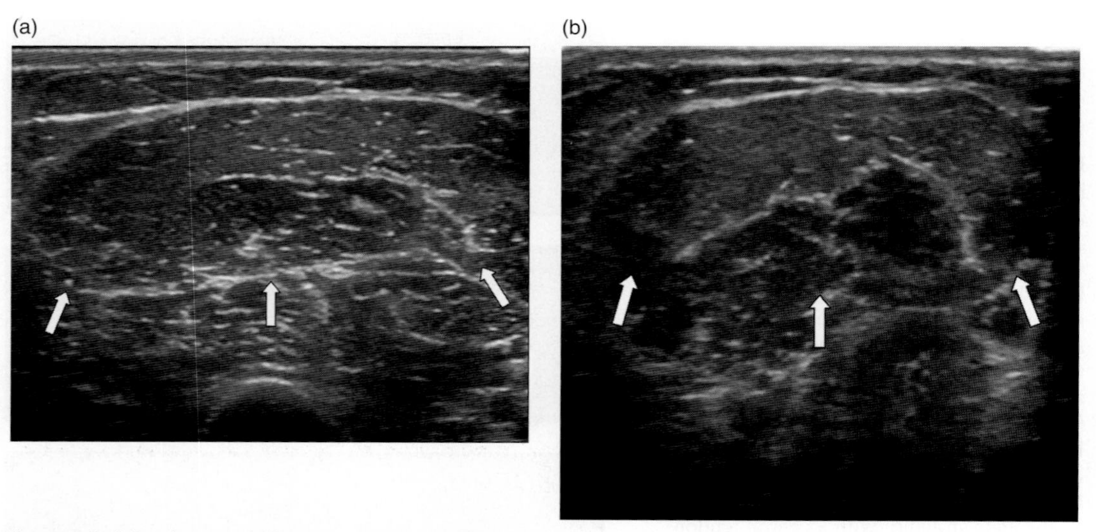

Figure 1.5. Muscle contraction: transverse ultrasound image of the anterior mid-arm biceps muscle, short and long heads (arrows) **(a)** pre- and **(b)** postmuscle contraction. In **(b)** there is an apparent increase in muscle bulk, and the hypoechoic fascicles appear thicker and slightly more hypoechoic.

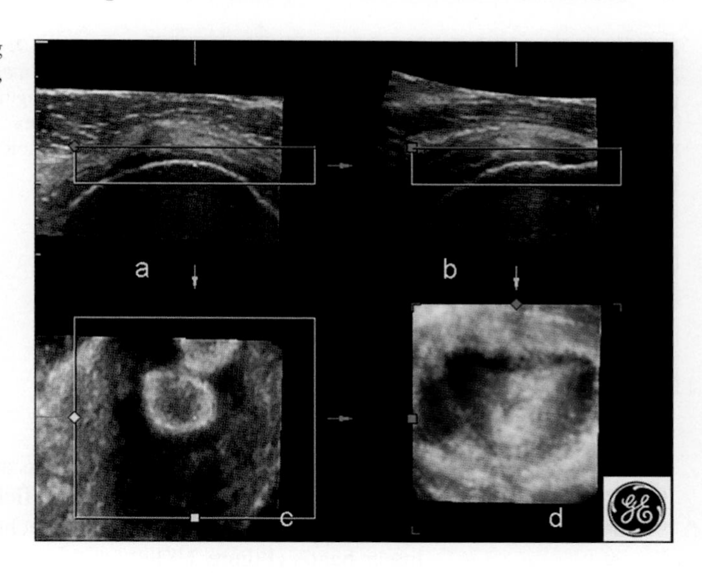

Figure 1.6. Supraspinatus tendon using 4-D transducer; (**a**) axial, (**b**) sagittal, (**c**) coronal, and (**d**) 3-D reconstruction.

one image. 3-D and 4-D are new applications that are in their early stages of development in musculoskeletal ultrasound (Figure 1.6). 3-D will allow multiplanar reformats and may allow better appreciation of the extent of pathology and surrounding anatomical relationships. This may be of particular benefit to referring clinicians not used to viewing ultrasound images.

The probe is held perpendicular to the axis of the muscle and scanned in the longitudinal and transverse planes. If the patient has significant point tenderness, we normally scan the area surrounding this point first until we identify a normal ultrasound appearance and then move slowly over the symptomatic region. Applying gel liberally and floating the probe over the area of interest to avoid compression are useful techniques in these circumstances. This allows the patient to relax and to tolerate a full study. Comparison to the contralateral side is helpful in delineating subtle abnormalities. If a muscle hernia is suspected, direct palpation over the suspected site of the hernia may allow the hernia to be felt as an intermittent soft tissue nodule that appears when the muscle contracts. On ultrasound, the hernia can be seen as a hypoechoic nodule extending through a defect in the fascia. Doppler may reveal the presence of a transversing blood vessel at the same point. Dynamic evaluation, with the patient actively contracting or the examiner passively moving and stretching the muscle of interest, can allow assessment of contraction patterns and aid in identifying the full extent of a muscle tear.

Fascia

Fasciae are divided into superficial and deep fasciae. The superficial fascia lies deep to the skin and is composed of fibroareolar tissue. It is of variable thickness and connects the skin to the deep fascia. It contains adipose tissue of various quantities except in a few areas, such as the eyelid, where it is absent.[8] Beneath this subcutaneous fat is the layer containing subcutaneous vessels and nerves. Collagen fibers within the superficial fascia become dense in the palms, soles of the feet, and the scalp. The superficial fascia may

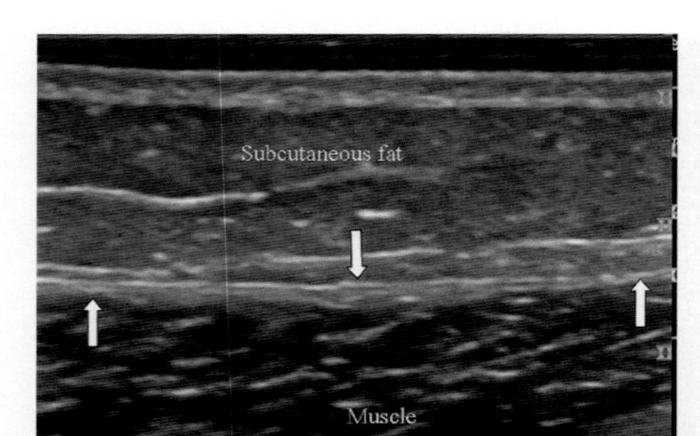

Figure 1.7. Fascia: longitudinal ultrasound image of the proximal thigh demonstrating the superficial fascia containing adipose tissue separated by thin hyperechoic linear bands. The deep fascia (arrows) is thin and hyperechoic, enclosing the deeper hypoechoic muscle.

contain superficial muscles or serve as attachment, e.g., platysma myoides. On **ultrasound,** the appearance of superficial fascia is determined by the content of adipose tissue. The latter is hypoechoic and separated by thin hyperechoic linear bands (Figure 1.7).

The deep fascia is a dense fibrous membrane that invests muscles and deeper structures. It is of variable thickness, becoming thicker on more exposed regions, e.g., it is thicker on the lateral aspect of the leg versus the medial aspect. It forms a sheath for muscles and occasionally as a site of attachment (Figure 1.7). It gives off the intermuscular septa, which separates various muscles and compartments and attaches to the periosteum. In the regions of joints, the deep fascia can become thickened to form retinaculae, as part of fibroosseous tunnels, maintaining the underlying tendons and nerves in place. On ultrasound, the deep fascia is hyperechoic with an identifiable fibrillar pattern of variable thickness. The hyperechoic intermuscular septae can be seen arising from the fascia.

Insider Information 1.2
The deep fascia helps form the muscle compartments and on ultrasound has a hyperechoic fibrillar pattern of variable thickness.

Tendon

Tendons are composed of tightly packed type I collagen fibers with intervening fibroblasts. Bundles of parallel fibers form primary (subfascicle), secondary (fascicle), and tertiary bundles. They are loosely bound in a loose connective tissue sheath, the endotendineum, and the peritendinal connective tissue. The latter encloses several subfascicles to form a fascicle. The peritendineum also contains the supplying blood vessels and nerves. The epitendineum is a thicker fibroelastic sheath surrounding the whole tendon. At the musculotendinous junction the sarcolemma intervenes, i.e., there is no direct continuity of muscle and tendon fibers. At the attachment site to bone, the tendon fibers attach to periosteum, fibrocartilage, or directly to bone. Tendons can also insert onto fascia.[8,9]

Tendons can be round, (e.g., biceps), oval (e.g., Achilles), or flattened (e.g., patellar tendon) in cross section (Figure 1.8). They are surrounded

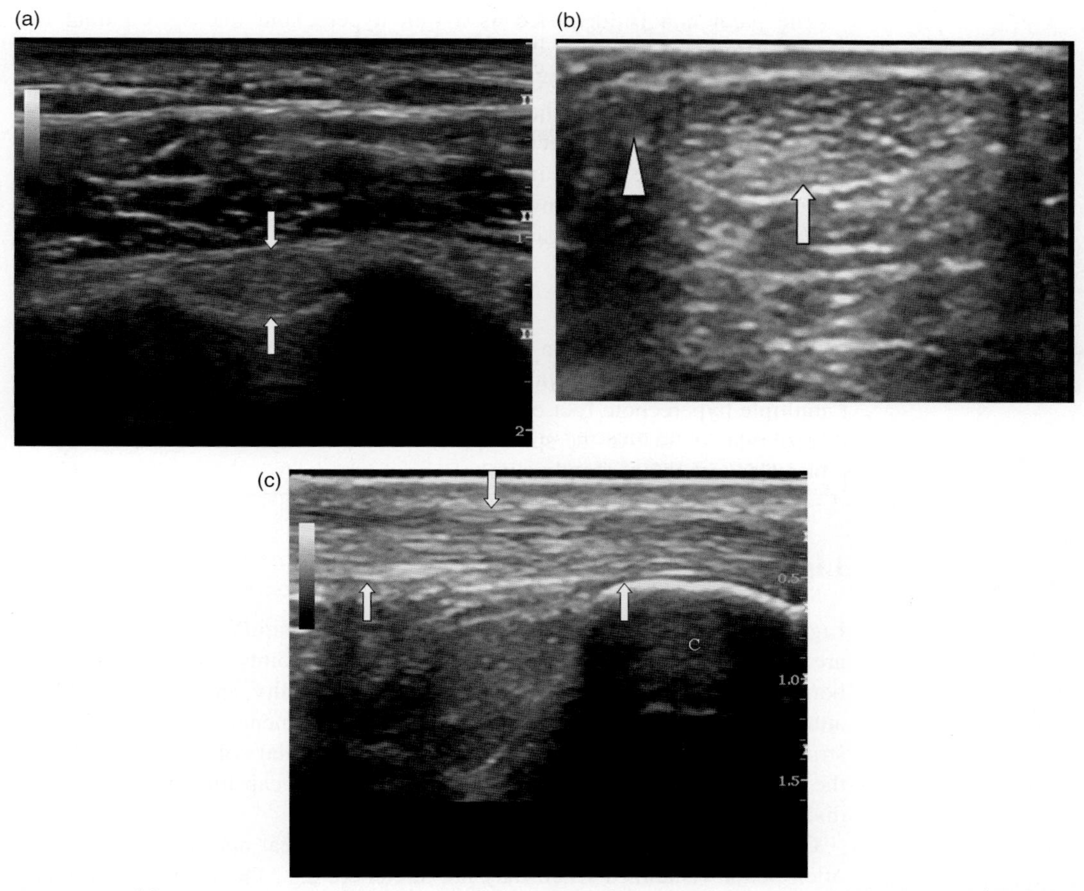

Figure 1.8. (**a**) Transverse ultrasound image of the hyperechoic round long head biceps tendon (arrowhead) within the bicipital groove. (**b**) Achilles tendon (AT) transverse ultrasound image of the oval AT: (arrows) and adjacent plantaris tendon (arrowhead) medially; the paratenon is identified as the thin hyperechoic rim surrounding the AT. (**c**) Longitudinal ultrasound at (arrows). C, calcaneus.

by a synovial sheath in areas where movement of the tendon would cause friction. The synovial sheath is composed of two layers, one of which is reflected along the surface of the tendon. The sheath contains synovium, which secretes a thick viscid fluid to reduce friction and encourage smooth gliding of the tendon. In areas where a synovial sheath is not required, the tendon is surrounded by the paratenon, a layer of loose connective tissue encasing the epitendineum (e.g., Achilles tendon) (Figure 1.8b).

On ultrasound, the tendon is composed of dense linear hyperechoic bands forming a fibrillar pattern when evaluated in the tendon's longitudinal axis (Figure 1.8c). On transverse images, the tendon is hyperechoic with multiple hyperechoic foci or dots (Figure 1.8b). The hyperechoic appearance is due to the specular reflections at the interface between the fascicles and the peritendineum.[10,11] Normal tendons are not compressible. Tendons are particularly prone to the artifact of anisotropy, discussed below, and the transducer must be maintained perpendicular to the axis of the tendon.

The paratenon is identified as a thin hyperechoic line surrounding the tendon (Figure 1.8b). The synovial sheath is best visualized when fluid is present between its layers. A small amount of fluid may normally be present. At the point of insertion, the tendon fibers often appear hypoechoic due to anisotropy as the fibers become curved. Realigning the transducer so it is perpendicular to the change in orientation will resolve most of the hypoechoic appearance in normal tendons; the remaining hypoechoic appearance is related to the interdigitating fibrocartilage.

Insider Information 1.3
On ultrasound, the tendon has a dense linear hyperechoic band pattern, fibrillar pattern, when evaluated in the tendon's longitudinal axis, and multiple hyperechoic foci or dots on the transverse axis. The hyperechoic appearance is due to the specular reflections at the interface between the fascicles and the peritendineum.

Ligament

Ligaments are fibrous structures with a histology similar to tendons. They are usually, but not exclusively, situated around joints and attach bone to bone, helping to maintain correct joint position, stability, and alignment. Their attachment to bone, like tendons, is an enthesis. Ligaments can be well-defined structures easily visualized on ultrasound, e.g., medial collateral ligament of the knee, or represent focal thickening of the joint capsule and may not be discernible as separate structures on ultrasound.

On ultrasound, ligaments have a hyperechoic linear appearance. They are often better visualized when they are stretched, e.g., the anterior talofibular ligament is stretched by mild plantar flexion foot and medial orientation forefoot (Figure 1.9).[13] Linear array transducers with high frequency are optimal. Smaller footpads allow for better manipulation of the transducer along the path of the ligament.

Insider Information 1.4
On ultrasound, ligaments are best evaluated when taut and display a hyperechoic linear appearance.

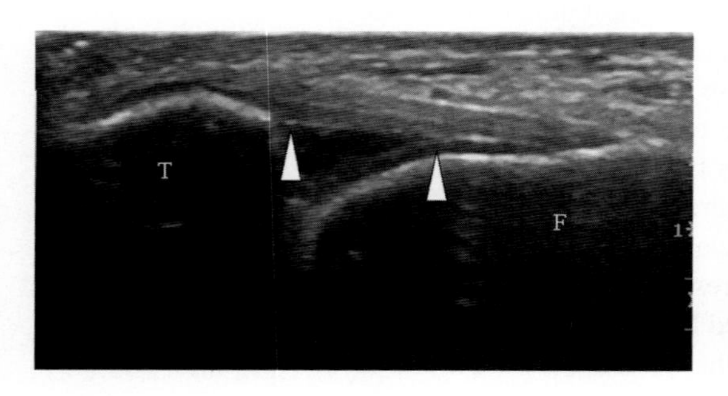

Figure 1.9. Transverse oblique ultrasound distal tibiofibular joint in the longitudinal axis of the anterior talofibular ligament.

Nerve

A peripheral nerve is a cordlike structure containing a large number of individual nerve fibers. The nerve fibers are grouped together into bundles known as fascicles (Figure 1.10). The fascicles are enclosed in a connective tissue sheath or membrane known as the epineurium. Each fascicle is in turn covered by a sheath of connective tissue, the perineurium. The individual nerve fibers within the fascicle are also enclosed by a sheath of connective tissue, the endoneurium. Extending inward from the epineurium is the interfascicular epineurium, which are thin septae adding further support to the nerve bundles and their vascular supply. Similar septae extend inward from the perineurium. The individual nerve fibers are continuous and do not branch or coalesce. The nerve may branch giving off one or more fasciculi and unite with other fasciculi.[8,9]

Ultrasound, in the longitudinal axis of the nerve, demonstrates a fascicular pattern of uninterrupted hypoechoic bands with intervening linear interrupted hyperechoic bands (Figure 1.11a). The hypoechoic bands represent the fasciculi and the hyperechoic bands the supporting interfascicular epineurium. The epineurium is hyperechoic and of similar appearance to perineural fat and may not be separable on ultrasound. On axial study, the nerve is composed of fasciculi seen as multiple hypoechoic dots, which may be of varying size, intermingled in a hyperechoic background of the supporting connective tissue (Figure 1.11b). Identification of individual fascicles will depend on a number of factors, including the depth of the nerve and the frequency of the transducer. In general, the greater the depth and the lower the frequency of the transducer, the lower the resolution. Nerves may become more uniformly hypoechoic when they pass through narrow passages, such as fibroosseous tunnels, with the fascicles becoming tightly packed and less intervening hyperechoic connective tissue.[10,14–16]

Tendons and nerves can have a similar appearance and size. Tendons have a fibrillar pattern versus the fascicular pattern of nerves, are more prone to the artifact of anisotropy, are not normally compressible, and demonstrate more motion on active movement of the adjacent muscles.[14] Small, hypoechoic perineural vessels can be distinguished from the adjacent nerve with color or power Doppler. When nerves pass through fibroosseous tunnels, they are held in place by retinaculae. Dynamic assessment is important to

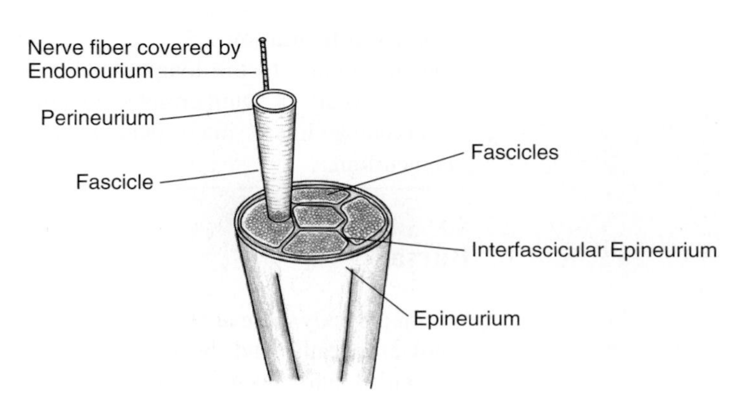

Figure 1.10. Peripheral nerve: cross section.

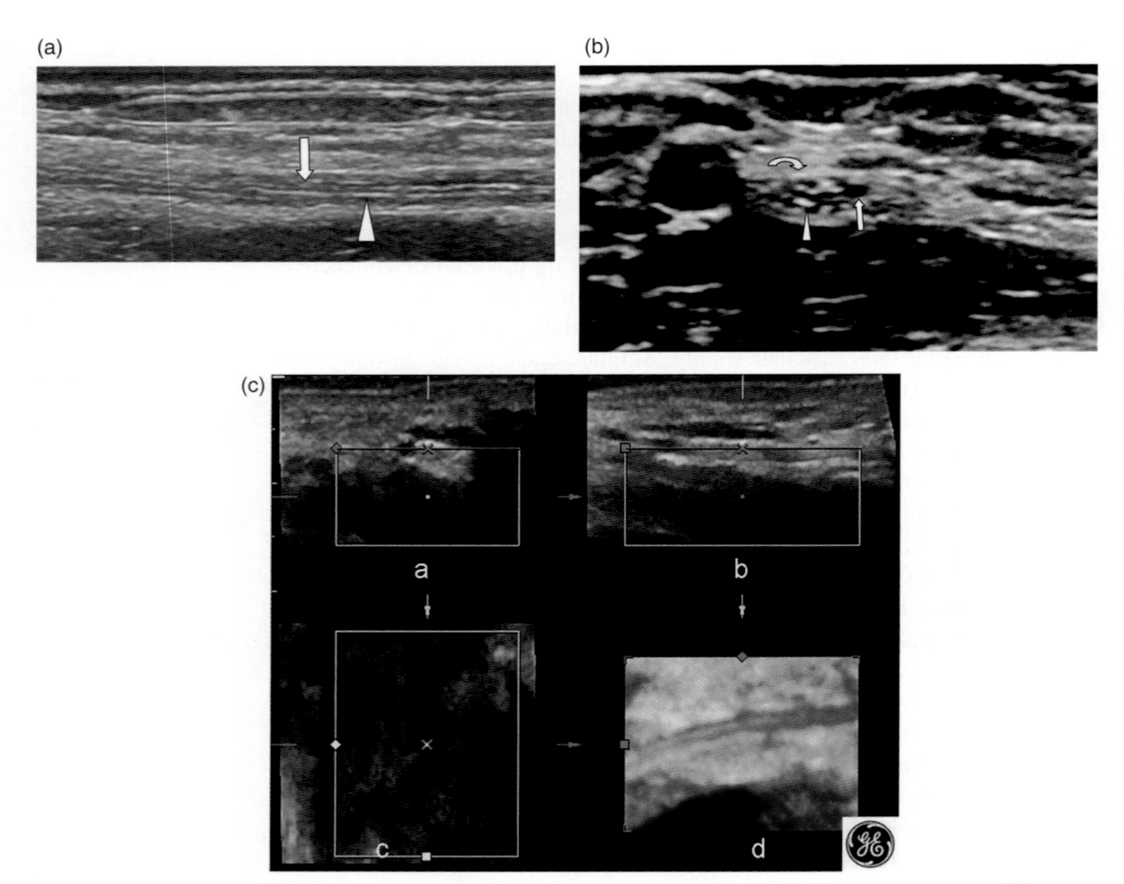

Figure 1.11. Peripheral nerve. (**a**) Longitudinal ultrasound of the medial nerve in the distal arm and (**b**) corresponding transverse image demonstrating the hypoechoic fasciculi (arrows) and the supporting hyperechoic interfascicular epineurium (arrowheads). The epineurium, seen on the axial image (curved arrow) as a thin hyperechoic rim of tissue around the periphery of the nerve, can be difficult to separate from perineural fat due to the same echotexture. (**c**) Ulnar nerve in Guyon's canal using 4-D transducer: (a) axial, (b) sagittal, (c) coronal, and (d) 3-D reconstruction.

exclude subluxation or dislocation of the nerve. A full discussion of dynamic maneuvers employed in this assessment is detailed in Chapter 12.

> **Insider Information 1.5**
> On ultrasound, in the longitudinal axis of a nerve, a fascicular pattern is composed of uninterrupted hypoechoic bands, the fasciculi, with intervening linear interrupted hyperechoic bands, the interfascicular epineurium.

Bursa

Within the body there are three subdivisions of synovial membranes: articular, synovial sheath, and bursal. The bursal synovial membrane is further subdivided into mucosae and synoviae. The former is present within the

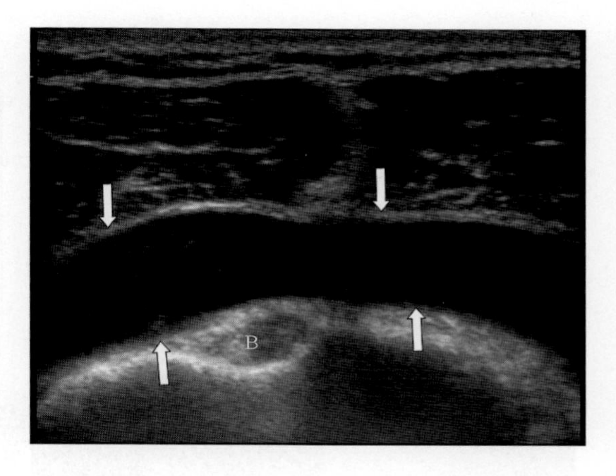

Figure 1.12. Bursa (B). Fluid distension of the subacromial-subdeltoid bursa, extending over the bicipital groove. The bursal capsule (arrows) and peribursal hyperechoic fat have a similar echogenicity and are difficult to separate.

subcutaneous tissue, between skin and underlying bony prominence (e.g., prepatellar bursa between the patella and skin). It becomes distended, for example, when there is increased friction between the bone and overlying soft tissue. Bursae synoviae are located deeper and lie between muscle or tendon and bone, and again serve to reduce friction. Occasionally, these deeper bursae will communicate with the joint, e.g., subscapularis bursa with the shoulder joint, and iliopsoas bursa with the hip joint.[8] Bursae are not usually discernible unless distended in part by fluid, with the fluid then appearing on ultrasound as anechoic between the hyperechoic tissue layers representing adjacent fat planes and capsule (Figure 1.12).

Bone

Although ultrasound has limitations when imaging bone, it does offer excellent anatomical detail of the cortical surface of superficial bone. The high resolution provided by ultrasound allows for the detection and assessment of subtle cortical changes. Fractures, e.g., scaphoid or Hill-Sachs, and erosions of superficial bones that sometimes are not visible on plain radiographs can be demonstrated on ultrasound (Figure 1.13). The cortical surface, however, is highly reflective on ultrasound. This causes the cortex to be visualized as a well-defined hyperechoic continuous line, but obscures the deeper medullary cavity. Deeper cortical surfaces, e.g., the posterior tibia in the calf, usually require a lower frequency transducer. The overlying normal periosteum is not normally identifiable separate from bone and the adjacent soft tissues.

Knowledge of the bony anatomy is essential in the full ultrasound evaluation of the musculoskeletal system. Bony landmarks will often form an easily identifiable location to assess the overlying soft tissues, e.g., Lister's tubercle and the third extensor compartment on the dorsal wrist (Figure 1.14).

Cartilage

Cartilage can be divided into hyaline cartilage, white fibrocartilage, and elastic or yellow fibrocartilage. The latter is present in only select regions, e.g., the auricle of the external ear. Articular cartilage, costal cartilage, and temporary

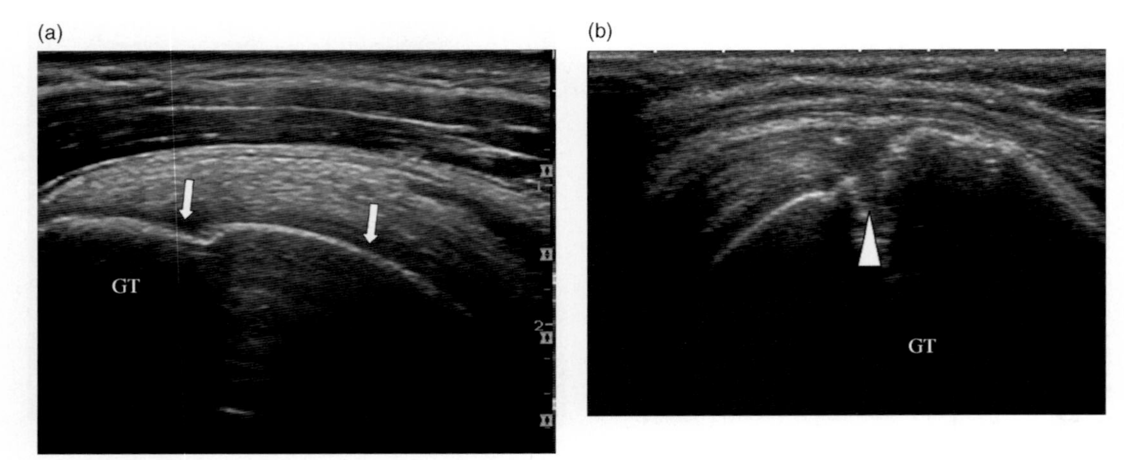

Figure 1.13. (**a**) Cortical bone: ultrasound of the normal greater tuberosity (GT) of the humerus demonstrating a smooth hyperechoic line consistent with cortex margin with posterior acoustic shadowing. (**b**) Fracture (arrowhead) GT with interruption of the normal smooth cortical line demonstrated in (**a**).

cartilage are composed of hyaline cartilage. With the exception of articular cartilage, cartilage is covered by perichondrium. Articular cartilage is of varying thickness, being thicker in points of greater stress and on convex rather than concave surfaces. It provides a degree of elasticity and shock absorption, as well as helping to dissipate stress across a joint.[8,9]

On ultrasound, it has a smooth, well-defined surface and border and is uniformly hypoechoic (Figure 1.15). In children, cartilaginous centers prior to ossification are not visible on plain radiographs, but are clearly visible on ultrasound as hypoechoic structures with early ossification beginning centrally as a zone of hyperechogenicity (Figure 1.16).

Fibrocartilage is a variable mixture of white fibrous tissue and cartilaginous tissue with a large component of collagen fibrils. It provides elasticity and flexibility. The menisci of the knee, temporomandibular and sternoclavicular

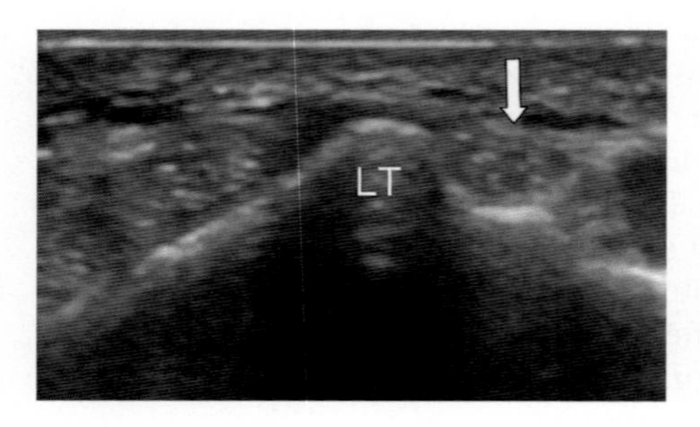

Figure 1.14. Lister's tubercle (LT) on the dorsal aspect of the distal radius is an important bone landmark in the assessment of the dorsal tendon compartments. The extensor pollicis longus tendon (arrow) lies on its ulnar aspect and is separated from the second compartment by LT.

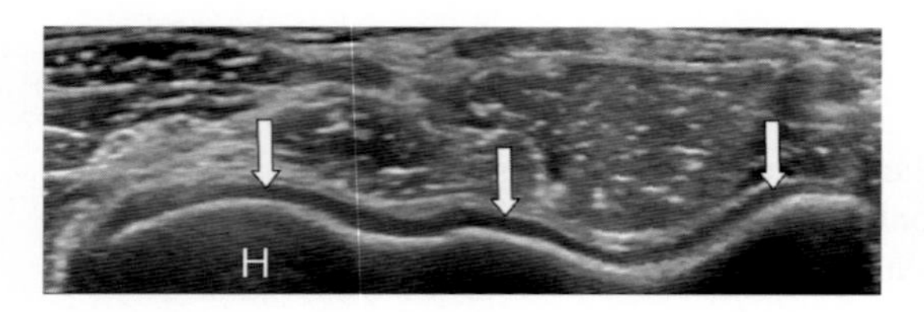

Figure 1.15. Articular cartilage: transverse ultrasound demonstrating the well-defined, uniformly hypoechoic normal articular cartilage (arrows) at the articulating surface of the distal humerus (H).

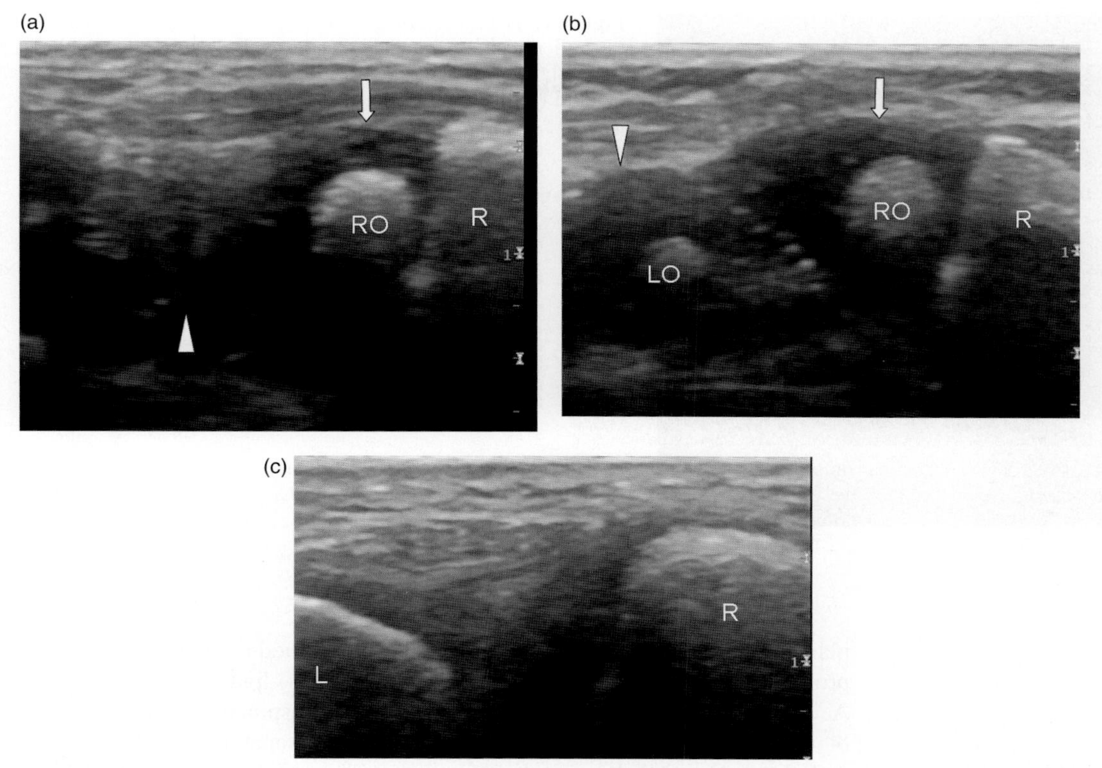

Figure 1.16. Cartilaginous centers prior to ossification are clearly visible on ultrasound as hypoechoic structures with early ossification beginning centrally as a zone of hyperechogenicity. (**a**) Longitudinal ultrasound of a 2-year-old girl demonstrating early ossification of the center distal radius (RO) surrounded by the hypoechoic cartilaginous center. No ossification has commenced within the lunate (arrowhead), which remains uniformly hypoechoic. (**b**) An early ossification center is now visible in the lunate (LO) in this 4-year-old boy. (**c**) Normal adult appearance.

joints, the glenoid and hip labra, and the triangular fibrocartilage of the wrist are composed of fibrocartilage. On ultrasound, fibrocartilage is hyperechoic with well-delineated borders. Because of its position within joints, it is not always fully accessible to a full ultrasound examination (Figure 1.17).

Insider Information 1.6
In children, cartilaginous centers, prior to ossification, are not visible on plain radiographs but are clearly visible on ultrasound as hypoechoic structures. Early ossification can be seen, beginning centrally, as a zone of hyperechogenicity.

Anisotropy

Anisotropy is one of the commonest, and probably the most important artifact, in musculoskeletal ultrasound imaging. Anisotropy is the different ultrasound echogenicity of normal tissue when the angle of insonation is not 90° to the

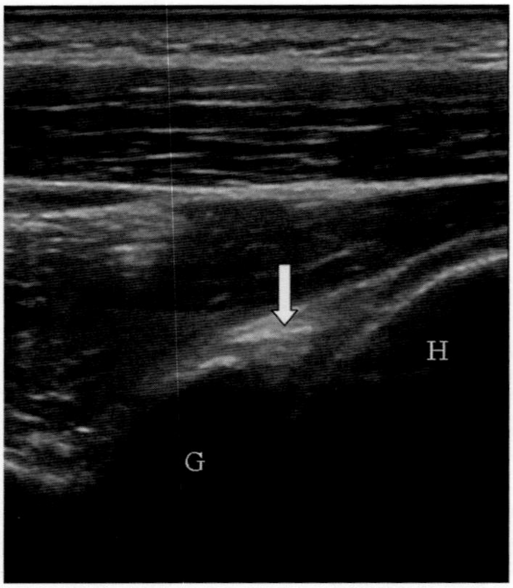

Figure 1.17. Fibrocartilage. The posterior glenoid labrum (arrow) is demonstrated here as a well-defined, hyperechoic triangular structure between the articulating surfaces of the glenoid (G) and humerus (H).

plane of the structure being imaged. It is best identified in tendons and is less pronounced in other soft tissues including muscles, ligaments, and nerves. A common site of occurrence is within the supraspinatus tendon because of its coronal oblique course and angulation. To separate anisotropy from pathology, the transducer is held in the same position but is angled until it is perpendicular to the tissue of interest, at which point the artifactual hypoechoic appearance will resolve in normal tendons and the tissue will be of homogeneous echogenicity (Figure 1.18).

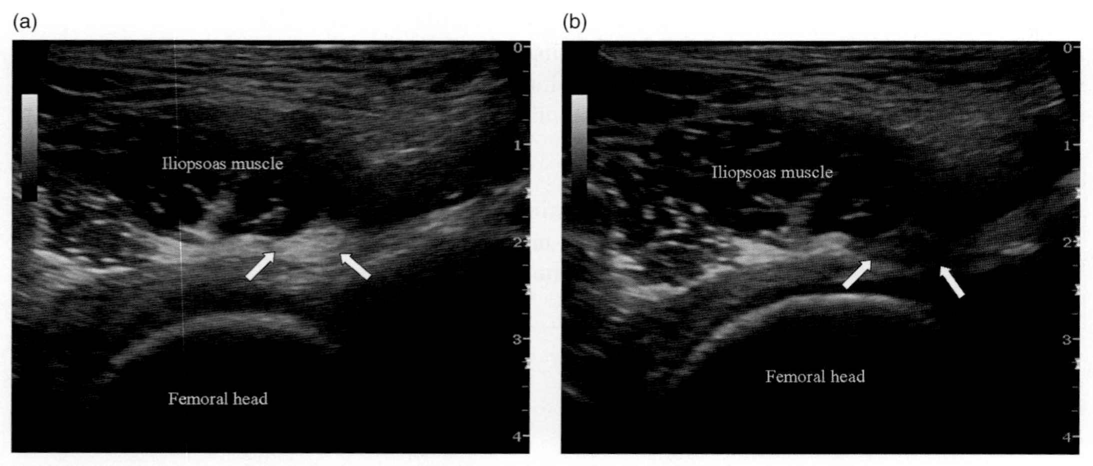

Figure 1.18. Anisotropy. The iliopsoas tendon (arrows) demonstrates a normal hyperechoic appearance in transverse ultrasound image **(a)**. By angulating the ultrasound beam 5° to 10°, so that the beam is no longer perpendicular to the hyperechoic tendon, the iliopsoas tendon becomes artifactually hypoechoic and simulates pathology **(b)**.

References

1. Kane D, Grassi W, Sturrock R et al. A brief history of musculoskeletal ultrasound: 'From bats and ships to babies and hips.' Rheumatology 2004;43:931–933.
2. Dussik KT, Fritch DJ, Kyriazidou M et al. Measurements of articular tissues with ultrasound. Am J Phys Med 1958;37:160–165.
3. Dussik KT. On the possibility of using ultrasound waves as a diagnostic aid. Z Neurol Psychiatr 1942;174:153–168.
4. McDonald DG, Leopold GR. Ultrasound B-scanning in the differentiation of Baker's cyst and thrombophelebitis. Br J Radiol 1972;45:729–732.
5. Graf R. The diagnosis of congenital hip-joint dislocation by the ultrasonic combound treatment. Arch Orthop Trauma Surg 1980;97:117–133.
6. De Flaviis L, Scaglione P, Nessi R et al. Ultrasonography of the hand in rheumatoid arthritis. Acta Radiol 1988;29:457–460.
7. Cooperberg PL, Tsang I, Truelove L et al. Gray scale ultrasound in the evaluation of rheumatoid arthritis of the knee. Radiology 1978;126:759–763.
8. Gray H. General anatomy or histology. In: The Complete Gray's Anatomy, 16th ed., pp. 1–72. London: Longman, Green, and Co., 1905.
9. Snell R. Basic anatomy. In: Clinical Anatomy, 7th ed., pp. 1–48. Philadelphia: Lippincott Williams & Wilkins, 2004.
10. Martinoli C, Bianchi S, Dahmane M. Ultrasound of tendons and nerves. Eur Radiol 2002;12:44–55.
11. van Holsbeeck M, Introcaso J. Sonography of tendons. In: Musculoskeletal Ultrasound, 2nd ed., pp. 77–81. St. Louis: Mosby, 2001.
12. Boehm T, Kirschner S, Mueller T. Dynamic ultrasonography of rotator cuff muscles. J Clin Ultrasound 2005;33:207–213.
13. Peetrons P, Creteur V, Bacq C. Sonography of ankle ligaments. J Clin Ultrasound 2004;32:491–499.
14. Silvestri E, Martinoli C, Derch L et al. Echotexture of peripheral nerves: Correlation between US and histologic findings and criteria to differentiate tendons. Radiology 1995;197(1):291–296.
15. Gruber H, Kovacs P. Sonographic anatomy of the peripheral nervous system. In: Peer S, Bodner G (eds.). High Resolution Sonography of the Peripheral Nervous System, 1st ed., pp. 28–32. New York: Springer, 2003.
16. Peer S. High-resolution sonography anatomy of the peripheral nervous system: General considerations and technical concepts. In: Peer S, Bodner G (eds.). High Resolution Sonography of the Peripheral Nervous System, 1st ed., pp. 1–11. New York: Springer, 2003.

Section 2

The Upper Limb

2

The Shoulder

John O'Neill

The shoulder joint is the commonest joint examined sonographically, and is often the first joint on which most imagers are introduced to musculoskeletal ultrasound. The shoulder is superficial and readily accessible to ultrasound assessment and is excellent for assessing the normal anatomy and pathology of the shoulder joint; it has sensitivities and specificities in assessment of the rotator cuff that are comparable to magnetic resonance imaging (MRI). Ultrasound offers excellent resolution, is multiplanar, accessible, and cost efficient. One of ultrasound's main strengths is its ability to image in real time the normal dynamic motion of joints and surrounding soft tissues. This dynamic component of the study may expose pathologies not apparent in a static examination. This feature is particularly important in assessing for subluxation of the biceps tendon or impingement syndromes, e.g., supraspinatus or subcoracoid impingement. In addition, ultrasound allows for a more complete functional assessment of the structure. This chapter will outline the clinical indications for shoulder ultrasound, discuss the transducers suited to the examination, and then review the normal anatomy of this region. Anatomy will include a brief overview of surface anatomy, which will allow the imager to identify key landmarks that can then be used to formulate a structured and reproducible approach to the study as detailed in the section on ultrasound technique.

Clinical Indications

The commonest indication is in the assessment of rotator cuff and biceps tendon pathology, including tendinosis, partial and full thickness tears, and impingement syndromes. Rheumatology referrals for joint effusion, synovial thickening, and erosions are increasing in number. Subtle nondisplaced fractures, particularly of the greater tuberosity, and Hill–Sachs defects, which may not be identified on plain radiographs, may be identified in a patient with persistent posttraumatic pain. Ultrasound can identify etiologies of nerve impingement, e.g., suprascapular nerve impingement and potential secondary findings such as atrophy and fatty infiltration of the supplied muscles. Labral injuries, particularly posterior labral tears with paralabral cyst formation, can be identified, although a full evaluation of the labrum requires MRI. Ultrasound is an important imaging modality in the primary imaging assessment of soft tissue masses, and is beneficial in assessing for solid/cystic components, internal and adjacent vascularity, and dynamic and functional components.

Interventional procedures include ultrasound-guided biopsy of soft tissue masses, arthrograms (e.g., in patients requiring MRI but who are allergic to iodine used in fluoroscopically guided injections), direct joint or tendon injections, joint aspiration, aspiration and dissolution of calcific tendinosis, and aspiration and injection of bursae and paralabral cysts.

The acromioclavicular joint can also be assessed at the same time for a wide range of local pathology including degeneration, inflammatory arthropathy, trauma, and joint sepsis. Interventional procedures include joint aspiration and injection.

Technical Equipment

High-resolution linear array transducers with a broad-bandwidth frequency between 7.5 and 12 MHz are generally preferred, with frequencies lower and higher required for deep and superficial structures, respectively. Linear array transducers lack divergent beam geometry, which accentuates anisotropy. Color and power Doppler are valuable in assessing hyperemia in inflammatory or reparative tissue and the vascularity of soft tissue masses, as well as in differentiating cystic lesions from vascular structures. Evaluation of deeper structures, depending on the patient's habitus, including the anterior labrum, may require a low-frequency curved array transducer.

Anatomy

Surface Anatomy

The clavicle is palpable, throughout its length, at the root of the neck. At its distal end it forms the articulation with the acromion, the acromioclavicular joint, which is felt as a change in the smooth contour of the clavicle. The acromion is the superolateral bony projection from the scapula directly over the glenohumeral joint. Anterior, lateral, and posterior to the acromion is the smooth soft tissue contour of the deltoid muscle that covers the glenohumeral joint and the humeral tuberosities. Anteriorly, a triangular depression is formed between the medial border of the deltoid and the pectoralis major: the deltopectoral angle. Within the lateral aspect of this triangle, a bony prominence can be felt on deep palpation: the coracoid process of the scapula (Figure 2.1). The anterior and posterior axillary folds are formed by the pectoralis major and latissimus dorsi muscles, respectively.[1] Posteriorly, extending from the acromion, a palpable bony ridge—the scapular spine—separates the supraspinatus and infraspinatus fossae. The soft tissue contour of the posterior aspect of the joint is formed in part by the supraspinatus and infraspinatus muscles as well as the overlying musculature, which includes the deltoid, trapezius, and latissimus dorsi muscles. Patients with atrophy of these muscles may have a visible loss of mass in this region when compared with a normal contralateral side (Figure 2.1).

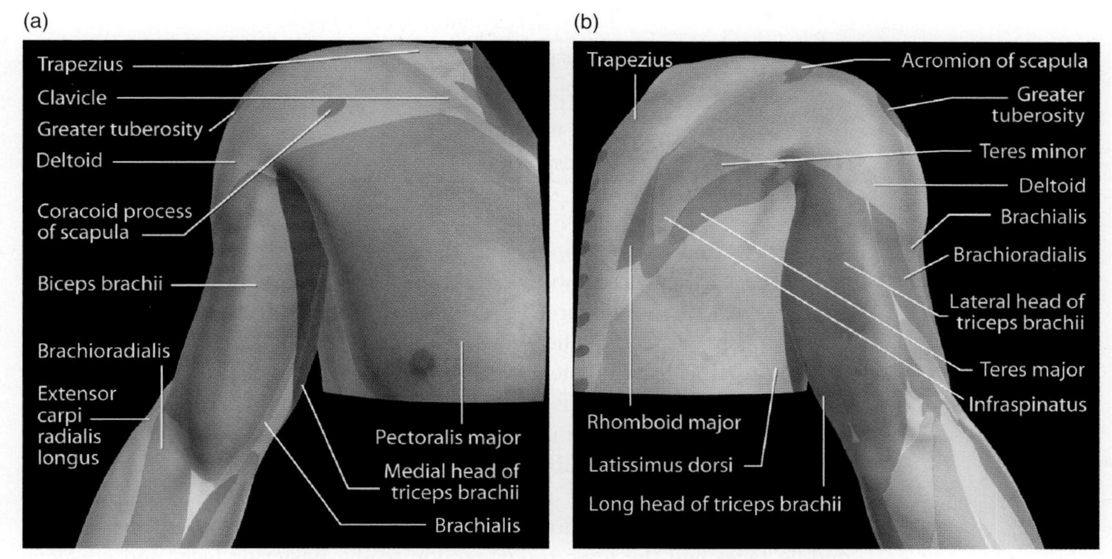

Figure 2.1. The surface anatomy of the shoulder: **(a)** anterior and **(b)** posterior views.

Bones

The glenohumeral joint is an enarthrodial, or ball-and-socket, joint with multidirectional capabilities (Figure 2.2).[2] This wide range of motion is facilitated by the shallow glenoid fossa of the scapula articulating with the significantly larger humeral head. This anatomical arrangement, however, predisposes the joint to dislocation, which in turn is counteracted by the support mechanism of the glenohumeral ligaments, the rotator cuff tendons (Table 2.1), and the glenoid labrum. The articulating surfaces of the humerus and glenoid are covered by articular cartilage, which is thin at the center of

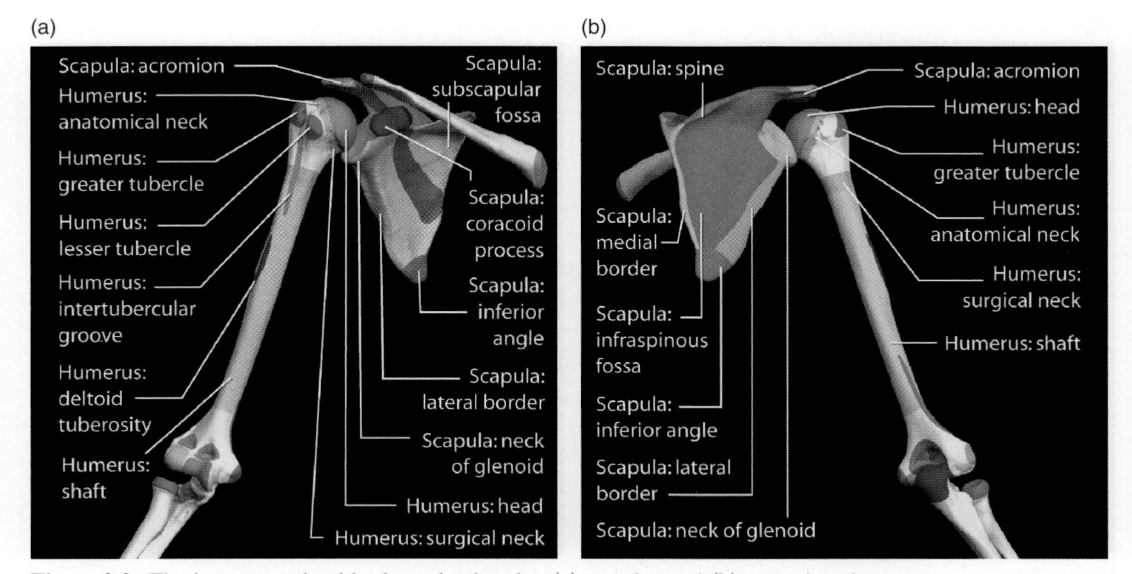

Figure 2.2. The important shoulder bony landmarks: **(a)** anterior and **(b)** posterior views.

Table 2.1. Rotator Cuff Muscles.

Supraspinatus
Infraspinatus
Teter minor
Subscapularis

the glenoid and thick peripherally; the opposite holds true for the humeral head. The cartilage is continuous except for a focal spot on the posterosuperior aspect of the humeral head, known as the bare area. On ultrasound, the peripheral aspect of the humeral articular cartilage is identifiable as a continuous thin hypoechoic covering of uniform thickness with the deeper cortical bone visualized as a smooth uninterrupted hyperechoic line with posterior acoustic shadowing.

The rounded greater tuberosity is lateral to the humeral head and has three facets. The anterior and middle facets serve as sites of attachment for the supraspinatus tendon; the infraspinatus tendon also attaches to the middle facet and the teres minor tendon to the posterior facet and adjacent humeral shaft (Figure 2.3). The lesser tuberosity is smaller, anteromedial, and separated from the greater tuberosity by the bicipital groove. The subscapularis tendon attaches to the lesser tuberosity and the adjacent humerus (Figures 2.2 and 2.3).

The acromion, meaning shoulder summit, is the termination of the scapular spine. It may be oblong or triangular in shape and has a smooth concave undersurface. It has three centers of ossification that usually unite by 22 years.[3] If nonunion persists, it is termed os acromiale, and is important to identify when present. Os acromiale occurs in approximately 5% of the population and is bilateral in up to 20% of cases. The fibrous capsule of the joint is lax, which allows for the wide range of motion, and is lined by a synovial

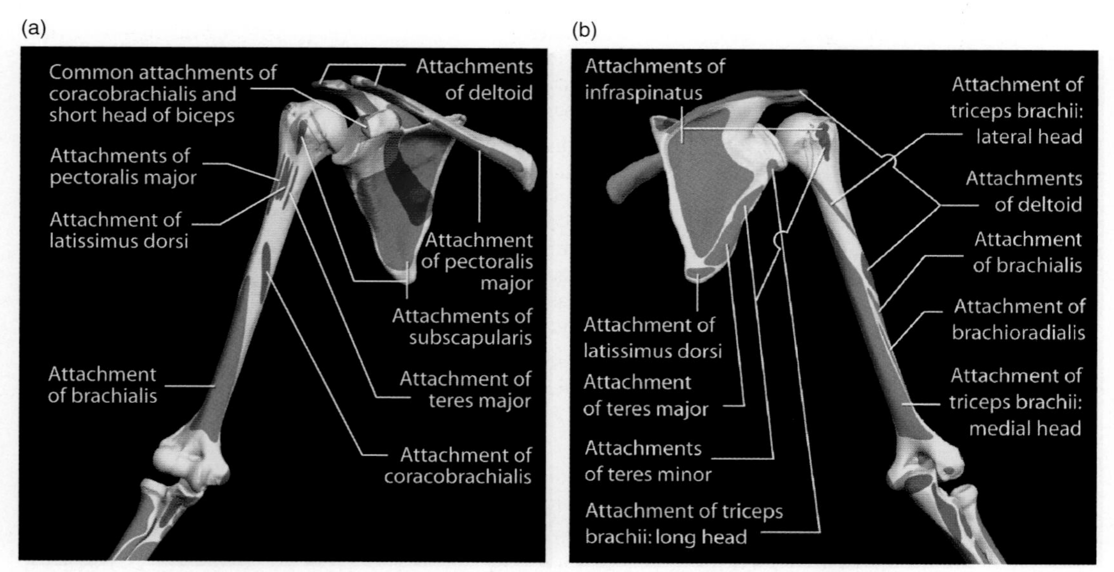

Figure 2.3. The muscle origin (red) and insertion (blue) points of the shoulder girdle muscles: **(a)** anterior and **(b)** posterior views.

membrane. The capsule attaches to the anatomical neck of the humerus and the circumference of the glenoid, posterior to the glenohumeral ligaments. It is strengthened by these ligaments, which are not usually identifiable on ultrasound, and by surrounding tendons including the subscapularis, the long head of the biceps, supraspinatus, infraspinatus, teres minor, long head triceps, and the coracohumeral ligament. Three main capsular openings may exist. The first is for the transmission of the long head of the biceps; the second is anterior and subcoracoid and communicates with the subscapularis bursa; the third, if present, lies posteriorly and communicates with the infraspinatus bursa.

Muscles and Tendons

The supraspinatus, infraspinatus, subscapularis, and teres minor muscles form the rotator cuff. Their origin, insertion, and actions are outlined in Table 2.2.[4] The supraspinatus, infraspinatus, and teres minor insert onto the greater tuberosity, from anterior to posterior, forming a continuous layer separating the subacromial bursa from the glenohumeral joint space and forming an important supporting mechanism for the joint capsule. In addition, they act as dynamic stabilizers of the glenohumeral joint and counteract the upward translation induced by the deltoid.[3] The muscles of the shoulder are shown in Figure 2.4.

Table 2.2. Shoulder Muscles.

Muscle	Origin	Insertion	Main action
Supraspinatus	Supraspinous fossa scapula	Greater tuberosity—anterior and middle facets	Shoulder/arm abduction
Infraspinatus	Infraspinous fossa scapula	Greater tuberosity—middle facet	External rotation, stabilizer
Subscapularis	Subscapular fossa scapula	Lesser tuberosity	Internal rotation, stabilizer
Teres minor	Dorsal surface axillary border scapula	Greater tuberosity—posterior facet and adjacent humeral shaft	External rotation, stabilizer
Biceps Long head	Supraglenoid tubercle scapula	Radial tuberosity and bicipital aponeurosis	Flexion and supination forearm
Short head	Apex coracoid process	Unites with long head to form a single tendon that inserts onto the radial tuberosity, bicipital aponeurosis	Flexion and supination forearm
Pectoralis major	Anteromedial aspect clavicle, sternum, and upper six costal cartilages	Lateral ridge of the bicipital groove	Adductor, medial rotator, and flexor arm
Pectoralis minor	Third to fifth ribs	Medial border; coracoid process	Protracts scapula
Deltoid	Anterolateral third clavicle, the acromion, and the spine of the scapula	Deltoid tuberosity (mid humerus)	Abducts arm to horizontal (anterior fibers); flexes and extends arm (posterior fibers)

(a)

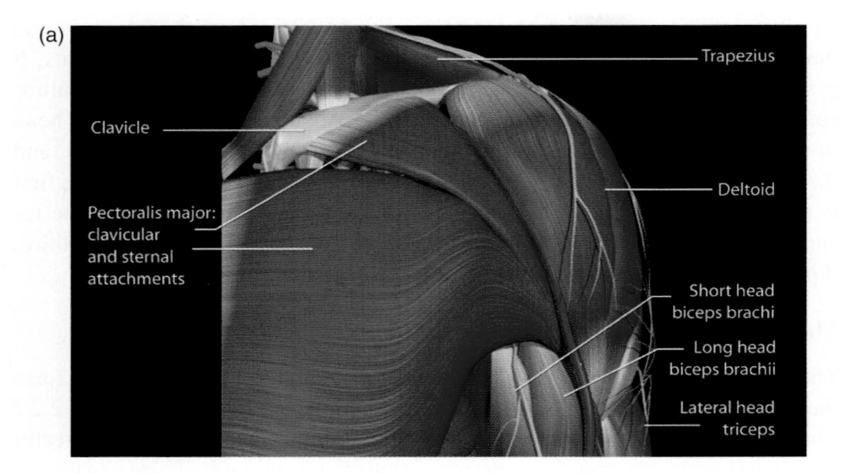

(b)

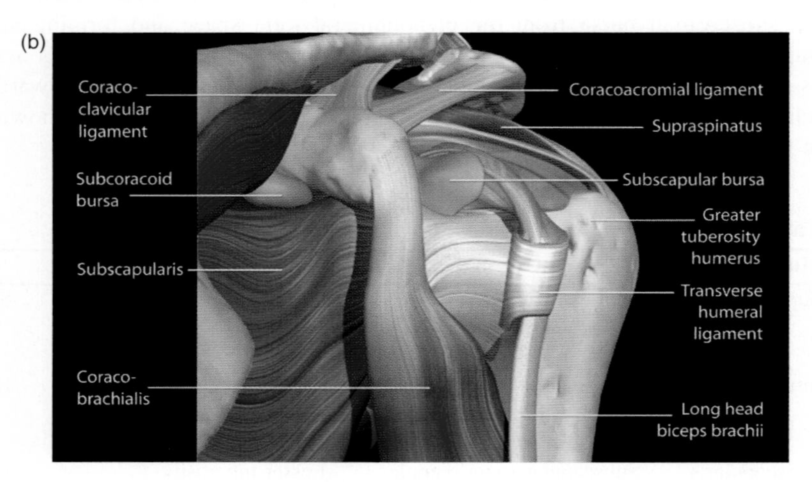

(c)

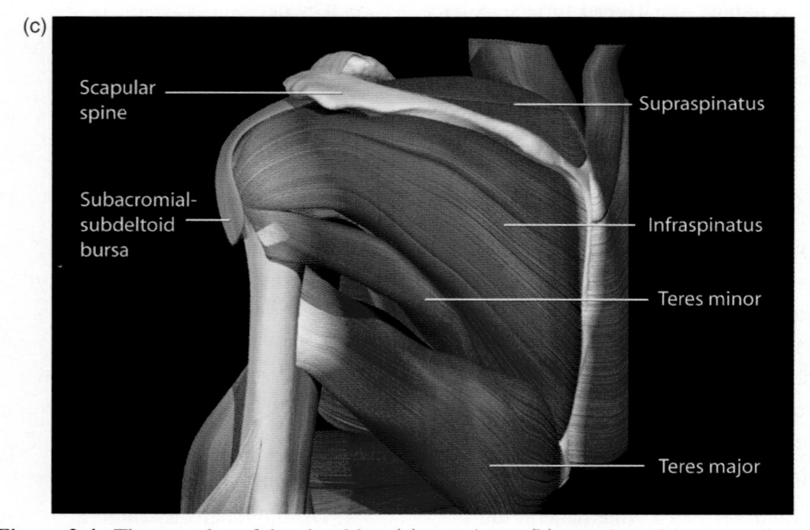

Figure 2.4. The muscles of the shoulder: **(a)** anterior c, **(b)** anterior with pectoralis and deltoid muscles removed, **(c)** posterior with deltoid and trapezius muscles removed.

(d)

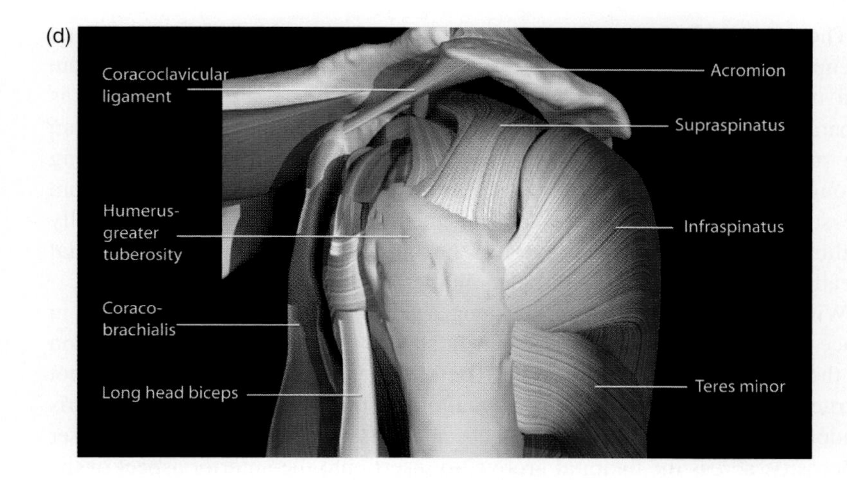

(e)

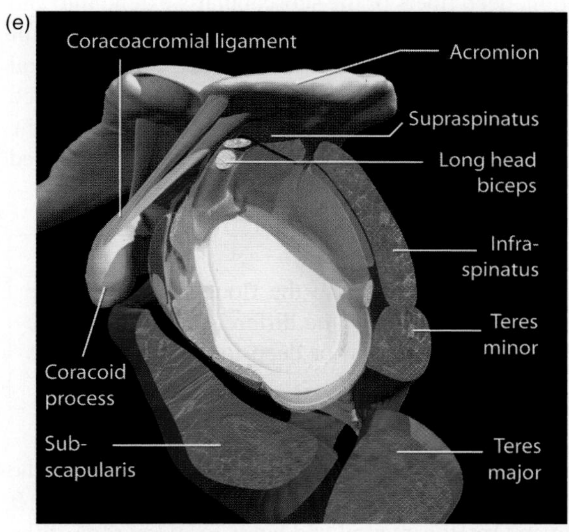

Figure 2.4. (*Continued*) The muscles of the shoulder: **(d)** lateral view with deltoid muscle removed, and **(e)** sagittal through shoulder joint with humerus removed.

The supraspinatus originates from the supraspinatus fossa of the scapula and adjacent scapular spine. The tendon has two components, ventral and dorsal, arising from the muscle and extending obliquely anteriorly, approximately 50° to the coronal plane, over the superior aspect of the humeral head to insert predominantly on the anterior and middle facets of the greater tuberosity.[5–7] The infraspinatus muscle arises from the internal two-thirds of the infraspinous fossa of the scapula and fascia. The tendon may be single or multipennate, and extends obliquely anterosuperiorly to insert onto the middle facet of the greater tuberosity. Occasionally a bursa, which can communicate with the glenohumeral joint, is present between the tendon and joint capsule. The teres minor is a smaller, elongated muscle that is in close contact with the infraspinatus, arising from the infraspinatus fascia and the axillary border of the scapula. It has a short tendon, which helps distinguish it from the infraspinatus, inserting onto the posterior facet of the greater tuberosity and adjacent humerus.

The subscapularis muscle is a large triangular muscle arising from and occupying the subscapularis fossa of the scapula. The tendon is multipennate and merges into a single tendon to insert onto the lesser tuberosity. It is separated from the neck of the scapula by the subscapularis bursa and from the supraspinatus, which lies laterally, by the rotator cuff interval. Passing through this interval is the long head of the biceps tendon, which arises from the supraglenoid tubercle. As the long head of the biceps courses distally within the intertubercular groove it is surrounded proximally by the bicipital sheath, a synovial recess of the glenohumeral joint.

Within the bicipital groove, the long head of the biceps tendon is held in place by the transverse humeral ligament superiorly and by a fibrous extension of the pectoralis major inferiorly. The transverse humeral ligament is not a true ligament, but rather a continuation of fibers from the subscapularis tendon.[8] Superficial fibers of the subscapularis tendon pass over the lesser tuberosity, across the bicipital groove, to insert onto the anterior aspect of the greater tuberosity. In addition, deep fibers of the subscapularis extend into and form a superficial layer to the floor of the bicipital groove, creating a sling of tissue around the biceps tendon. The supraspinatus tendon and coracohumeral ligament lend fibers, deep to the superficial band of the subscapularis, which help to form the roof of the bicipital groove. This anatomy accounts for the pattern of biceps dislocation. Inferiorly, the roof of the groove is maintained by the pectoralis major tendon.

Insider Information 2.1

The subscapularis tendon contributes fibers to the floor and roof of the bicipital groove. This anatomy accounts for the different positions of the dislocated biceps tendon, superficial, within or deep to the subscapularis tendon and muscle.

The coracohumeral ligament is composed of two bands extending from the base of the coracoid process to the lesser and greater humeral tuberosities. It reinforces the joint capsule and rotator interval and helps form the roof of the bicipital groove.[3]

The following muscles and tendons are included for completeness, as pathology within them may present with shoulder symptoms. The short head of the biceps is extraarticular, arising from the apex of the coracoid process in union with the coracobrachialis tendon. The short and long heads of the biceps continue into adjacent but separate muscle bellies that unite only in the distal arm as the distal biceps tendon. The pectoralis major muscle arises from a broad attachment from the anteromedial aspect of the clavicle, sternum, and upper six costal cartilages to insert onto the lateral ridge of the bicipital groove. The tendon is broad and bilaminar. The pectoralis minor lies deep to the pectoralis major, arises from the third through fifth ribs, and inserts on the medial border of the coracoid process.

The deltoid is a large muscle that covers the anterior, lateral, and posterior aspect of the shoulder and imparts a rounded appearance to it. It receives its name from its resemblance to the inverted Greek letter delta: Δ. It has an extensive origin from the anterolateral third clavicle, the acromion, and the spine of the scapula, and inserts as a thick tendon onto the deltoid tuberosity in the mid humerus. It abducts the arm to a horizontal position. The anterior fibers flex and the posterior fibers extend the arm.[4]

The ultrasound appearance of muscle and tendons is reviewed in detail in Chapter 1. The normal size of the above muscles and tendons is related to the patient's age and physical activity. Correlation with the contralateral shoulder is advised. In general, the rotator cuff tendons measure between 5 and 10 mm in thickness and the biceps less than 5 mm.

Bursae

The subacromial-subdeltoid (SASD) bursa is the largest bursa in the body. It lies deep to the deltoid muscle and the acromion process, being attached to the periosteal undersurface of the acromion. It extends laterally beyond the attachment of the rotator cuff by up to 3 cm, medially to the acromioclavicular joint, anteriorly to overlie the bicipital groove, and posteriorly over the rotator cuff. It does not normally communicate with the shoulder joint. The normal ultrasound appearance is of two opposing hyperechoic layers formed by fibroadipose tissue and capsule with an intervening hypoechoic layer representing the viscous fluid within the bursa. The bursa normally measures less than 2 mm in thickness.[7]

Insider Information 2.2
The subcoracoid bursa may communicate with the SASD bursa.

The subcoracoid bursa lies between the subscapularis and coracoid process. It may communicate with the SASD bursa but does not normally communicate with the shoulder joint. The subscapularis bursa lies between the subscapularis tendon and joint capsule and normally communicates with the shoulder joint; it may be better described as a recess.

Multiple other bursae are seen around the shoulder joint (Table 2.3). These include the infraspinatus bursa, between the infraspinatus and joint capsule, which may communicate with the joint. The supraacromial bursa lies within the subcutaneous tissues superficial to the acromion. The teres major bursa lies between the teres major and humerus. Two latissimus dorsi bursae are present, one lying anterior and the other posterior to its tendon.

Table 2.3. Bursae around the Shoulder.

Subacromial-subdeltoid
Subcoracoid
Subscapularis[a]
Infraspinatus[a]
Supraacromial
Teres major
Coracobrachialis
Anterior latissimus dorsi
Posterior latissimus dorsi

[a]Indicates bursae that normally communicate with the glenohumeral joint.

Rotator Cuff Interval

The rotator cuff interval is a triangular space between the subscapularis and the supraspinatus tendons. The base is formed by the coracoid process and the apex by the transverse humeral ligament. It is a dynamic space whose area decreases significantly in internal rotation, less so in external rotation, and is maximal in the neutral position.[9] The long head of the biceps passes through the interval, separated from the supraspinatus and subscapularis by up to 3 mm. Overlying the interval, from superficial to deep, is skin, subcutaneous tissue, the deltoid muscle, a fibrofatty layer, the coracohumeral ligament, the joint capsule, the superior glenohumeral ligament, and the long head of the biceps tendon.

Coracoacromial Arch

This arch is formed by the coracoid process, the acromion, and the connecting coracoacromial ligament (Figure 2.5). This ligament is triangular with the base attached to the lateral coracoid margin and the apex attached to the anterior margin of the acromion. It may consist of two bands and an intermediate band that may in turn be absent as a normal variant with the pectoralis minor inserting onto the joint capsule. Deep to the coracoacromial ligament lie the supraspinatus, the superior aspect of the subscapularis tendon, and the anterior fibers of the infraspinatus tendon. Supraspinatus impingement between the acromion and greater tuberosity can occur, due to the restricted space of the coracoacromial arch. Impingement is most prevalent in 60° forward flexion, abduction, and internal rotation.[10]

Acromioclavicular Joint

The acromioclavicular joint (ACJ) is a diarthrodial joint between the distal end of the clavicle and the medial aspect of the acromion. The articular surfaces are covered by fibrocartilage. An articular fibrocartilage disc is usually present, although it may often be incomplete. Degeneration of both disc and joint occurs early and may be seen as early as the second decade of life.[11–13] A lax capsule,

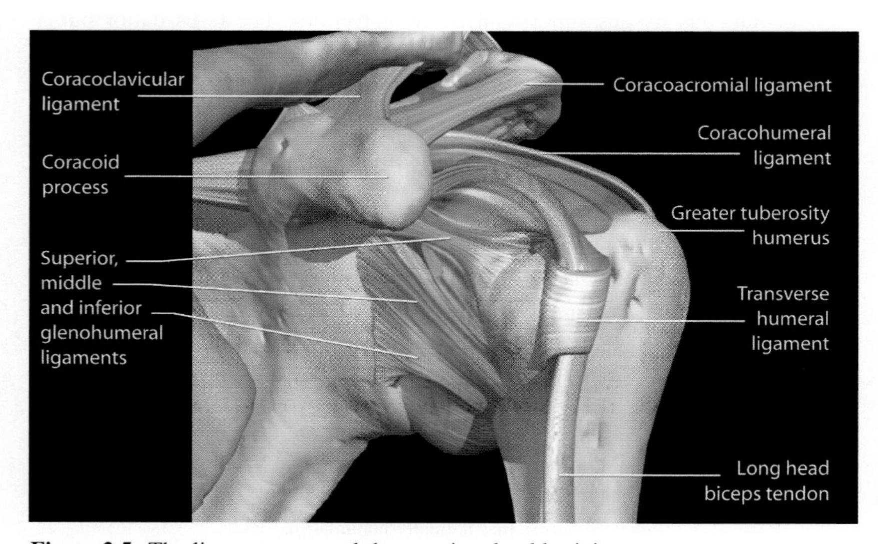

Figure 2.5. The ligaments around the anterior shoulder joint.

lined by synovium, is supported by the acromioclavicular (AC) ligaments: anterior, posterior, inferior, and superior. The strong superior AC ligament interlaces with fibers from the overlying deltoid and trapezius. The weaker inferior ligament and joint are in direct contact inferiorly with the SASD bursa.

This joint is further supported by two additional ligaments, the coracoclavicular and the coracoacromial ligaments, which do not belong to the AC articulation but form an additional support mechanism for the joint (Figure 2.5). The former is in turn composed of two ligaments, the conoid and the trapezoid, which extend between the lateral aspect of the clavicle and the coracoid process of the scapula. The trapezoid attaches to the oblique line on the inferior aspect of the clavicle. The conoid component extends from the base of the coracoid to the conoid tubercle on the clavicular undersurface. The coracoacromial ligament is detailed in the previous section.

Labrum

The glenohumeral joint has the widest range of motion of all joints and combined with an articulating humeral head almost four times the size of the glenoid cavity is predisposed to instability. This instability is counteracted in part by the glenoid labrum. The labrum is composed of fibrous tissue, hyaline cartilage, and fibrocartilage and forms a rim around the glenoid (Figure 2.6).[14] It serves as a site of attachment for the glenohumeral ligaments, and the resulting labral-ligamentous complex is an important component in stabilizing the joint. The labrum is subject to many anatomical variations in size and shape, particularly anteriorly. It has a triangular appearance and is most commonly hyperechoic and homogeneous on ultrasound with the base attaching to the glenoid rim.[15–17] The shape of the posterior labrum changes from a triangular structure in internal rotation of the shoulder to a slightly buckled appearance in external rotation.[18] The same maneuver gives the anterior labrum a more pointed form.[19] It can be divided into 12 segments, extending in a clockwise fashion from the 12 o'clock position at the biceps anchor. Alternatively, it can also be divided into four quadrants: anterosuperior (1-3), anteroinferior (3-6), posteroinferior (6-7), and posterosuperior (9-12), with the equivalent 12-segment classification given in parentheses.

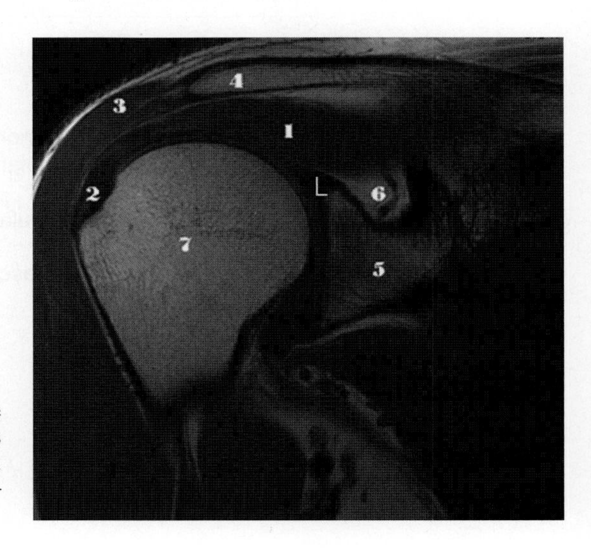

Figure 2.6. Coronal T1-weighted magnetic resonance (MRI) anatomy mid-shoulder joint: 1–supraspinatus muscle, 2–supraspinatus tendon, 3–deltoid muscle, 4–acromion, 5–glenoid, 6–spinoglenoid notch, 7–humerus, L-labrum.

Insider Information 2.3
The shape of the posterior labrum changes from triangular in internal rotation to a more buckled appearance in external rotation.

Scapular Notches and the Suprascapular Nerve

The suprascapular nerve arises from the upper trunk of the brachial plexus, C5–6. It contains motor and sensory fibers and supplies both the supraspinatus and infraspinatus muscles with articular branches to the glenohumeral joint and acromioclavicular joints. From its origin, it passes posterior to the trapezius and omohyoid to enter the supraspinous fossa via the suprascapular notch. The suprascapular notch is converted into a fibroosseous tunnel by the transverse or suprascapular ligament. This ligament attaches to the base of the coracoid process and to the inner aspect of the scapular notch. The suprascapular vessels pass over this foramen. The suprascapular nerve passes on the scapular aspect of the supraspinatus muscle, which it supplies, and courses inferiorly through the spinoglenoid notch.[20] The spinoglenoid notch connects the supraspinous and infraspinous fossae between the lateral margin of the scapular spine and the medial margin of the glenoid (Figure 2.7). It is bounded posteriorly by the spinoglenoid ligament and transmits the suprascapular nerve and vessels. Inferiorly, it supplies the infraspinatus. Knowledge of the different levels of innervation will allow an understanding of entrapment neuropathies and their subsequent imaging findings. Pathology affecting the suprascapular nerve above the spinoglenoid notch involves the innervation to both the supraspinatus and infraspinatus and, at or below this level, the infraspinatus. The teres minor is supplied by the axillary nerve.

Insider Information 2.4
Pathology of the suprascapular nerve at or below the spinoglenoid notch affects the infraspinatus muscle. More proximal pathology will also affect the supraspinatus muscle. The teres minor muscle is supplied by the axillary nerve.

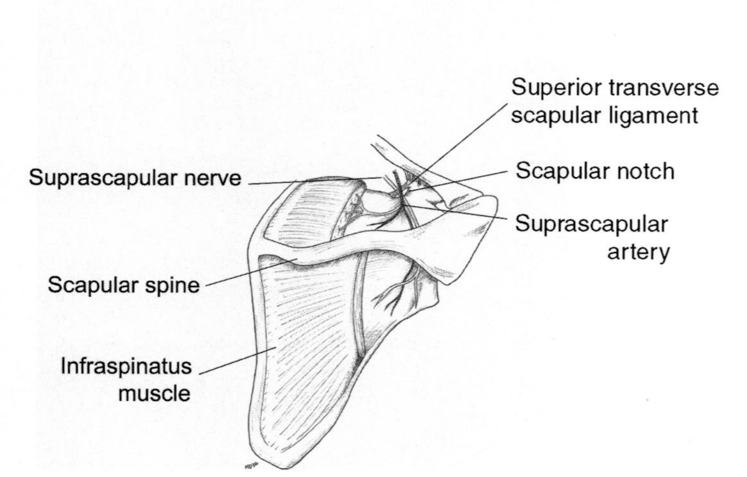

Figure 2.7. The posterior surface of the scapula demonstrating the suprascapular nerve and the spinoglenoid notch.

Technique

The patient sits on a revolving stool with the shoulder exposed; this allows for easy access to the anterior and posterior aspects of the shoulder and for the required positional changes. A pertinent history should be obtained from the patient, especially as symptoms may have changed since clinical referral. The examiner can either sit or stand in front or behind the patient. I prefer to perform the examination while standing behind the patient. This allows me to directly face the monitor and keep the transducer below the level of my own shoulder. This puts less stress on my own rotator cuff, particularly if I need to perform multiple similar examinations in the same session. The examination can be focused on a specific pathology or require a full routine evaluation, which will be described here. All tendons are assessed in their orthogonal planes. A summary of positions in which the individual tendons are evaluated is provided in Table 2.4. "Longitudinal" and "axial" refer to the axis of the structure being imaged.

Long Head Biceps

The long head of the biceps tendon and sheath are evaluated in a neutral position with the arm in supination resting on the ipsilateral thigh (Figure 2.8a). This position places the bicipital groove anteriorly. Transverse and longitudinal views are obtained from the proximal aspect of the bicipital groove distally to the musculotendinous junction (Figures 2.8b and c and 2.9). On the longitudinal view, the fibrillar pattern of the biceps tendon may appear hypoechoic in part, but by gently pressing on the inferior aspect of the transducer the fibrillar pattern will, in normal tendons, become homogeneous. This is termed the heel–toe effect (Figure 2.9).

Table 2.4. Ultrasound Evaluation: Position of the Shoulder Muscles.

Muscle	Position examined	Muscle	Position examined
Supraspinatus	Crass position Middleton position	Long head biceps	Elbow flexed to 90°, arm supinated and hand resting on ipsilateral thigh
Infraspinatus	Ipsilateral hand on contralateral arm/shoulder	Short head biceps	Elbow flexed to 90°, arm supinated and hand resting on ipsilateral thigh
Subscapularis	Elbow flexed to 90°, arm supinated resting on ipsilateral thigh, dynamic with internal and external rotation	Pectoralis major	Elbow flexed to 90°, arm supinated and hand resting on ipsilateral thigh
Teres minor	Ipsilateral hand on contralateral arm/shoulder	Pectoralis minor	Arm adducted in relaxed state
Deltoid	Arm adducted in relaxed state		

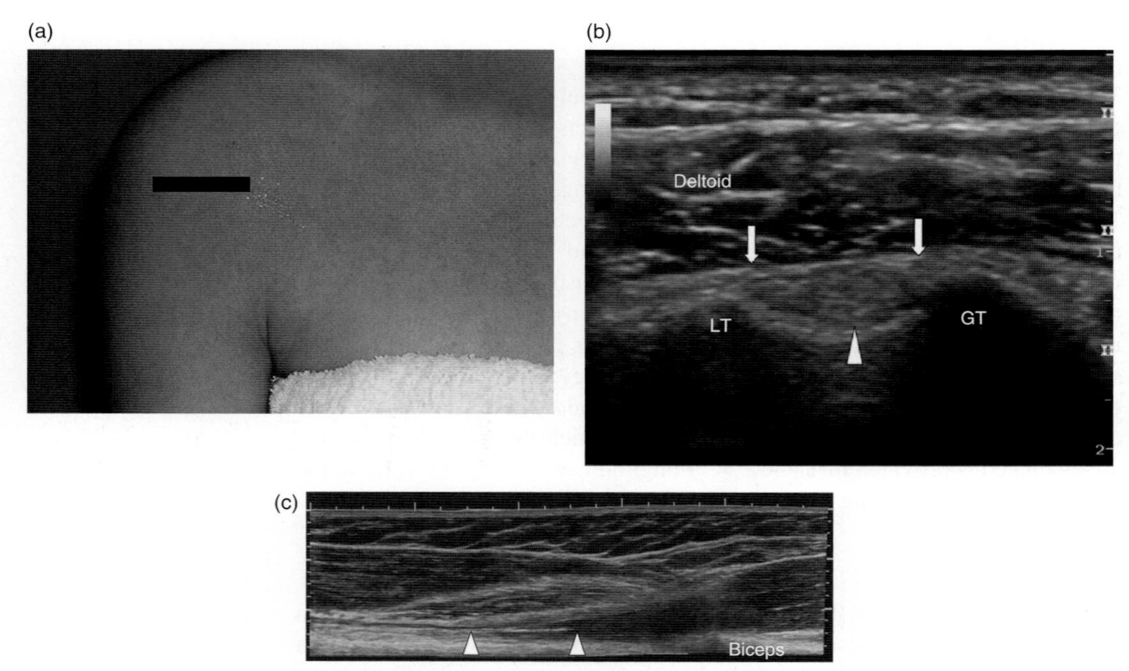

Figure 2.8. Long head biceps tendon (LHBT): **(a)** transducer position and corresponding **(b)** transverse ultrasound image of the hyperechoic oval LHBT (arrowhead) within the bicipital groove. **(c)** Longitudinal ultrasound image of the LHBT at its musculotendinous junction (curved arrow). LT, lesser tuberosity; GT, greater tuberosity; arrows, transverse humeral ligament.

Insider Information 2.5
Perform the heel–toe effect in the longitudinal assessment of the long head of the biceps tendon. The intraarticular portion of the biceps tendon can be evaluated with the arm in external rotation.

The hyperechoic transverse humeral ligament (THL), essentially a continuation of fibers from the coracohumeral ligament, the subscapularis, and supraspinatus tendons, is seen spanning the intertubercular groove (Figure 2.8b). A dynamic examination should then be performed with internal and external rotation of the shoulder, maintaining the elbow by the side, to assess the integrity of the transverse humeral ligament and for biceps tendon subluxation. The biceps tendon should normally be maintained within the groove (Figure 2.10). Subluxation and dislocation may become apparent only on this dynamic component of the study.[21]

The superior intraarticular portion of the long head of the biceps, within the rotator interval, can be further evaluated by externally rotating the shoulder, keeping the elbow by the side, and maintaining the transducer in a longitudinal plane to the biceps within the bicipital groove. Moving the transducer superiorly, in the longitudinal axis of the biceps, allows visualization of its proximal component and occasionally the bicipital anchor (Figure 2.11).

The bicipital groove, between the greater and lesser tuberosities, is deep and narrow superiorly, becoming wider and shallower inferiorly (Figure 2.8b).[22] It contains the biceps tendon and a branch of the anterior circumflex artery.

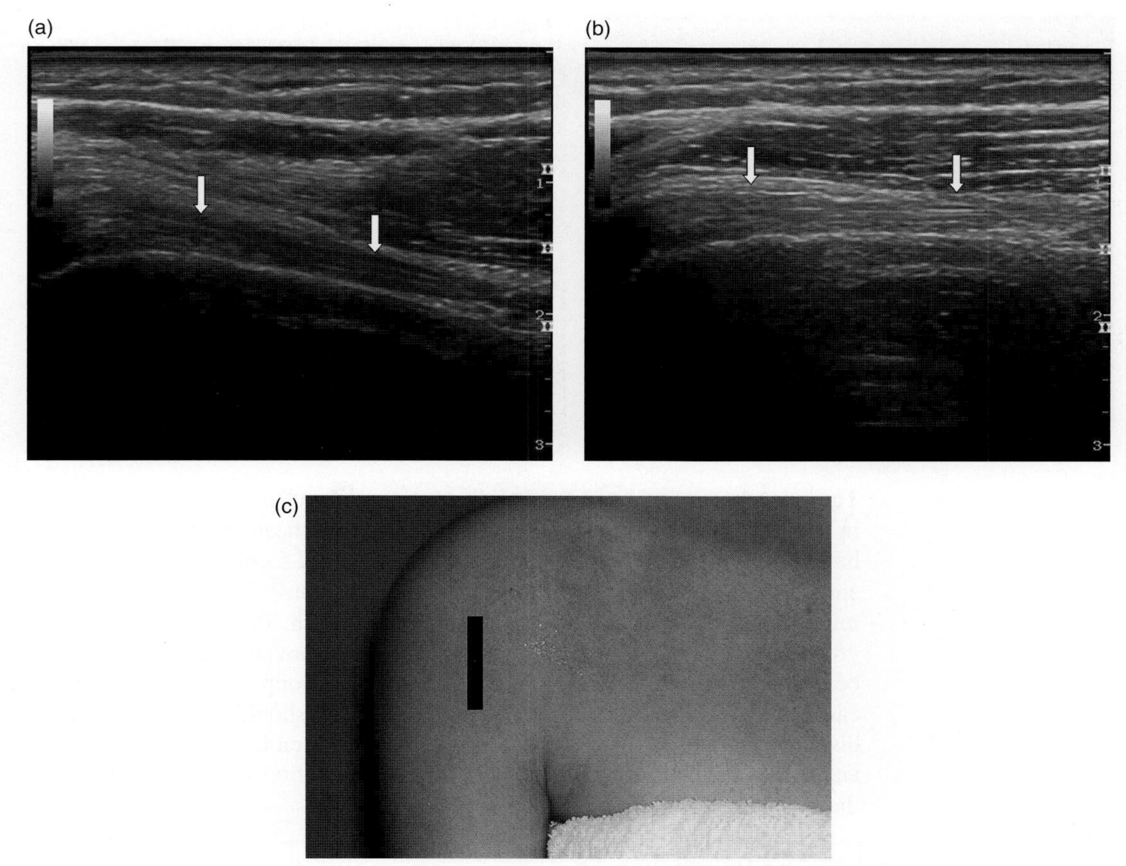

Figure 2.9. Long head of the biceps tendon: longitudinal ultrasound image demonstrating the "heel–toe" effect. **(a)** Pre heel–toe the fibrillar pattern of the tendon is not clearly discerned. **(b)** Post heel–toe. By gently depressing the distal margin of the transducer the fibrillar pattern of the normal tendon is clearly seen. **(c)** Corresponding photograph of the transducer position.

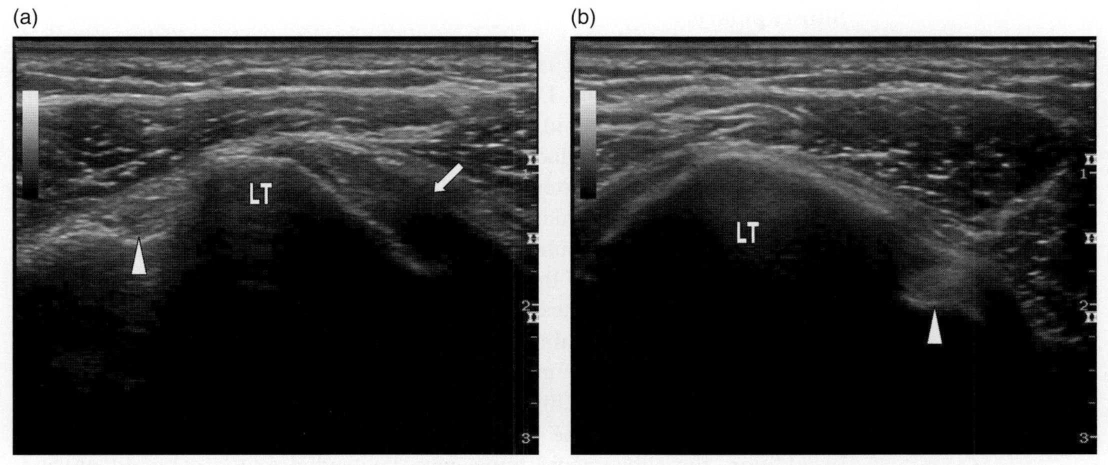

Figure 2.10. Transverse ultrasound image of the hyperechoic long head biceps tendon (arrowhead) within the bicipital groove on **(a)** internal rotation and **(b)** external rotation. LT, lesser tuberosity; arrow, subscapularis tendon.

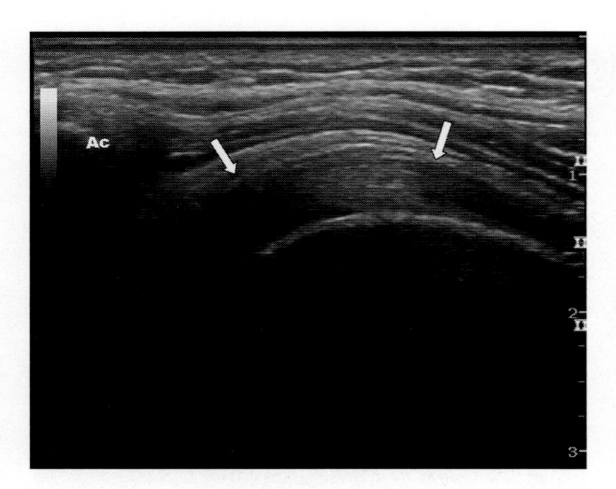

Figure 2.11. Longitudinal ultrasound image of the intraarticular portion long head biceps tendon (arrows). Ac, acromion.

The smooth, continuous, hyperechoic bony contour of the groove is best seen in the axial plane as in the assessment of the long head biceps. The groove has a width of approximately 10 mm and a length of 5 cm. A shallow groove and medial wall are predispositions to subluxation.[15] There is normally a minimal amount of fluid within the bicipital sheath. Proximally within the groove, the bicipital sheath is encompassed by a synovial sheath. This should be evaluated for thickening or internal flow on Doppler, as may occur in cases of synovial proliferation. The bicipital sheath should be evaluated to its distal aspect. Due to gravity, this is the point of accumulation of joint fluid and, occasionally, intraarticular bodies. The evaluation of the short head of the biceps is detailed in Chapter 3.

Insider Information 2.6
Evaluate the bicipital sheath to its inferior-most extent; this is a common location for intraarticular bodies to gravitate.

Subscapularis

The subscapularis tendon is assessed with the arm both in neutral and in external rotation positions. Longitudinal assessment in the plane of the tendon demonstrates its subcoracoid position and attachment onto the lesser tuberosity (Figure 2.12). The transducer should be moved superiorly and inferiorly to encompass the full extent of the tendon. The axial scan best demonstrates its multipennate structure with the multiple proximal tendon slips seen as hyperechoic foci surrounded by the hypoechoic muscle (Figure 2.12c).[7] Maintaining the elbow by the side and abducting and adducting the forearm allows for a dynamic assessment. This is an important component of the study that can help discriminate anisotropy, focal tendinosis, and partial tears. Reposition the transducer medially so that it overlies the coracoid process and repeat the above dynamic study (Figure 2.13). This may reveal subcoracoid impingement of the subscapularis tendon or the subcoracoid bursa. In addition, the subcoracoid bursa may lie medial to the coracoid process on a static study and extend to the lateral aspect of the coracoid only when assessed dynamically.

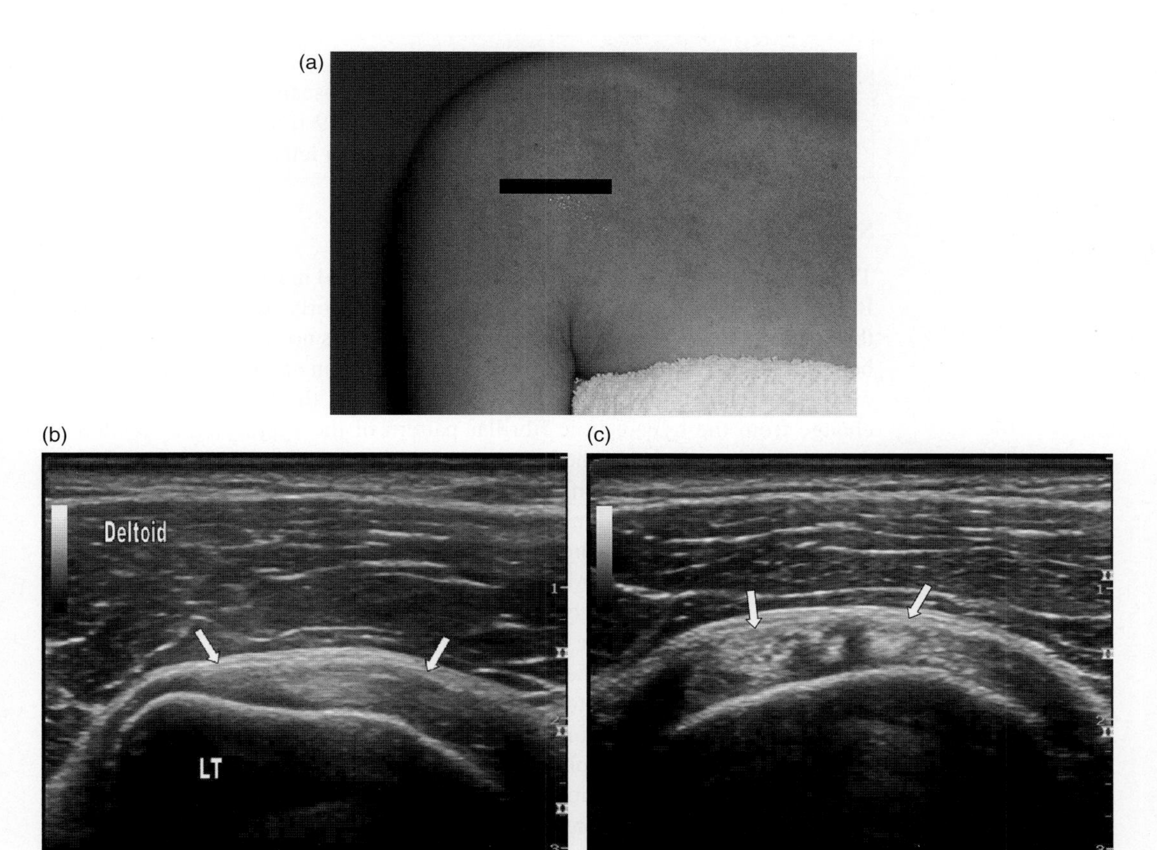

Figure 2.12. Subscapularis tendon (arrows). (**a**) Transducer position and corresponding (**b**) longitudinal ultrasound image. (**c**) Subscapularis in the transverse plane demonstrating the normal appearance of the multipennate hyperechoic tendons. LT, lesser tuberosity.

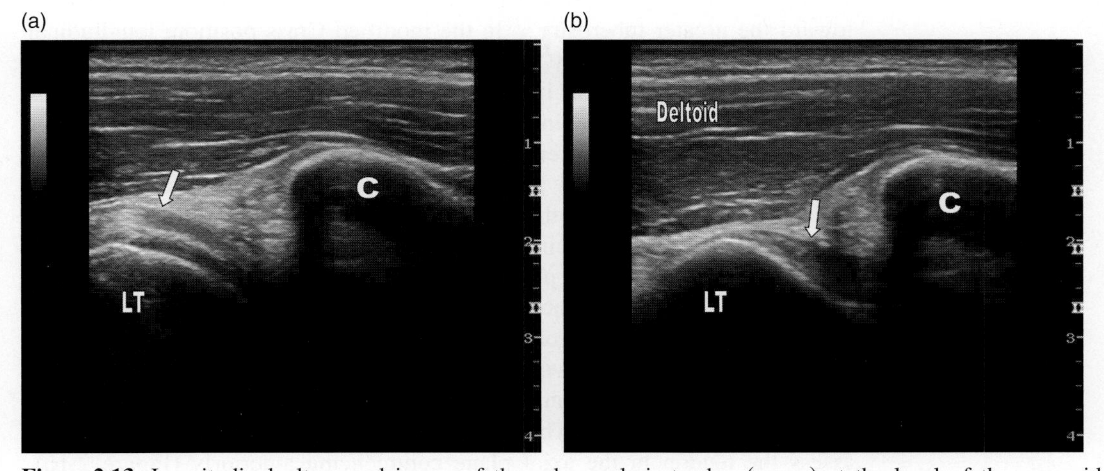

Figure 2.13. Longitudinal ultrasound image of the subscapularis tendon (arrow) at the level of the coracoid process (C). (**a**) External rotation and (**b**) internal rotation. LT, lesser tuberosity.

> **Insider Information 2.7**
> Insertional measurements of the rotator cuff: subscapularis 40 × 20 mm, supraspinatus 23 × 16 mm, infraspinatus 29 × 19 mm, teres minor 29 × 21 mm [anterior to posterior (length) × medial to lateral (width)].[24]

Supraspinatus

The supraspinatus is the commonest tendon involved in rotator cuff pathology. It is clearly separated from the subscapularis anteriorly by the rotator interval through which the biceps passes. Posteriorly, there is no clear anatomical plane between it and the infraspinatus; however, there is an extensive interdigitation of fibers between the tendons.[23] On ultrasound, this region is seen as a change from the hyperechoic fibrillar pattern of the supraspinatus tendon to the lower echogenicity of the infraspinatus. The supraspinatus tendon extends for approximately 2.5 cm in the anteroposterior direction.[5,24]

The supraspinatus tendon is normally partially obscured by the overlying acromion process. To overcome this, the supraspinatus tendon should be viewed in full internal rotation and hyperextension with the forearm behind the back, palm facing posteriorly, overlapping the scapular tip while maintaining the elbow by the side, the Crass position (Figure 2.14a). This places the tendon under stress and hence accentuates tears.[25] Examination is repeated in the modified Crass/Middleton position with the upper arm extended and the shoulder in a neutral position, elbow flexed and pointing directly posteriorly, and the palm of the hand placed forward against the ipsilateral back pocket (Figure 2.14b). This position allows for visualization of the supraspinatus tendon immediately adjacent to the bicipital interval, an area often obscured by the acromion in the Crass position. This anterior region, just proximal to the distal fiber insertion, is known as the "critical zone." It is important to keep the elbow adducted.[26]

The supraspinatus tendon has two visible main components, as described in the anatomy section. On ultrasound they appear as a cone of tendinous bundles anteriorly and a flatter posterior tendon. A hypoechoic band of intervening muscle may be present medially, but fades as one extends laterally toward the greater tuberosity.[27] In the modified Crass position, longitudinal images are obtained first by visualizing the intraarticular portion of the long head of the biceps tendon in the longitudinal plane (Figure 2.15a); this is equivalent to the longitudinal plane of the supraspinatus. The transducer is then slowly moved posteriorly in the plane of the supraspinatus, 45° to 50° to the coronal oblique plane (Figure 2.15b). This plane can be better understood by visualizing the supraspinatus fossa and mentally drawing a line from the fossa to the point of insertion, i.e., along the plane of the muscle fibers. In the longitudinal plane, the tendon fibers have a smooth convex upper border, which is noncompressible, and insert into the raised cortical surface of the greater tuberosity, which appears like a shelf. The insertional tendon fibers are also known as the tendon footprint, or footplate. Note that the articular cartilage extends only to the base of the shelf of the greater tuberosity (Figure 2.15b). The transducer is rotated 90° counterclockwise to assess the tendon in the axial plane commencing anteriorly (Figure 2.16). In this position, the coracoid process can be identified medially, but the subscapularis is poorly visualized as it is now subcoracoid. The biceps tendon

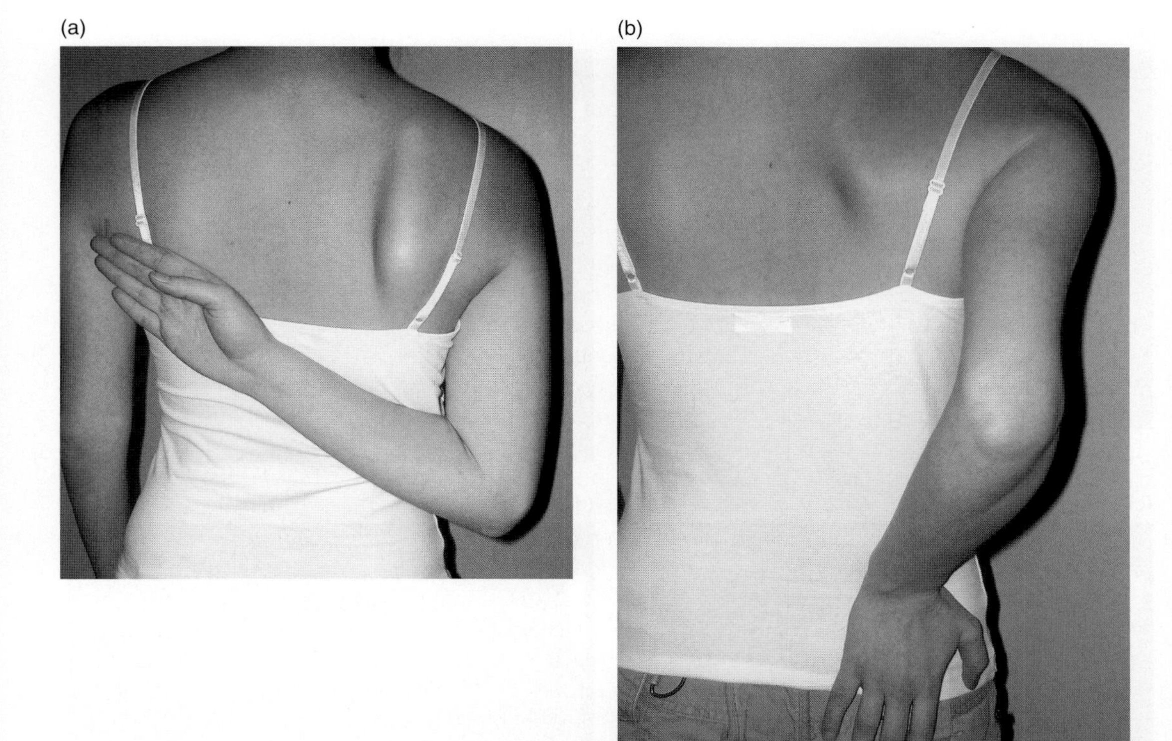

Figure 2.14. Supraspinatus tendon: positions for ultrasound evaluation: **(a)** Crass and **(b)** Middleton (modified Crass).

is noted as a hyperechoic oval structure. Lying just lateral to the biceps is the anterior aspect of the supraspinatus. The transducer is maintained in this plane and moved posteriorly to encompass the whole of the supraspinatus tendon. In the Crass position, the subscapularis and occasionally the biceps may not be identified as they are in a subcoracoid position. The transducer is positioned in the plane of the longitudinal axis of the supraspinatus tendon as described above and placed over the coracoid process. This is now used as our anterior marker if we do not identify the long head of the biceps tendon e.g., in a complete biceps rupture (Figure 2.17). The transducer is then slowly moved posteriorly, carefully maintaining it in the longitudinal axis of the supraspinatus tendon, and then evaluated in the transverse plane. It is important to use both the Crass and modified positions for a complete study.

Where there is limited range of movement, the supraspinatus tendon is examined in as much internal rotation and hyperextension as possible. It may occasionally be easier for the patient and the examiner if the examiner moves the arm back and forth in this position to unroof as much of the supraspinatus tendon from under the acromion as possible, while also assessing the dynamic motion of the fibers. The layers of structures, from deep to superficial in the longitudinal plane, are the hyperechoic humeral cortex, hypoechoic thin

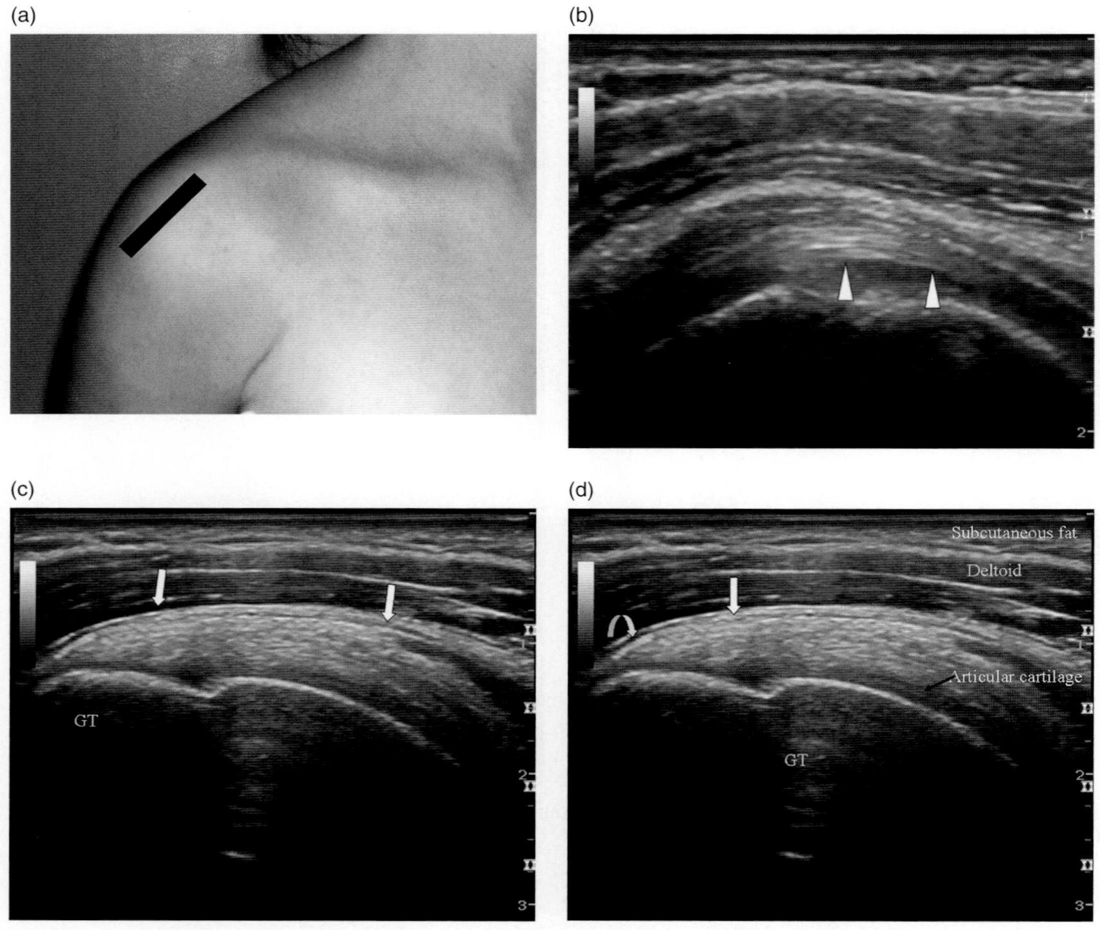

Figure 2.15. Supraspinatus tendon (arrows): **(a)** transducer position and corresponding **(b)** longitudinal ultrasound image of the intraarticular portion long head of the biceps tendon (arrowheads) at the rotator cuff interval. **(c)** The longitudinal ultrasound image demonstrating the hyperechoic fibrillar pattern of the supraspinatus is achieved by slowly moving the transducer posteriorly in the same plane. **(d)** Surrounding structures. GT, greater tuberosity; black arrow, articular cartilage; curved arrow, hypoechoic SASD bursa and adjacent hyperechoic capsule and peribursal fat.

rim articular cartilage, hyperechoic supraspinatus tendon, peribursal hyperechoic fat and bursal capsule layers with intervening hypoechoic fluid within the SASD bursa, the hypoechoic deltoid muscle, subcutaneous fat, and skin (Figure 2.15). Once the SASD bursa is identified, it should be followed in the anterior, posterior, medial, and lateral direction. This is important as significant distention with fluid may be visualized in only one region; this is usually lateral to the greater tuberosity as this is a low pressure zone. An alternative position for examination of the supraspinatus has been described whereby the patient lies supine with the shoulder at the edge of the bed, arm and elbow extended with the forearm pronated.[27]

The supraspinatus muscle is evaluated in the suprascapular fossa (Figure 2.18). This is performed to assess muscle mass and fatty infiltration. The transducer is aligned with the muscle fibers, perpendicular to

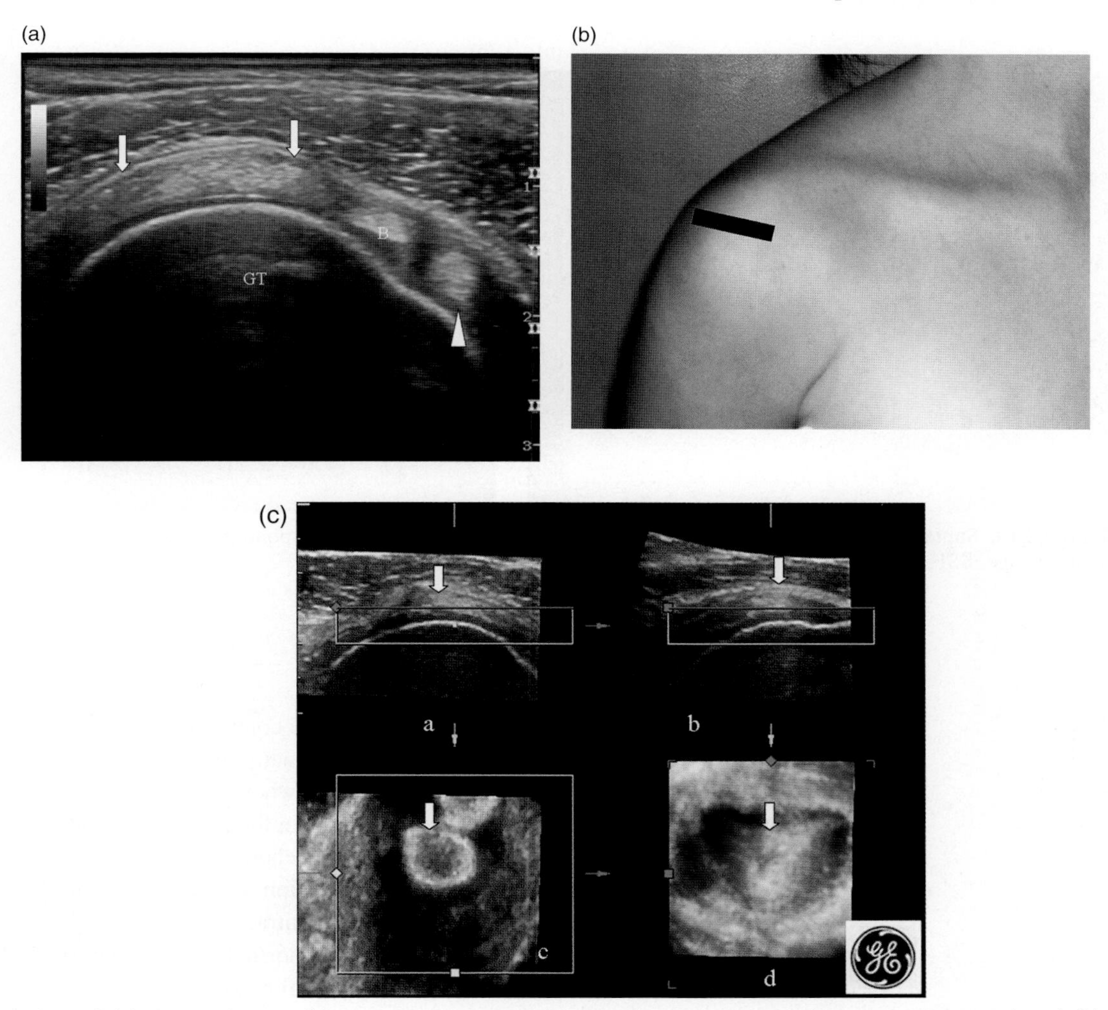

Figure 2.16. Supraspinatus: **(a)** transverse ultrasound image demonstrating the rotator cuff interval and **(b)** corresponding transducer position. **(c)** Ultrasound of the supraspinatus tendon using 4-D transducer: a, axial, b, sagittal, c, coronal, and d, 3-D reconstruction. Arrows, supraspinatus tendon; GT, greater tuberosity; B, long head biceps tendon; arrowhead, subscapularis.

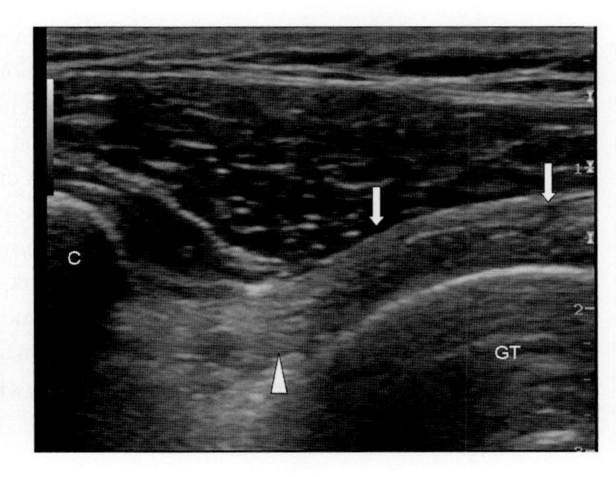

Figure 2.17. Ultrasound image of the transverse plane supraspinatus tendon in a modified Crass (Middleton) position. Arrows, supraspinatus tendon; arrowhead, long head biceps tendon; GT, greater tuberosity; C, coracoid process.

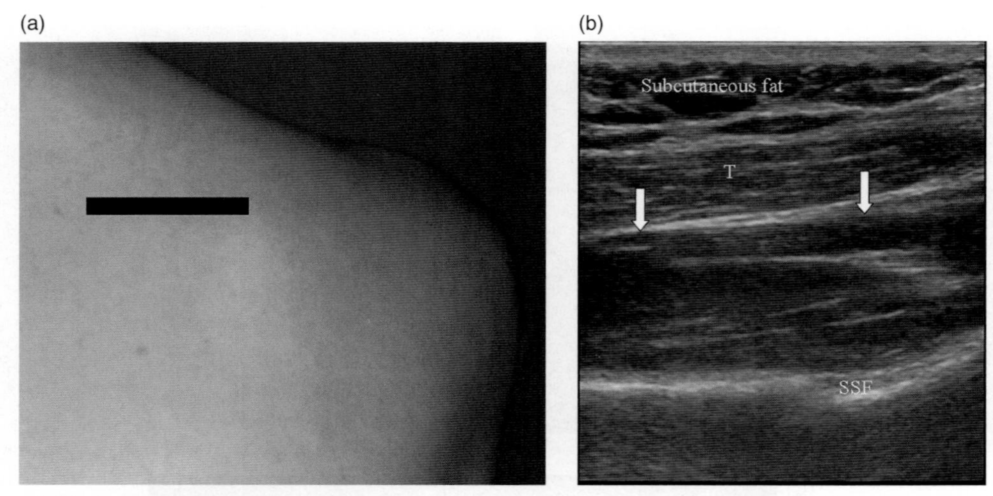

Figure 2.18. Supraspinatus muscle (arrows): **(a)** transducer position and **(b)** corresponding longitudinal ultrasound image. SSF, suprascapular fossa; T, trapezius.

the skin. The trapezius muscle is superficial, and the continuous hyperechoic cortical line of the scapula is deep to the supraspinatus muscle. Abnormal fatty infiltration is noted as increased echogenicity when compared with the contralateral side. Assessment should be performed in the relaxed state of the muscle being investigated. Contraction decreases echotexture and increases the apparent mass. New studies of dynamic evaluation during active muscle contraction have been performed to assess the contraction patterns of the supraspinatus and infraspinatus in normal and abnormal states. Abnormal contraction patterns may explain different functional capabilities in patients with similar pathology.[28] Further clinical studies are required to assess these contraction patterns and clinical significance.

Anisotropy

This is the commonest artifact in musculoskeletal ultrasound and it is essential to be able to recognize both its presence and its remedy. Anisotropy is the different ultrasound echogenicity of normal tissue when the angle of insonation is not 90° to the plane of the structure being imaged. It is most pronounced in tendons, but can be seen in other soft tissues such as ligaments and nerves. A common site of occurrence is within the supraspinatus tendon due to its coronal oblique course and angulation. To separate anisotropy from pathology, the transducer is held in the same position but is angled until it is perpendicular to the tissue of interest. When this position is achieved, the apparent hypoechoic region will resolve and the tissue, if normal, will be of homogeneous echogenicity (Figure 2.19). The tissue will remain hypoechoic if pathology is present.

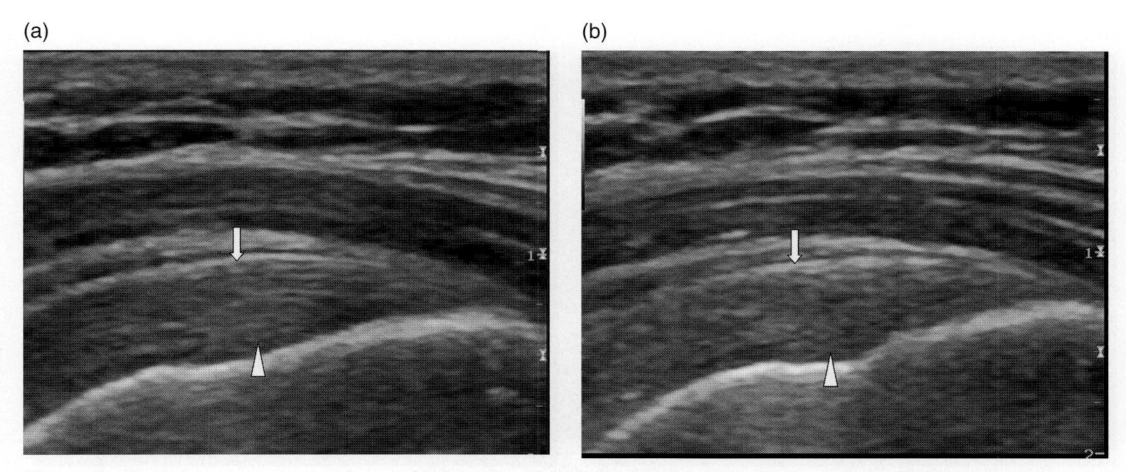

Figure 2.19. Anisotropy: supraspinatus (SS) tendon. **(a)** Normal longitudinal hyperechoic ultrasound appearance of the SS tendon. **(b)** Same position as **(a)** with transducer angled 5–10°. Hypoechoic areas appear when the transducer is no longer perpendicular to the tendon fibers and simulate pathology. Arrowhead depicts hyperechoic fibers perpendicular to the supraspinatus consistent with the rotator cable.

> **Insider Information 2.8**
> Anisotropy is the different ultrasound echogenicity of normal tissue when the angle of insonation is not 90° to the plane of the structure being imaged.

Infraspinatus and Teres Minor

The infraspinatus and teres minor tendons are evaluated with the forearm placed across the chest and the palm of the hand placed against the contralateral shoulder (Figure 2.20a). The infraspinatus is larger and lies superior to the teres minor (Figure 2.20b). Differentiation is easily achieved at

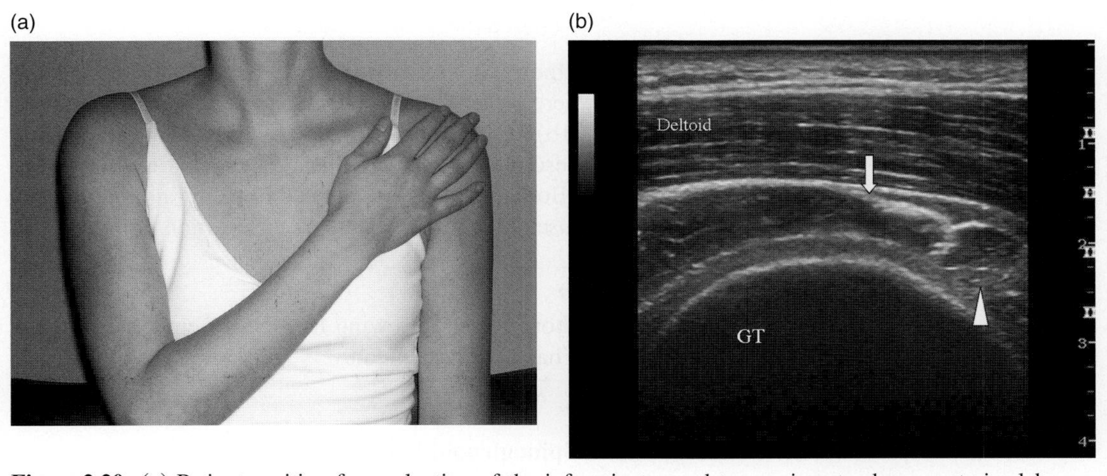

Figure 2.20. **(a)** Patient position for evaluation of the infraspinatus and teres minor tendons, posterior labrum, and spinoglenoid notch and **(b)** transverse ultrasound image of the junction of the inferior border infraspinatus (arrow) and superior border teres minor (arrowhead) muscles. GT, greater tuberosity.

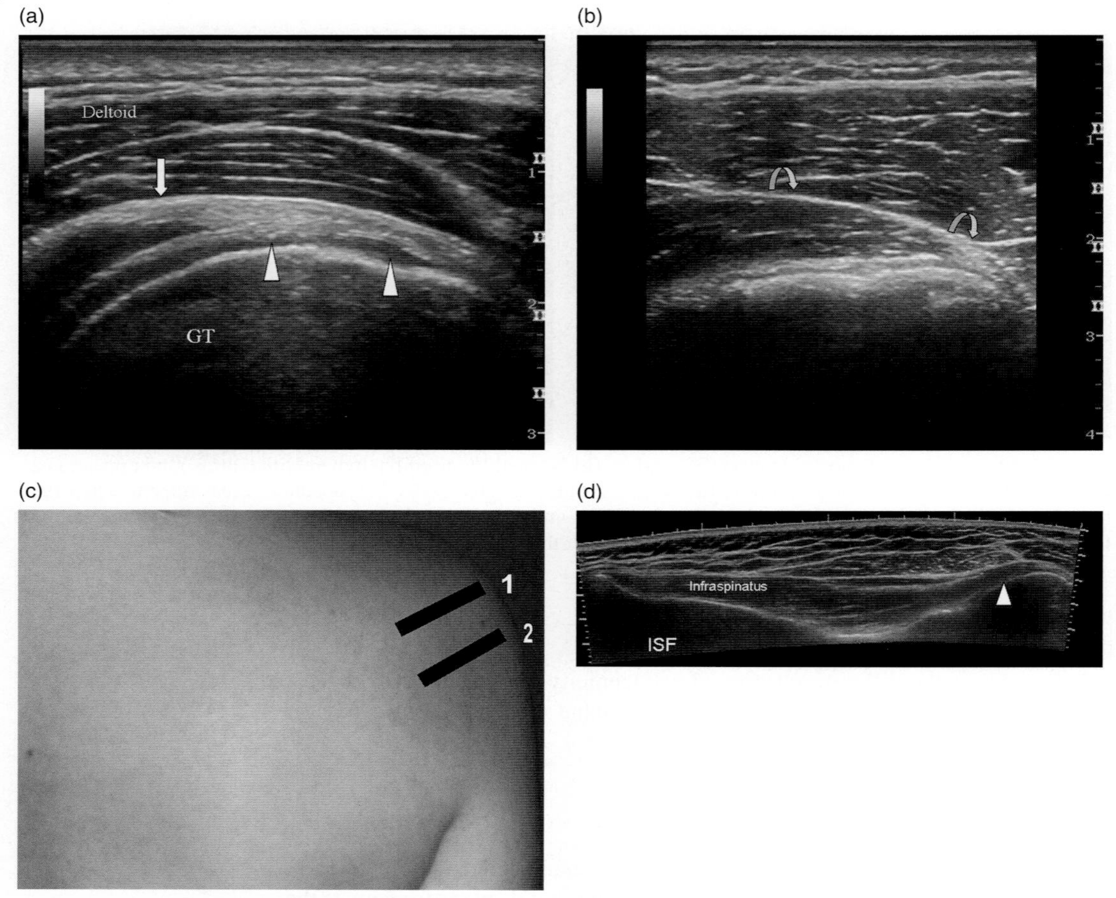

Figure 2.21. Longitudinal ultrasound of **(a)** infraspinatus tendon (arrowheads) and musculotendinous junction (arrow) and **(b)** teres minor (curved arrows). Note the short hyperechoic tendon of the teres minor, which can be used to differentiate from the infraspinatus. **(c)** Transducer positions. **(d)** Extended field of view ultrasound of the infraspinatus. 1, infraspinatus; 2, teres minor; GT, greater tuberosity; ISF, infraspinous fossa scapula.

their site of insertion onto the greater tuberosity as the infraspinatus has a long tendon (Figure 2.21a), whereas the teres minor has a short tendon, measuring only 1–2 cm (Figure 2.21b). The separation between the supraspinatus and infraspinatus tendons is described previously in the ultrasound evaluation of the supraspinatus tendon. Both tendons are evaluated in their longitudinal and transverse planes from musculotendinous junctions to insertion points.

Insider Information 2.9
The teres minor has a short tendon, allowing it to be differentiated from the infraspinatus, which has a longer tendon.

Posterior Labrum and Spinoglenoid Notch

The posterior labrum and spinoglenoid notch are viewed with the arm maintained in the same position as that for the infraspinatus. The transducer is moved transversely, perpendicular to the glenoid, and medially to overlie the

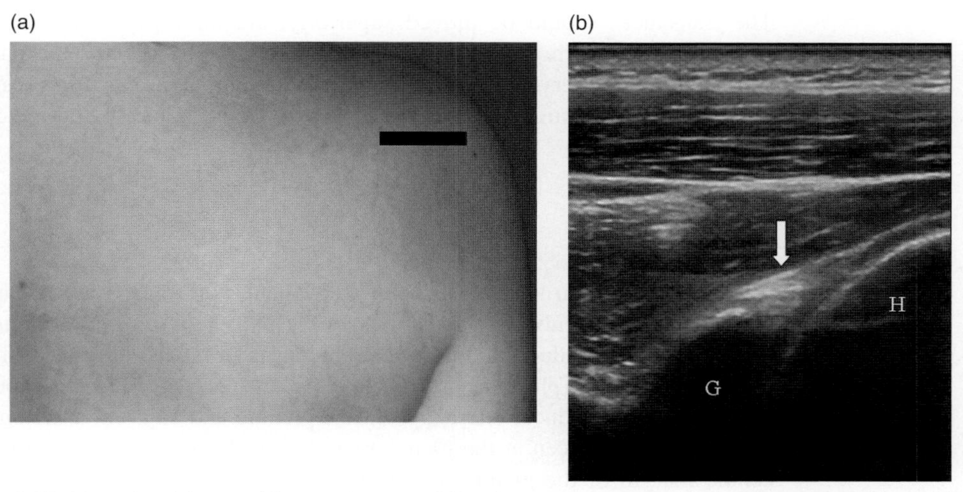

Figure 2.22. Posterior labrum: (**a**) transducer position for evaluation of the posterior labrum and (**b**) corresponding ultrasound image demonstrating the hyperechoic triangular labrum (arrow) between the humeral head (H) and glenoid (G).

posterior aspect of the glenohumeral joint (Figure 2.22a). The hyperechoic triangular labrum, the commonest morphology, lies between the hyperechoic cortical surfaces of the humeral head and the bony glenoid (Figure 2.22b).[15,16] Ask the patient to gently tap the ipsilateral hand on the contralateral shoulder. This movement will allow easier identification of joint fluid within the posterior recess as it extends between the labrum and humeral head. No fluid should normally extend through the labrum; if present, this would indicate a tear of the labrum. If fluid is identified, adjacent and posterior to the labrum, this may represent a paralabral cyst and as such will not change configuration on the dynamic motion described above. Moving the transducer medially, in the same plane, the spinoglenoid notch can be identified as a focal bony depression outlined by a continuous hyperechoic cortical line (Figure 2.23).

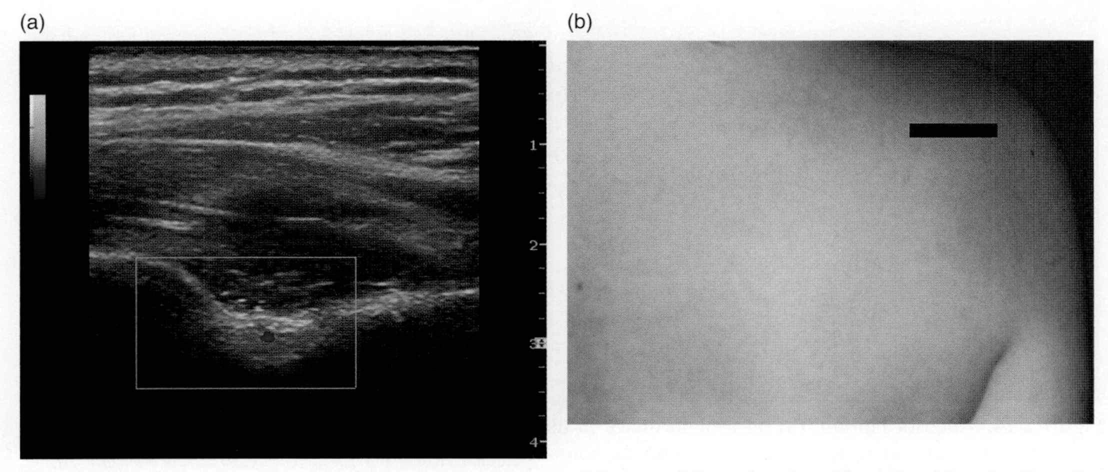

Figure 2.23. Spinoglenoid notch: (**a**) transverse ultrasound image of the spinoglenoid notch with color Doppler demonstrating the suprascapular artery and (**b**) the corresponding transducer position.

The transducer should be moved superiorly and inferiorly in a transverse plane to evaluate the full extent of the notch, which contains the suprascapular nerve, artery, and vein. With power Doppler, the suprascapular vessels can be identified and distinguished from the adjacent suprascapular nerve.

Anterior Labrum

The anterior labrum is more difficult to evaluate than the posterior labrum, particularly in patients of large habitus, and usually requires a low-frequency curved array transducer. Once the coracoid process is identified in the deltopectoral angle, place the transducer in a plane parallel to the subscapularis and move the transducer laterally until the glenoid and adjacent anteromedial humeral head are seen at the glenohumeral joint. Projecting from the hyperechoic margin of the glenoid is a triangular hyperechoic body, the anterior labrum (Figure 2.24). There may be a hypoechoic line seen at the base of the labrum; this line should normally measure less than 2 mm. A hypoechoic line wider than 2 mm has been reported to be diagnostic of a labral tear.[29] The transducer is then moved inferiorly to evaluate the remainder of the labrum. The arm is then moved in internal and external rotation.

On external rotation, the labrum is partly compressed by the humeral head and adapts a more rounded appearance.[30] The overlying capsule may be seen as a thin echogenic line interposed between the more superficial subscapularis and deeper labrum. As in the posterior labral study, this will contribute to the evaluation of the anterior recess and for joint effusion. Evaluation of the anterosuperior labrum is limited due to the overlying coracoid process. We do not normally perform an assessment of the anterior labrum as part of our standard study of the shoulder.

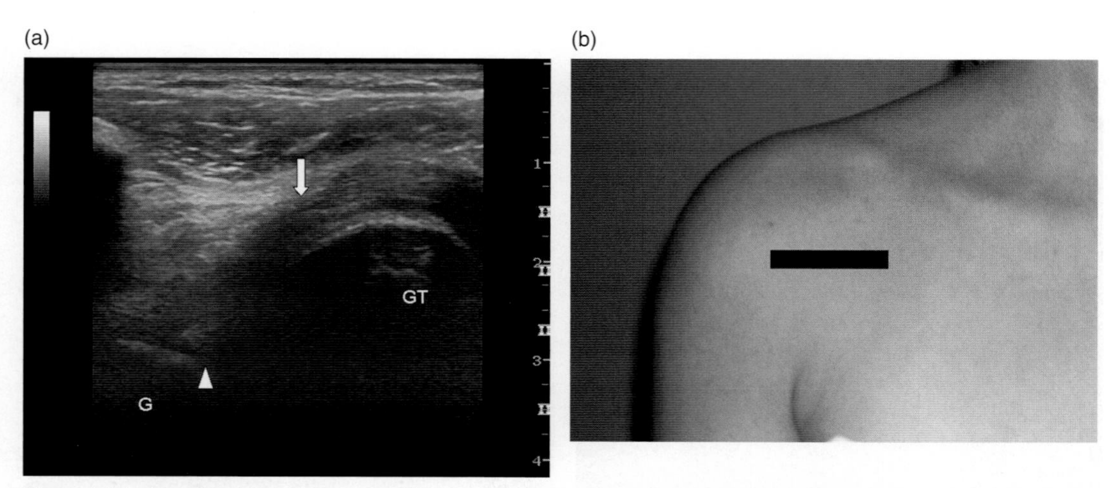

Figure 2.24. Anterior labrum: **(a)** ultrasound image in the long axis of the subscapularis muscle demonstrating the anterior labrum (arrowhead) deep to the subscapularis tendon and **(b)** the corresponding transducer position. LT, lesser tuberosity; G, glenoid.

Acromioclavicular Joint and Acromion

The acromioclavicular joint is assessed in the sagittal and coronal planes, with the arm in a neutral position by the patient's side (Figure 2.25). In the coronal position, the clavicle usually lies at a slightly higher position than the acromion. The capsule is convex at, or just above, the hyperechoic cortical line of the adjacent clavicle. The transducer is then moved from anterior to posterior, noting that the joint space is wider anteriorly. Joint width is compared with the contralateral side. Dynamic assessment can be performed by abducting and adducting the arm.[12] If acromioclavicular instability is suspected clinically, measurement of acromioclavicular separation before and after attachment of weights to each wrist or hand, with contralateral comparison, has been shown to correlate with radiographic measurements.[31]

Coracoclavicular distance can be assessed by placing the base of the transducer in a coronal plane on the tip of the coracoid process and the tip on the clavicle. Measurements are taken from the superior border of each; these measurements have also been shown to be accurate and reliable when compared to radiographic evaluation.[32] The acromion is evaluated initially in a coronal plane, anterior to posterior. It is necessary to assess for the presence of an os acromiale, which can be identified as a break in the linear cortical line (Figure 2.26), presuming there is no history of acromial fracture. The patient's age should be noted because the acromion fuses late, around the 22nd year. The subacromial space can be measured, though we do not routinely perform this component of the study, by aligning the transducer in a coronal plane to the acromion with the upper margin of the transducer on the acromion and the lower margin overlying the humeral head.[33]

Ligaments

The ultrasound appearance of ligaments is outlined in detail in Chapter 1. Ligaments have a homogeneous hyperechoic appearance with a fibrillar pattern. The ligaments of the shoulder and acromioclavicular joints are summarized in Table 2.5. The transverse humeral ligament is assessed

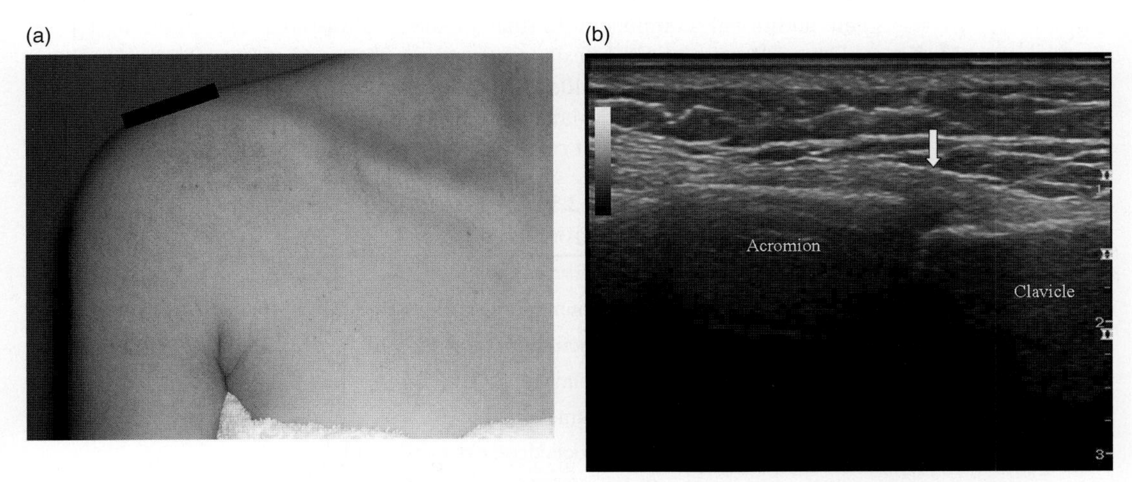

Figure 2.25. Acromioclavicular joint: **(a)** transducer position and **(b)** corresponding ultrasound image in the coronal axis. Arrow, joint capsule and superior acromioclavicular ligament.

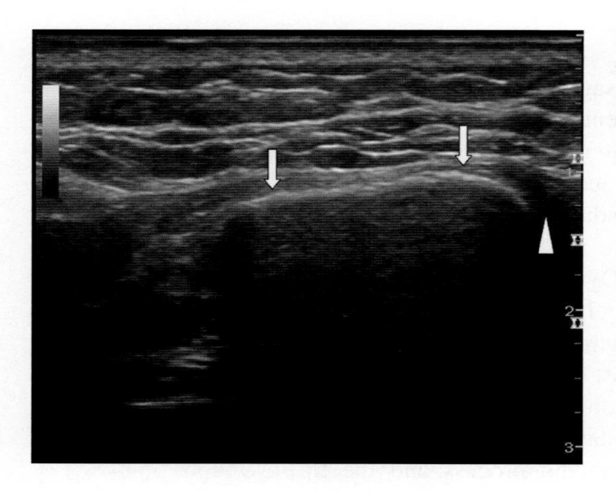

Figure 2.26. Acromion: coronal ultrasound with the transducer maintained in the same plane as Figure 2.25a, but moved slightly laterally from the acromioclavicular joint (arrowhead).

when evaluating the biceps tendon as described previously. The remaining ligaments, which are not routinely assessed, include the coracohumeral (C-H) ligament, which is visualized with the arm in the neutral position, as described in the assessment of the long head biceps tendon, with the medial aspect transducer on the coracoid process and the lateral aspect on the greater tuberosity (Figure 2.27). Rotating the transducer superiorly so the lateral edge lies on the acromion brings the coracoacromial ligament into view (Figure 2.28). Occasionally the rotator cable, a fibrous sheath that extends from the coracoacromial ligament to envelop the supraspinatus and infraspinatus, can be identified. Its fibers pass perpendicular to those of the supraspinatus and can be seen as a thin hyperechoic fibrillar structure medial to the greater tuberosity. The fibers are prone to anisotropy and it is important not to misinterpret this appearance as pathology of the articular fibers of the supraspinatus (Figure 2.19a).[34] The glenohumeral ligaments are not routinely identifiable with ultrasonography.

Subacromial Impingement

Dynamic assessment of possible subacromial impingement has become an additional component to the shoulder ultrasound examination. Up to eight different clinical tests are used in the assessment of supraspinatus impingement.[35] The shoulder is adducted in internal rotation, and the transducer is placed over the lateral margin of the acromion in a coronal plane (Figure 2.29a). Movement of the supraspinatus tendon and overlying bursa is

Table 2.5. Ligaments of the Shoulder and Acromioclavicular Joints.

Ligament
Transverse humeral[a]
Coracohumeral[a]
Coracoacromial[a]
Coracoclavicular
Glenohumeral (3)
Acromioclavicular (superior[a]) (4)
Suprascapular

[a]Can normally be visualized on ultrasound.

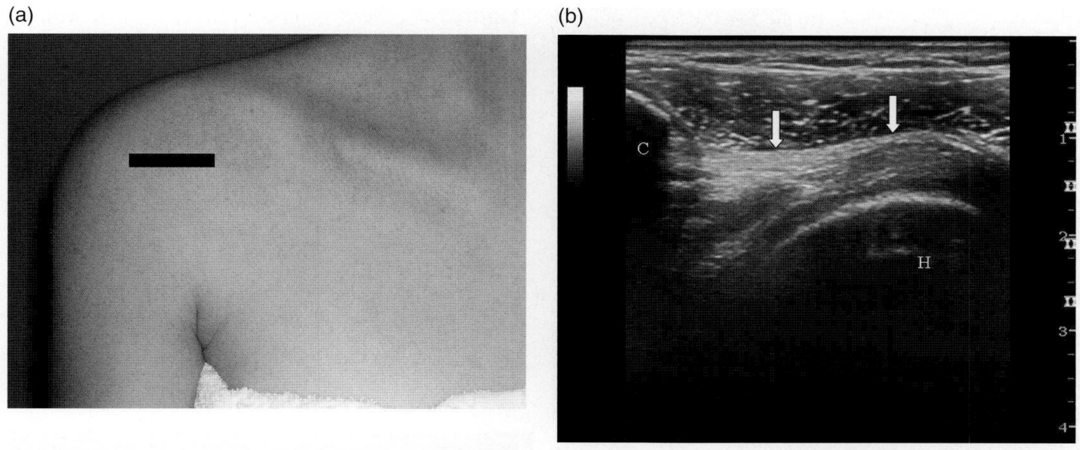

Figure 2.27. Coracohumeral ligament (arrow): (**a**) transducer position and (**b**) corresponding ultrasound image. C, coracoid process; H, humerus.

assessed during abduction (Figure 2.29b). The tendon may be better visualized with the transducer in an oblique coronal plane anterior to the acromion and acromioclavicular joint. The transducer is then placed in a sagittal plane with its posterior margin upon the anterior aspect of the acromion, and the arm is then flexed in internal rotation. The supraspinatus tendon and the SASD bursa normally move smoothly under the acromion, without bunching of the fibers of the tendon or lateral distention of the bursa. The patient should not have limitation of motion or pain.[36] Alternative etiologies, if the SASD bursa is significantly distended and impinges on dynamic assessment, need to be excluded, e.g., inflammatory arthropathy.[37] In these alternate pathologies, the supraspinatus tendon should not impinge.

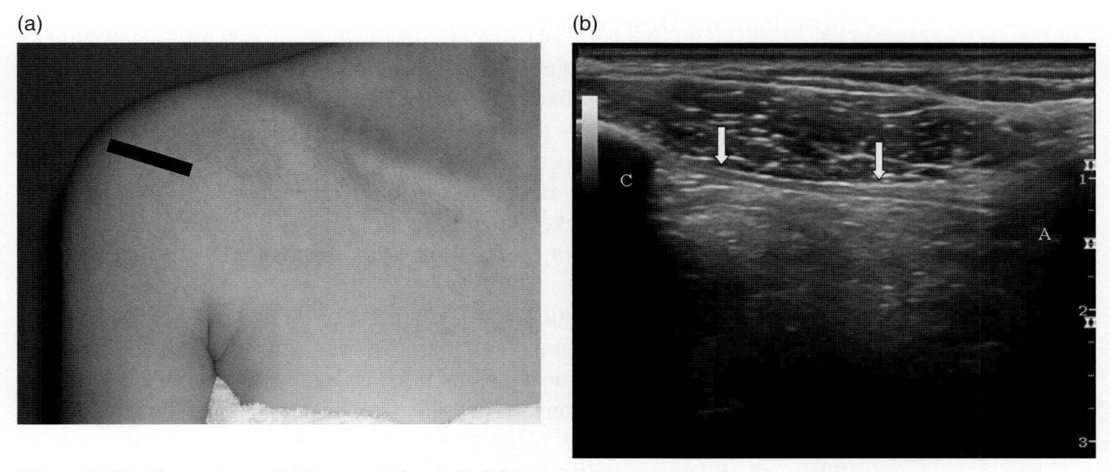

Figure 2.28. Coracoacromial ligament (arrow): (**a**) transducer position and (**b**) corresponding ultrasound image. C, coracoid; A, acromion.

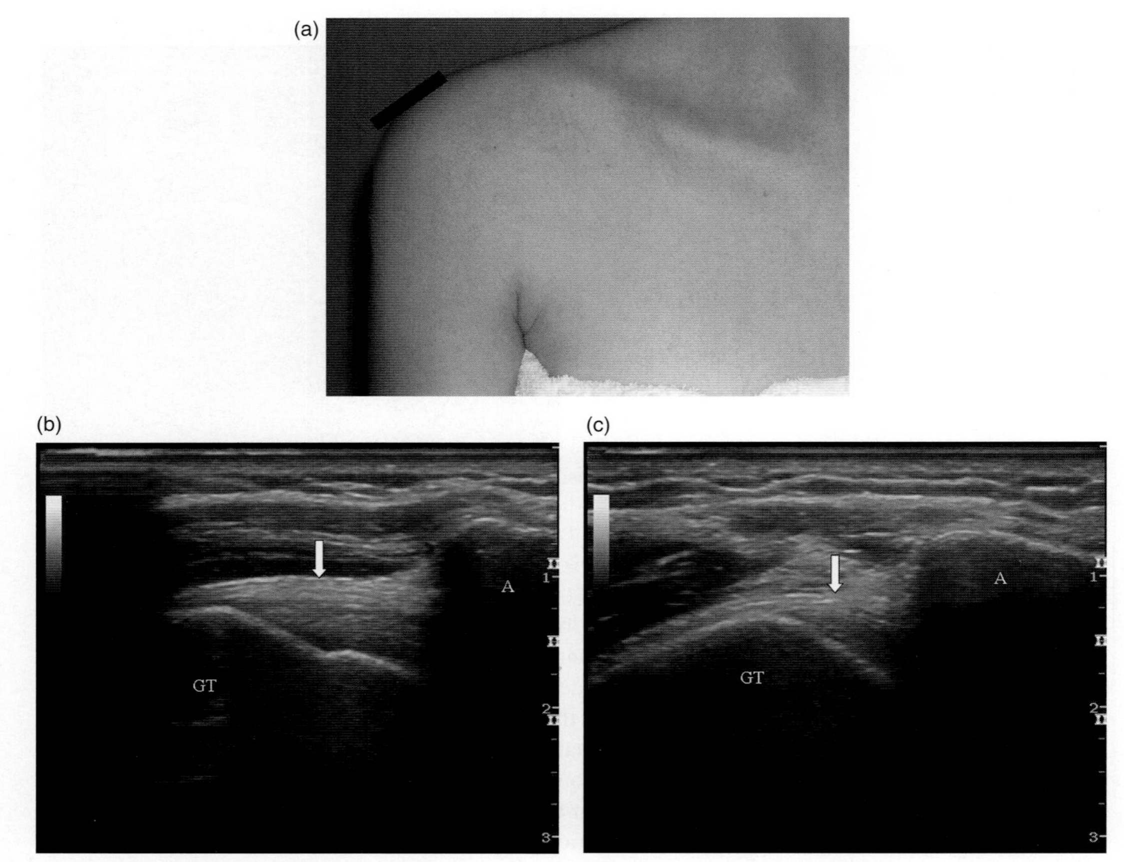

Figure 2.29. Supraspinatus dynamic impingement test: **(a)** transducer position and **(b)** corresponding ultrasound image in the longitudinal plane of the tendon in the neutral position and **(c)** in abduction. The supraspinatus tendon should move smoothly under the acromion without bunching of its fibers, lateral distention of the overlying SASD bursa, or superior translation of the humeral head. A, acromion; GT, greater tuberosity.

Miscellaneous Observations

The cortical surface of the humeral head normally appears as a smooth, hyperechoic, continuous line and is evaluated initially with the arm by the side in a neutral position followed by internal and external rotation. The bare area, on the posterosuperior humeral head, is identified as a small focal depression and lies directly deep to the infraspinatus (Figure 2.30). It should not be mistaken for early erosion or a small Hill–Sachs defect; if there is concern, correlation with the contralateral side can be performed.

The deltoid is not routinely evaluated, but is imaged if the patient is symptomatic in this region or if there is a history of trauma including postsurgical dehiscence and contracture. The three anatomical components of the deltoid—anterior, intermediate, and posterior—are evaluated separately in a transverse plane from origin to insertion onto the deltoid tuberosity. Fiber orientation is posterior oblique, vertical, and anterior oblique, respectively.

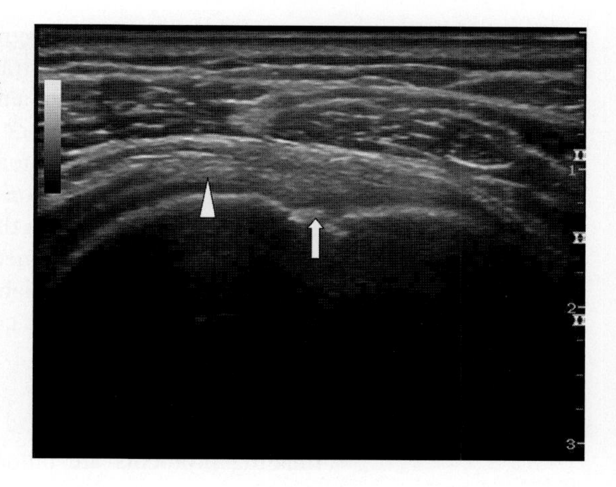

Figure 2.30. Ultrasound image: "bare area" demonstrated as focal cortical irregularity on the posterosuperior aspect greater tuberosity (arrow), with overlying infraspinatus tendon (arrowhead).

Occasionally, pathology within the pectoralis major may present with shoulder symptoms. The patient is examined in the long head of the biceps position with the transducer in the axial plane to the body, longitudinal to tendon, overlying the mid and distal bicipital groove (Figures 2.31). The muscle has an extensive origin, and it is important to evaluate the tendon from its superior to inferior border. In addition, we perform a dynamic test by externally rotating the arm, keeping the elbow by the side. Anterior shoulder instability, which accounts for 95% of shoulder instability, can be assessed on ultrasound.[30] Ultrasound examination is often limited, however, in the assessment of the anterior labrum, the underlying bony glenoid, and anterior capsule, but can usually clearly visualize a Hill–Sachs defect of the humeral head. The glenohumeral ligaments are not normally visible on ultrasound.

Sonoarthrography, wherein a standard shoulder arthrogram is performed and then evaluated with ultrasound, has been studied.[38] In the study, sonoarthrography exhibited similar sensitivity and specificity to standard ultrasound in the diagnosis of rotator cuff tears. It is our practice that patients

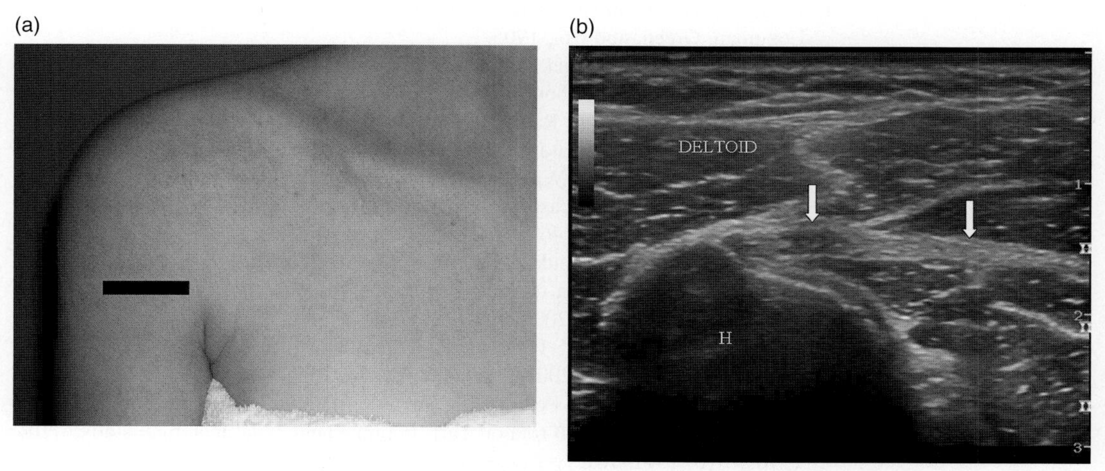

Figure 2.31. Pectoralis major: **(a)** transducer position and **(b)** corresponding ultrasound image of the longitudinal plane tendon at the humeral insertion. H, humerus.

proceed to an MRI arthrogram, the imaging gold standard for rotator cuff pathology, if a standard ultrasound examination is inconclusive in the appropriate clinical setting. Patients who fail to complete MRI arthrogram, e.g., those with claustrophobia or for whom it is contraindicated, would normally proceed to a computed tomography (CT) arthrogram in our institution. Anterior shoulder translation measurements can be performed in patients with anterior instability,[39] but in the author's opinion, this adds little to information that already has been obtained by clinical examination. Underlying pathology, such as disruption of the labrum and bony defects such as a Bankart lesion or a Hill–Sachs deformity, can be evaluated as described above.

Imaging Protocols

Imaging protocols are tailored to the clinical question. We will routinely include any new area of symptoms that have developed in the region of the shoulder since the previous clinical review. All patients with a clinical question of pathology related to a single or all components of the rotator cuff or proximal biceps will undergo a standard study of the shoulder as outlined in the Appendix. Assessments for joint effusion or synovitis receive a dedicated study of the joint space, recesses, and bursae, including Doppler, and an examination of the visible glenoid and humeral cortex for erosions. Posttraumatic patients are evaluated as per standard protocol, in addition to the area of symptoms. Patients suspected of neural impingement, e.g., within the spinoglenoid notch, will receive a standard study with special focus on the nerve in question and its region of innervation.

References

1. Snell R. The upper limb. In: Clinical Anatomy, 7th ed., pp. 570–572. Philadelphia: Lippincott Williams & Wilkins, 2004.
2. Gray H. The Complete Gray's Anatomy, 16th ed., pp. 378–383. London: Longman, Green, and Co., 1905.
3. Resnick D. Internal derangements joints. In: Diagnosis of Bone and Joint Disorders, 4th ed., pp. 3068–3146. Philadelphia: Saunders, 2002.
4. Gray H. The Complete Gray's Anatomy, 16th ed., pp. 502–513. London: Longman, Green, and Co., 1905.
5. Vahlensieck M, an Haack K, Schmidt H. Two portions of the supraspinatus muscle: A new finding about the muscles macroscopy by dissection and magnetic resonance imaging. Surg Radiol Anat 1994;16:101–104.
6. Zlatkin M. Shoulder anatomy. In: MRI of the Shoulder, 2nd ed., pp. 85–116. Philadelphia: Lippincott Williams & Wilkins, 2003.
7. van Holsbeeck M, Introcaso J. Sonography of the shoulder. In: Musculoskeletal Ultrasound, 2nd ed., pp. 463–516. St. Louis: Mosby, 2001.
8. Gleason P, Beall D, Sanders T. The transverse humeral ligament: A separate anatomical structure or a continuation of the osseous attachment of the rotator cuff? Am J Sports Med 2006;34(1):72–77.
9. Plancher K, Johnston J, Peterson R. The dimensions of the rotator interval. J Shoulder Elbow Surg 2005;14(6):620–625.
10. Brossmann J, Preidler K, Pedowitz R. Shoulder impingement syndrome: Influence of shoulder position on rotator cuff impingement—an anatomic study. AJR 1996;167(6):1511–1515.
11. Buttaci C, Stitik T, Yonclass P et al. Osteoarthritis of the acromioclavicular joint. Am J Phys Med Rehabil 2004;83:791–797.

12. Ferri M, Finlay K, Popowich T et al. Sonographic examination of the acromioclavicular and sternoclavicular joints. J Clin Ultrasound 2005;33:345–355.
13. Shaffer B. Painful conditions of the acromioclavicular joint. J Am Acad Orthop Surg 1999;7:176–188.
14. Mosely HF, Overgaard B. The anterior capsular mechanism in recurrent anterior dislocation of the shoulder. J Bone Joint Surg 1962;44B:913–927.
15. Taljanovic M, Carlson K, Kuhn J et al. Sonography of the glenoid labrum: A cadaveric study with arthroscopic correlation. AJR 2000;174:1717–1722.
16. Schydlowsky P, Strandberg C, Galatius S et al. Ultrasonographic examination of the glenoid labrum of healthy volunteers. Eur J Ultrasound 1998;8:85–89.
17. Schydlowsky P, Strandberg C, Tranum-Jensen J. Post-mortem ultrasonographic assessment of the anterior glenoid labrum. Eur J Ultrasound 1998;8:129–133.
18. Bouffard J, Lee S, Dhanju J. Ultrasonography of the shoulder. Semin Ultrasound CT MRI 2000;21(3):164–191.
19. Prescher A. Anatomical basics, variations, and degenerative changes of the shoulder joint and shoulder girdle. Eur J Radiol 2000;35(2):88–102.
20. Plancher k, Peterson R, Johnston J. The spinoglenoid ligament. Anatomy, morphology, and histological findings. J Bone Joint Surg Am 2005;87:361–365.
21. Farin PU, Jaroma H, Harju A. Medial displacement of the biceps brachii tendon: Evaluation with dynamic sonography during maximal external shoulder rotation. Radiology 1995;195(3):845–848.
22. Itamura J, Dietrick T, Roidis N. Analysis of the bicipital groove as a landmark for humeral head replacement. J Shoulder Elbow Surg 2002;11(4):322–326.
23. Clark J, Harryman D. Tendons, ligaments and capsule of the rotator cuff. J Bone Joint Surg Am 1992;74:713–726.
24. Curtis AS, Burbank KM, Tierney JJ et al. The insertional footprint of the rotator cuff: An anatomic study. Arthroscopy 2006;22(6):603–609.
25. Crass J, Craig E, Feinberg S. The hyperextended internal rotation view in rotator cuff ultrasonography. J Clin US 1987;6:416–420.
26. Middleton W, Teefey S, Yamaguchi K. Sonography of the shoulder. Semin Musculoskelet Radiol 1998;2(3):211–222.
27. Turrin A, Capello A. Sonographic anatomy of the supraspinatus tendon and adjacent structures. Skeletal Radiol 1997;26:89–93.
28. Boehm T, Kirschner S, Mueller T. Dynamic ultrasonography of rotator cuff muscles. J Clin Ultrasound 2005;33:207–213.
29. Hammar M, Wintzell G, Astrom K et al. Role of US in the preoperative evaluation of patients with anterior shoulder instability. Radiology 2001;219:29–34.
30. Rasmussen O. Anterior shoulder instability: Sonographic evaluation. J Clin Ultrasound 2004;32:430–437.
31. Kock H, Jurgens C, Hirche H. Standardised ultrasound examination for evaluation of instability of the acromioclavicular joint. Arch Orthop Trauma Surg 1996;115:136–140.
32. Sluming V. Technical note: Measuring the coracoclavicular distance with ultrasound—a new technique. Br J Radiol 1995;68(806):189–193.
33. Azzoni R, Cabitza P, Parrini M. Sonographic evaluation of subacromial space. Ultrasonics 2004;42:683–687.
34. Morag Y, Jacobson J, Lucas R et al. US appearance of the rotator cable with histiologic correlation: Preliminary results. Radiology 2006;241(2):485–491.
35. Park H, Yokota A, Gill H. Diagnostic accuracy of clinical tests for the different degrees of subacromial impingement syndrome. J Bone Joint Surg Am 2005;87(7):1446–1455.
36. Farin P, Jaroma H, Harju A et al. Shoulder impingement syndrome: Sonographic evaluation. Radiology 1990;176:845–849.

37. Hollister M, Mack L, Patten R et al. Association of sonographically detected subacromial/subdeltoid bursal effusion and intra-articular fluid with rotator cuff tear. AJR 1995;165:605–608.
38. Lee H, Joo K, Park C et al. Sonography of the shoulder after arthrography (arthrosonography): Preliminary results. J Clin Ultrasound 2002;30(1):23–32.
39. Krarup A, Court-Payen M, Skjoldbye B. Ultrasonic measurement of the anterior translation in the shoulder joint. J Shoulder Elbow Surg 1999;8(2):136–141.

3

The Arm

Karen Finlay

The arm is that part of the upper extremity between the shoulder and the elbow. Important proximal muscles acting on the shoulder and elbow joint are present, along with terminal branch nerves of the brachial plexus. The muscle compartments are easily divided into flexor and extensor groups. Knowledge of these structures and muscle groups is important for the assessment of local pathology and also for tracing pathology proximal and distal to the more commonly imaged shoulder and elbow joints.

Imaging Indications

Sonographic evaluation of the arm can easily be incorporated into the study of the adjacent joints, particularly if there is extension of pathology. Alternatively, the examination can be restricted to the arm to investigate specific regional pathology. Specific indications for dedicated ultrasound of the arm include regional muscle pathology, such as trauma and suspected muscle or tendon injury, as well as investigation of soft tissue masses. Important nerves are present in the arm. For a thorough investigation of focal pathology, the course of these nerves should be familiar and their relationship to adjacent abnormalities explored. This assists in assessing and describing the relationship of traumatic injuries or masses to adjacent anatomical structures. In addition, knowledge of the flexor and extensor compartments, the location of muscle groups, as well as the course of important nerves helps in determining an appropriate needle course if aspiration or biopsy is undertaken.

Technical Review

The technical requirements of the arm examination are frequently similar to those of the shoulder and elbow joint study. Multifrequency linear array probes are utilized, with optimal frequency selected based on body habitus, nature of specific pathology, and depth of region of interest. Generally this is between 7 and 12 MHz. It is important to utilize color or power Doppler, particularly if focal pathology is adjacent to regional arteries or veins, in order to confirm anatomical relationships. This can also assist in determining the extent of hyperemia or vascularity of regional masses or abnormalities. Dynamic imaging can also be employed: e.g., in the evaluation of a soft tissue intramuscular mass the position and relationship of the mass to surrounding structures may change with flexion, extension, and compression with the transducer and may reveal information not available from a static study.

Anatomy

Surface Anatomy

The humerus is almost completely surrounded by muscles (Figure 3.1). The epicondyles at the elbow represent the only subcutaneous portions of this

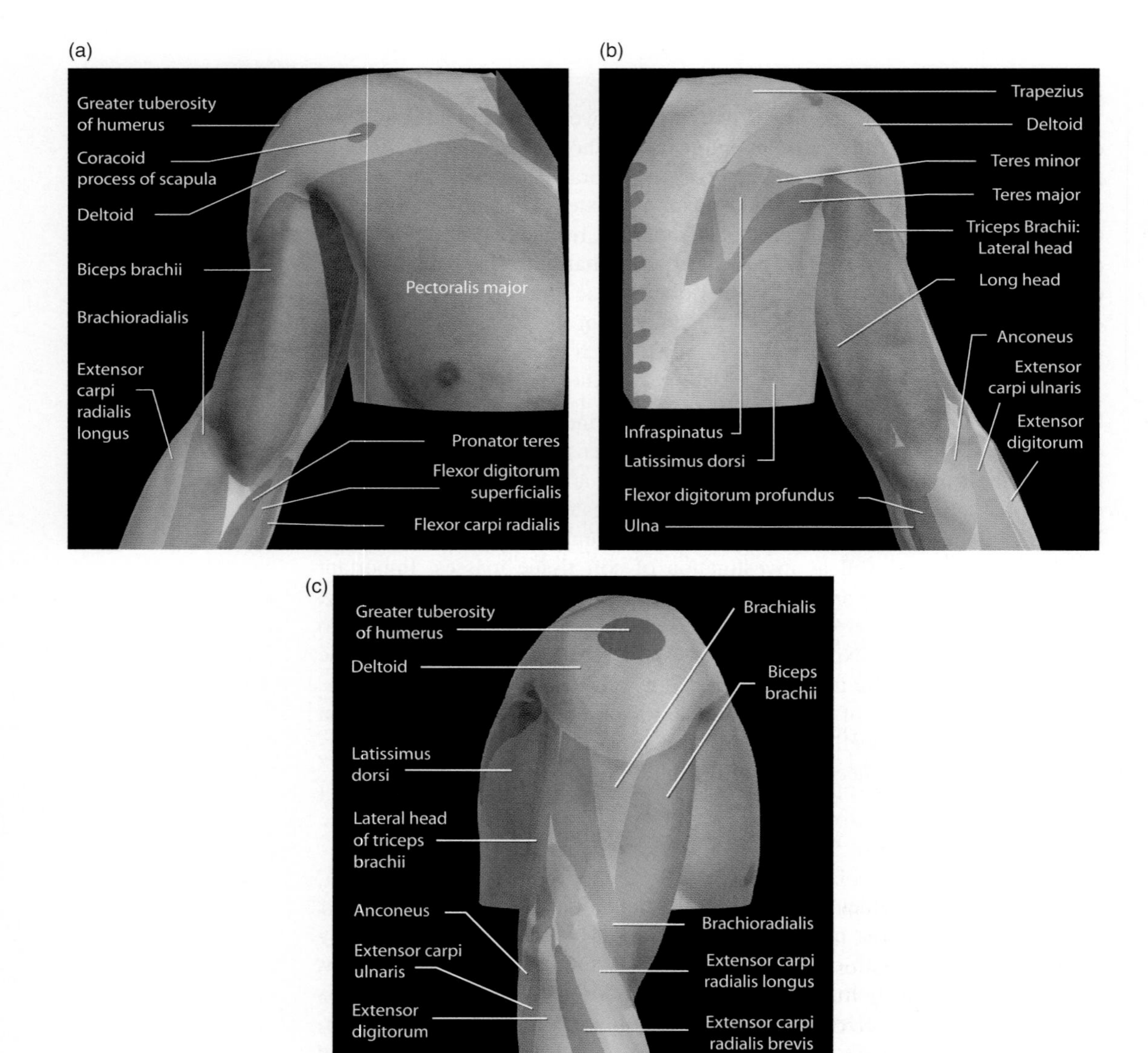

Figure 3.1. The surface anatomy of the arm: **(a)** anterior, **(b)** posterior, and **(c)** lateral views.

long bone, with the medial epicondyle more prominent than the lateral. The greater and lesser tuberosities are palpable proximally; however, much of the surface anatomy of the proximal arm is due to the overlying and dominant deltoid muscle. The deltoid muscle forms the smooth, rounded contour of the shoulder that is fuller on the anterior than the posterior surface. The insertion of the deltoid onto the lateral aspect of the mid arm is sometimes visible as a distinct elevation. At the anterior aspect of the arm, the biceps brachii is visible as an elongated muscle with lateral and medial depressions at its margins. It forms the rounded contour of the anterior arm. With flexion or contraction, the biceps is identified as a discrete, elongated muscle mass. While the proximal tendons of the long and short head of the biceps are obscured, the distal tendon is visible crossing the elbow joint when the elbow is flexed.

In the lower arm, just proximal to the elbow, the brachialis muscle is visible, with the lateral border visible extending along the proximal arm and the medial aspect forming some fullness above the elbow joint. Posteriorly and below the deltoid, the triceps muscle appears as a longitudinally oriented structure, extending inferiorly to a flattened tendon, which inserts onto the olecranon process.

Bones

The humerus is the single long bone of the arm. The proximal aspect consists of a head, anatomical neck, greater and lesser tuberosities, as well as the proximal shaft. The spherical humeral head is covered with hyaline cartilage and articulates with the glenoid cavity of the scapula. The greater and lesser tuberosities are separated from the head by the anatomical neck. The tuberosities represent important bony prominences that are landmarks for the insertion sites of the rotator cuff tendons. The intertubercular sulcus, or biceps groove, is identified anteriorly between the two tuberosities and delineates the course along which the long head of biceps brachii exits the shoulder joint. The proximal half of the humeral shaft is cylindrical; the distal half expands in transverse diameter to become triangular. The deltoid tuberosity is an important proximal landmark, which is identified anterolaterally on the humerus and represents a focal elevation of variable prominence at the insertion site of the deltoid tendon (Figure 3.2). It is important to recognize this normal physiological landmark on the humeral surface in order to avoid misdiagnosing it as an abnormal finding. The radial groove is present on the posterior surface of the humerus. The radial nerve courses along this important groove, with the groove oriented in an inferolateral direction. Distally, the lateral and medial epicondyles represent important palpable landmarks. Prominent supracondylar ridges are identified on either side of the humerus, running proximal from both the lateral and medial epicondyle.

The anterior border of the humerus commences at the level of the greater tuberosity and extends distally along the length of the bone. The posterior surface is the most extensive and is closely related to the medial head of the triceps.[1] The medial and lateral borders are best delineated distally where the edges are more distinct or roughened. Occasionally, a supracondylar process is identified emanating from the anteromedial surface of the distal humerus, approximately 5 cm proximal to the medial epicondyle.[1] This process may be 5 to 20 cm in length, curving in an anterior and inferior direction, and represents a normal congenital variant.

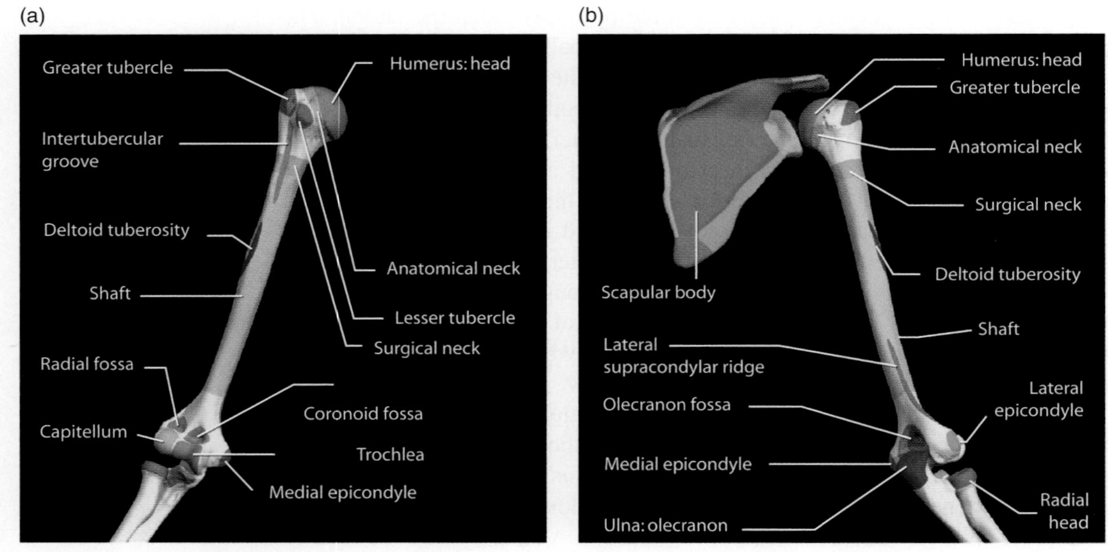

Figure 3.2. The important bony landmarks of the humerus: **(a)** anterior and **(b)** posterior views.

Muscles and Tendons

The muscles of the arm are listed in Table 3.1. The deltoid muscle is a large multipennate muscle that forms the characteristic round contour of the shoulder. Proximally, the muscle has attachments to the distal clavicle, acromion, and spine of the scapula. The distal portion attaches to a rough

Table 3.1. Arm Muscles: Origin, Insertion, and Action.

Muscle	Origin	Insertion	Main action
Deltoid	Lateral one-third of clavicle Acromion Spine of scapula	Mid humerus—deltoid tuberosity	Shoulder abduction Anterior fibers: flexion and medial arm rotation Posterior fibers: extension and lateral arm rotation
Biceps brachii—long head	Supraglenoid tubercle scapula	Radial tuberosity and bicipital aponeurosis	Forearm supination Elbow flexion
Biceps brachii—short head	Coracoid process of scapula	Joins with long head to insert onto radial tuberosity and bicipital aponeurosis	Forearm supination Elbow flexion
Coracobrachialis	Coracoid process of scapula	Medial aspect midshaft of humerus	Arm flexion and adduction
Brachialis	Anterior surface, lower one-half of humerus	Coronoid process of ulna	Forearm flexion
Triceps brachii—long head	Infraglenoid tubercle of scapula	Olecranon process of ulna	Adducts arm, extends shoulder
Triceps brachii—lateral head	Posterolateral aspect of humerus	Olecranon process of ulna	Extends forearm at elbow
Triceps brachii—medial head	Lower one-half of posteromedial humerus	Olecranon process of ulna	Extends forearm at elbow

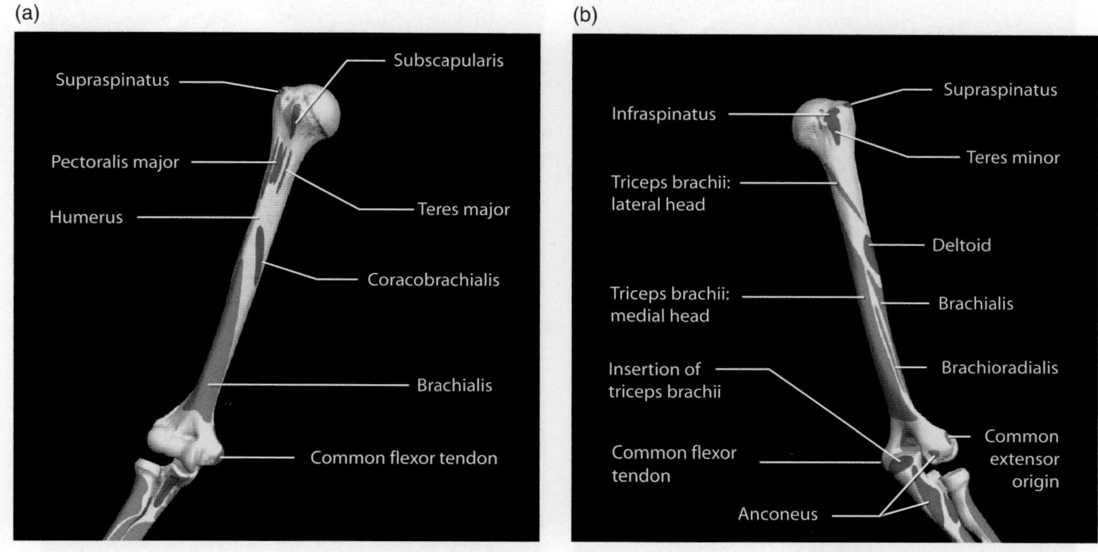

Figure 3.3. The muscle origin (red) and insertion (blue) points of the humerus: **(a)** anterior and **(b)** posterior views.

elevated area on the humerus (Figure 3.3), known as the deltoid tuberosity, that is located midway down the lateral aspect of the humerus. The deltoid has three discrete components, consisting of anterior, intermediate, and posterior fibers (Figure 3.4). It is the main abductor of the shoulder, produced with action of the acromion or intermediate deltoid fibers. The anterior deltoid fibers act to flex the shoulder; the posterior fibers contribute to shoulder extension.[1]

Insider Information 3.1
The deltoid muscle has three components, each with a different function:
Anterior—shoulder flexion
Intermediate—shoulder abduction
Posterior—shoulder extension

Muscle Compartments
The remaining muscles of the arm are easily separated into anterior (flexor) and posterior (extensor) muscle compartments (Table 3.2 and Figure 3.5). These are separated from one another by the humerus and the medial and lateral intermuscular septa.[2]

Insider Information 3.2
The lateral and medial intermuscular fascia separates the arm into anterior and posterior muscle compartments. This is an important consideration when approaching any procedure or biopsy.

Anterior Compartment: The anterior compartment consists of the biceps brachii, coracobrachialis, and brachialis muscles, which are supplied by the

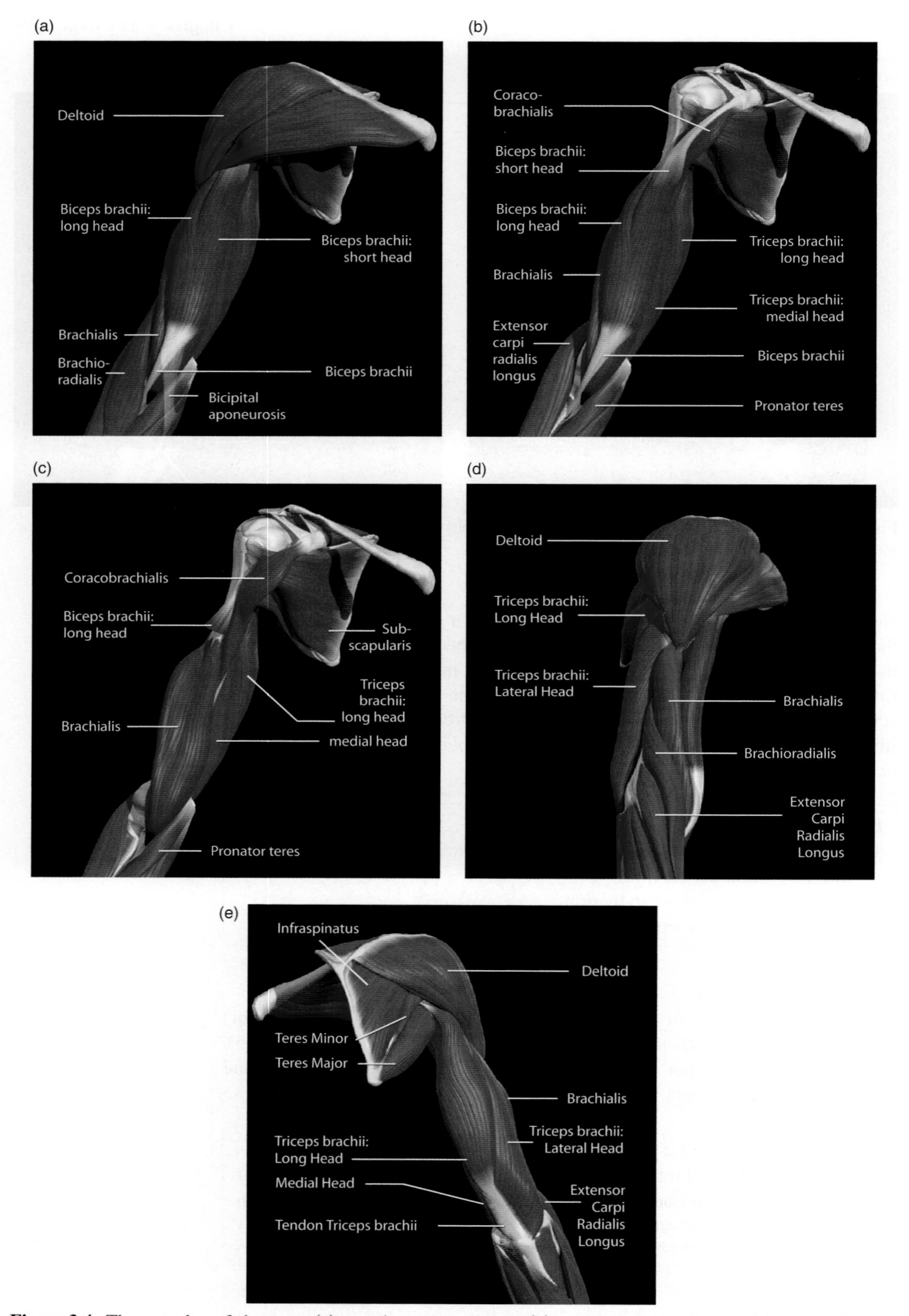

Figure 3.4. The muscles of the arm: **(a)** anterior compartment, **(b)** anterior compartment with pectoralis and deltoid muscles removed, **(c)** anterior compartment with biceps removed, **(d)** lateral view, and **(e)** posterior view.

Table 3.2. Muscle Compartments of the Arm.

Anterior compartment	Posterior compartment
Biceps brachii	Triceps
Long head	Long head
Short head	Lateral head
Coracobrachialis	Medial head
Brachialis	

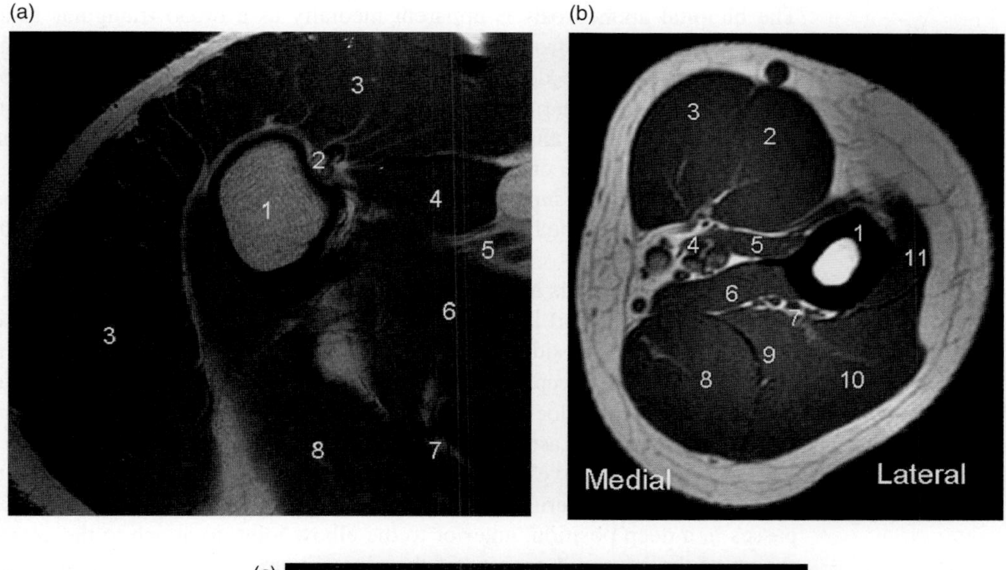

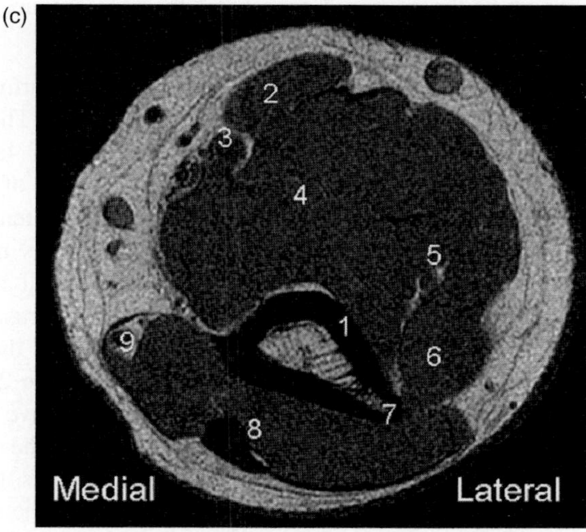

Figure 3.5. Axial T1-weighted MRI anatomy of the arm. **(a)** Proximal arm: 1–proximal humeral shaft, 2–biceps: long head, 3–deltoid, 4–coracobrachialis, 5–axillary vessels, 6–subscapularis, 7–scapula: inferior aspect, 8–teres minor. **(b)** Mid arm: 1–humerus, 2–biceps: short head, 3–biceps: long head, 4–brachial artery, median and ulnar nerves, 5–brachialis, 6–coracobrachialis, 7–radial nerve and vessels, 8–triceps: long head, 9–triceps: medial head, 10–triceps: lateral head, 11–deltoid. **(c)** Distal arm: 1–humerus, 2–biceps, 3–median nerve and brachial vessels, 4–brachialis, 5–radial nerve, 6–extensor carpi radialis longus, 7–humerus, lateral epicondyle, 8–triceps, 9–ulnar nerve.

musculocutaneous nerve. The two heads of the biceps brachii part proximally, with the short head identified medially, originating from the apex of the coracoid process of the scapula (Figure 3.4b). The long head has an origin at the supraglenoid tubercle of the scapula and leaves the shoulder joint via the intertubercular sulcus of the proximal humerus. The short and long head of the biceps brachii, commonly known as the biceps muscle, closely approximate within the arm and form a common tendon distally, which rotates or spirals as it approaches its distal insertion (Figure 3.4). This distal tendon crosses the elbow joint to insert onto the radial tubercle, with the proximal anterior fibers rotating laterally just prior to insertion.[1] The bicipital aponeurosis is apparent medially as a broad triangular fascial expansion extending from the biceps tendon across the brachial artery and cubital fossa into the deep fascia of the forearm.[1] The biceps is a strong supinator of the forearm, flexor of the elbow, and weaker flexor of the shoulder.[1,2] There are anatomical variations to the biceps muscle and tendons. In approximately 10% of the population, a third head of the biceps is present, originating from the superomedial aspect of the brachialis, with the fibers attaching distally to the bicipital aponeurosis and medial aspect of the tendon insertion.[1]

The coracobrachialis has a proximal attachment to the coracoid process, in common with the short head of the biceps (Figure 3.4). Distally, this muscle attaches to the medial side of the humeral shaft, near its midpoint, between the attachments of the triceps and brachialis (Figure 3.3a). This muscle, which is pierced by the musculocutaneous nerve, functions to weakly flex and adduct the shoulder joint.[2] Lastly, the brachialis muscle lies in a deep position in the arm, with extensive proximal attachment to the anterior surface of the distal half of the humerus and intermuscular septa (Figure 3.3a). This muscle passes in a deep position, anterior to the elbow joint, to attach to the anterior aspect of the coronoid process of the ulna (Figure 3.4c). The brachialis acts as a powerful flexor of the elbow joint.

Posterior Compartment: The posterior compartment contains the triceps muscle, which is supplied by the radial nerve. The triceps fills most of the extensor compartment of the arm (Figures 3.3, 3.4e, 3.5, and 3.6). This large muscle is named secondary to its three heads of origin: long, lateral, and medial. The long head originates as a flattened tendon from the infraglenoid tubercle of the scapula. In the arm it descends medial to the lateral head and superficial to the medial head. The lateral head arises as a flattened tendon from the posterior surface of the humerus, above the radial groove. The medial head has an extensive origin from the posterior surface of the humerus, inferior to the radial groove, to within 2.5 cm from the trochlea.[1] The three components of the triceps muscle have a common insertion onto the olecranon process of the ulna. Some of the medial head fibers reach the olecranon process directly.[1] The triceps is the chief extensor of the forearm. Other functions include extension of the shoulder and adduction of the arm.

The anconeus muscle is also identified posteriorly, partially blending with the triceps muscle. This muscle arises as a separate tendon from the posterior surface of the humerus, at the level of the lateral epicondyle, and traverses the posterior aspect of the annular ligament, attaching to the lateral aspect of the olecranon process. The anconeus assists the triceps in elbow extension.

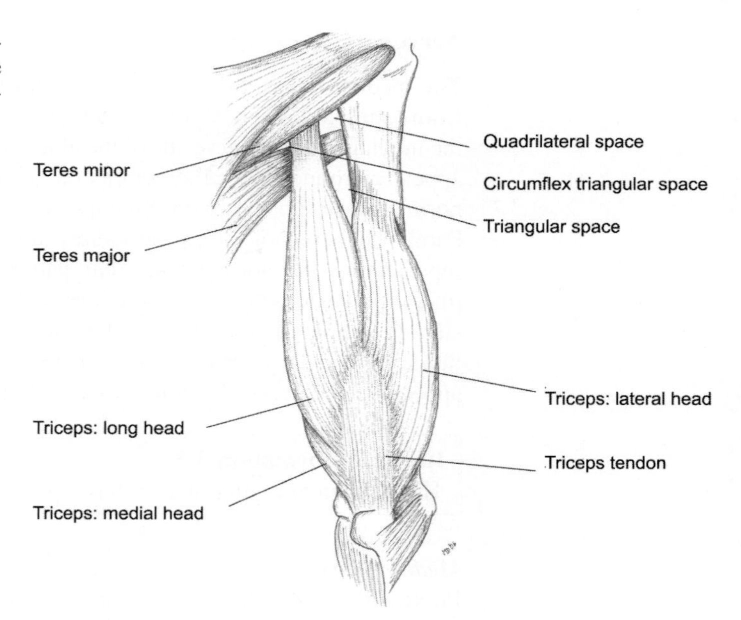

Figure 3.6. Quadrilateral and triangular spaces. Illustration of the posterior arm, demonstrating intermuscular spaces.

Spaces

Quadrilateral Space

This posterior anatomical space is bordered by the teres minor superiorly, teres major inferiorly, long head triceps medially, and humerus laterally (Figure 3.6). These structures define the quadrilateral shape of this space. The subscapularis lies at the anterior aspect. Important structures traversing within the space are the axillary nerve and posterior humeral circumflex artery and vein (Chapter 12, Figure 12.3b).

Triangular Space

This posterior space, also known as the triangular interval, lies below the quadrilateral space.[1] It is bordered superiorly by the subscapularis at its anterior aspect and by the teres major at its posterior aspect. The long head of the triceps forms the medial border and lateral head of the triceps forms the lateral border. The margins of these structures create the triangular configuration of this space (Figure 3.6). The radial nerve and profunda brachii vessels traverse through this anatomical space. It should be noted that a second triangular intermuscular space lies medial to the quadrilateral space, with the long head of the triceps forming its lateral border and transmitting the circumflex scapular artery.

Fascia

Superficial and Deep

The brachial fascia encloses the structures of the arm.[3] This fascia is continuous proximally with the pectoral and axillary fascia, as well as the fascia covering the deltoid and latissimus dorsi muscles.[3] Distally, the fascia attaches to the humeral epicondyles and the olecranon process. It is also continuous with the deep fascia of the forearm. The medial and lateral intermuscular septae separate the arm into anterior and posterior fascial compartments, each with its own muscles, nerves, and vessels (Figure 3.5). The septae extend from the brachial fascia and attach to lateral and medial ridges of the humerus.[3]

Nerves

The median, ulnar, and radial nerves traverse the length of the arm, arising from terminal branches of the brachial plexus. No branches arise from either the median or ulnar nerve above the elbow joint. On ultrasound, normal nerves appear as round or oval structures on short axis orientation. Longitudinally, normal nerves appear as cordlike hypoechoic structures of uniform thickness. Parallel hyperechoic linear structures are identified throughout their course, representing the normal fascicular pattern of nerve fibers.[4] On transverse imaging, the background echotexture is hypoechoic, with multiple, discrete, slightly echogenic foci dispersed evenly throughout that represent the nerve fascicles in cross section.[5,6] As a result of this microanatomy, the ultrasound appearance of nerves is more hypoechoic than tendons.

Insider Information 3.3
The median and ulnar nerves have no branches in the arm.

Median Nerve

Proximally within the arm, the median nerve lies in a lateral position relative to the axillary artery (Chapter 12, Figure 12.3a). Beyond the axillary artery, the median nerve is identified at the medial aspect of the arm, lateral to the brachial artery. Near the level of the coracobrachialis insertion, at the middle of the arm, the median nerve moves anterior and subsequently medial to the brachial artery, contacting the brachialis muscle. From this position, the median nerve descends into the cubital fossa, where it is positioned deep to the bicipital aponeurosis.

Ulnar Nerve

Proximally, the ulnar nerve is positioned medially, adjacent to the axillary artery, and, as the nerve moves distally, the brachial artery (Chapter 12, Figure 12.3a and b). Approximately halfway down the arm, the nerve pierces the intermuscular septum and moves posterior, descending between the septum and the medial head of the triceps.[3] At the elbow joint, the nerve is adjacent to the posterior aspect of the medial epicondyle. At this level, the ulnar nerve is superficial and palpable (Chapter 12, Figure 12.3c).

Radial Nerve

The radial nerve is positioned at the posterior aspect of the upper arm. It is identified posteriorly and superiorly as it emerges from the inferior margin of the teres major muscle. It is positioned behind the brachial artery, medial to the humerus and anterior to the long head of the triceps. At the level of the deltoid tuberosity, the radial nerve courses around the humerus, along a spiral groove on the bony surface (Chapter 12, Figure12.3b). It is important to recognize this anatomical arrangement because the radial nerve is vulnerable to injury associated with fractures and pathology of the humerus. Distal to the spiral groove, the radial nerve pierces the lateral intermuscular septum and descends inferiorly toward the elbow, between the brachialis and brachioradialis muscles.[3] Both the close relationship of the radial nerve to the humerus and its fixed position with penetration of the intermuscular septum make the radial nerve vulnerable to injury or compression.[7] Just proximal to the elbow joint, at the level of the lateral epicondyle, it divides into superficial and deep branches.

Insider Information 3.4
The radial nerve is vulnerable to injury, given its intimate course, around the spiral groove of the humerus.

Technique

For examination of the arm, the patient is usually seated, facing the examiner, with the arm in the neutral position and the elbow flexed (Table 3.3). The patient can also be examined supine or semireclined;[8] however, imaging of the posterior arm requires repositioning of the patient and arm, or use of a pillow to elevate the arm. A patient seated on a rotating chair or stool is easy to reposition for evaluation of the anterior and posterior aspects of the arm. Typically, in the arm, ultrasound evaluation is targeted to a specific clinical question or area of focal pathology; hence, the extent to which individual muscles, tendons, and nerves are evaluated can vary.

Deltoid

For evaluation of the deltoid muscle, the arm is positioned at the patient's side with the elbow either flexed or extended. Given the different orientation of the muscle fibers, the three portions of the deltoid (anterior, intermediate, and posterior) can be discriminated by ultrasound.[9] The muscle can be imaged systematically, with transverse scanning from proximal to distal. For evaluation of the intermediate fibers, the origin at the lateral acromial edge is identified (Figure 3.7a and b), with muscle fibers followed to insertion onto the deltoid tuberosity (Figure 3.7c). This evaluation should proceed from the anterior to posterior aspect of the intermediate bundle. After completing the longitudinal imaging, the muscle is reevaluated in transverse orientation, from proximal to distal aspect (Figure 3.8). The anterior fibers, from the origin of the distal clavicle, as well as posterior fibers, from the lateral edge of the scapular spine, can be examined in a similar fashion.[9] It is important to recognize the breadth of this muscle in order to image it completely. Distally, the deltoid tuberosity may be appreciated as a subtle elevation on the lateral humeral surface. It is important to observe a normal appearance of the deltoid fascial planes and tendons, as well as normal muscle architecture.

Table 3.3. Muscles and Tendons: Position for Ultrasound Examined.

Muscle	Position examined
Deltoid	Arm adducted, in neutral and relaxed position
Biceps brachii—long head	Elbow flexed, forearm supinated
Biceps brachii—short head	Elbow flexed, forearm supinated
Coracobrachialis	Mild arm abduction
Brachialis	Elbow flexed
Triceps brachii—Long head	Posterior approach, elbow flexed, arm abducted
Lateral head	
Medial head	

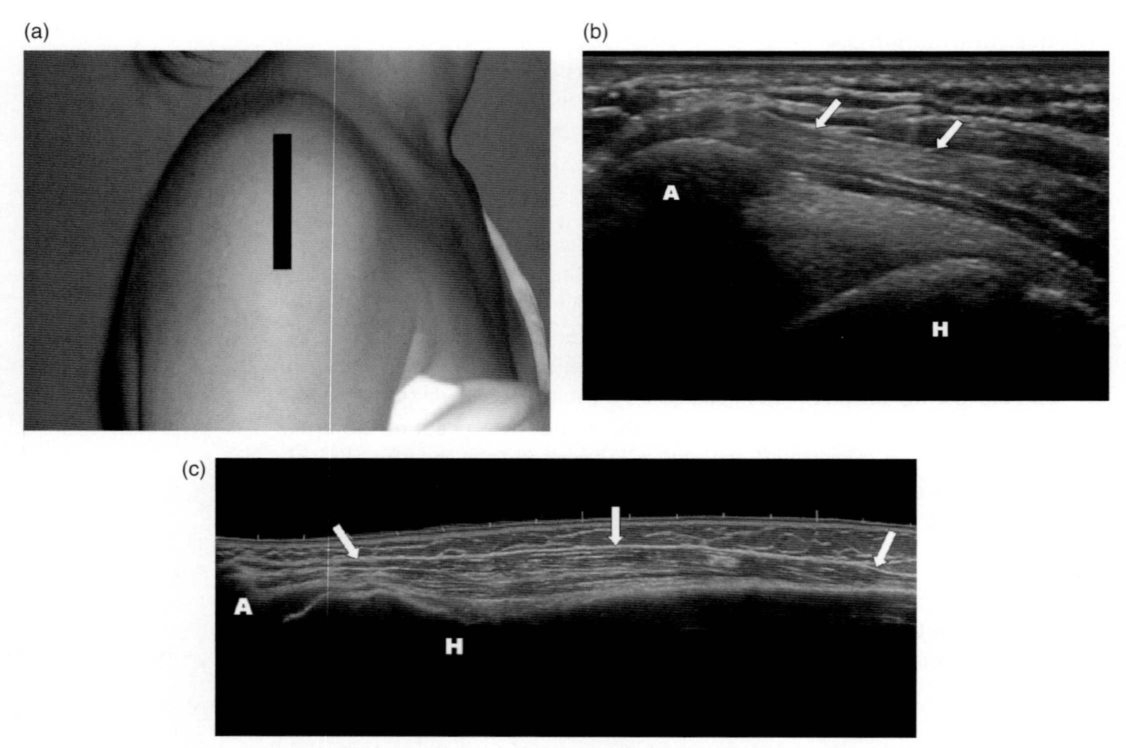

Figure 3.7. **(a)** The positioning of an ultrasound probe for evaluation of the proximal deltoid tendon fibers, as they originate from the acromion process. **(b)** Longitudinal ultrasound image of the proximal deltoid intermediate tendon fibers (arrows), as they originate from the acromion process (A), overlying the lateral aspect of the humeral head (H). **(c)** Extended longitudinal field of view image of the deltoid muscle (arrows), demonstrating the longitudinal course of the intermediate fibers, from the acromion process (A) to distal insertion on the humerus (H), at the level of the deltoid tuberosity (not shown).

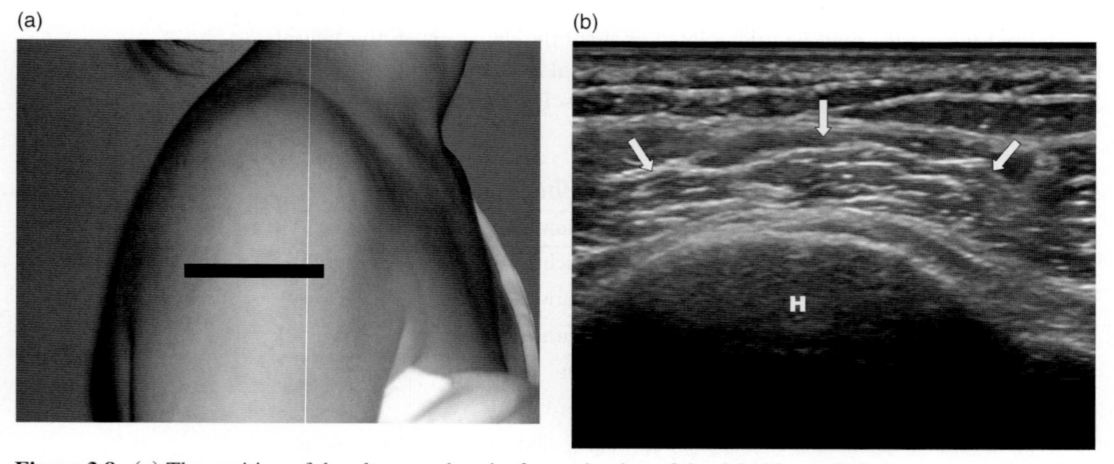

Figure 3.8. **(a)** The position of the ultrasound probe for evaluation of the deltoid muscle in transverse orientation. **(b)** Transverse image of the proximal deltoid muscle (arrows) overlying the lateral aspect of the proximal humeral shaft (H).

Anterior Compartment

The biceps brachii is the commonest muscle evaluated in the anterior compartment. The tendon of the long head of the biceps brachii is easily identified proximally, lying within the intertubercular groove of the proximal humerus. This tendon should be evaluated in both transverse and longitudinal orientation (Chapter 2). It is important to recognize the distal course of the long head, which is positioned adjacent to the anterior humerus, in a more shallow indentation on the humerus surface (Figure 3.9a), as compared with the deeper intertubercular groove proximally. Longitudinally, the tendon is coursing to the musculotendinous junction and into the proximal biceps muscle belly (Figure 3.9b). Upon completion of the long head tendon examination, the short head of the biceps brachii is identified at its origin on the coracoid process. To follow its course, the ultrasound probe is positioned in a slightly oblique orientation, with the proximal probe end positioned at the coracoid process and the distal end of the probe oriented slightly lateral, off the true sagittal plane, along the longitudinal plane of the tendon (Figure 3.10). These two tendons closely approximate in the arm, with the normal bulk of the biceps brachii muscle evaluated at this level in both transverse and longitudinal planes (Figure 3.10c). The distal biceps tendon follows a slightly oblique course, as it crosses the elbow joint to insert onto the radial tuberosity. Evaluation of this tendon is described in more detail in Chapter 4. The distal tendon examination requires careful technique and positioning of the patient.

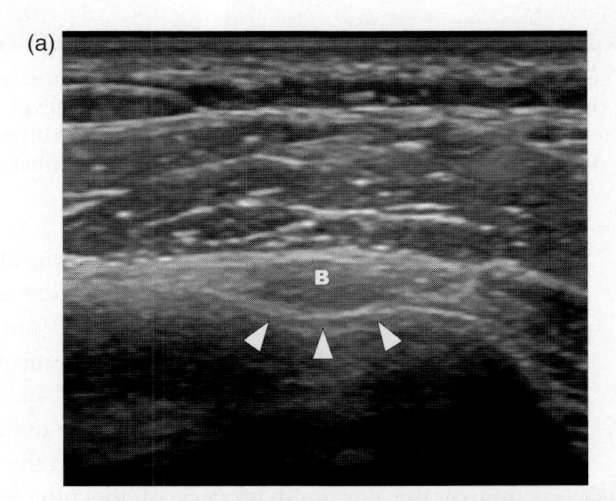

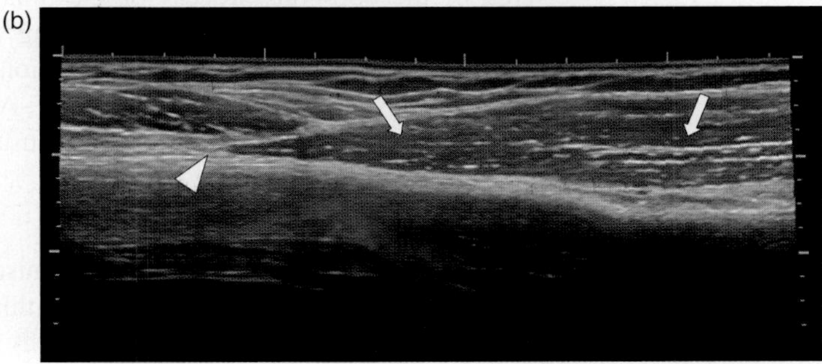

Figure 3.9. **(a)** Transverse ultrasound image of the long head biceps tendon (B), lying within the more shallow distal biceps groove (arrowheads). **(b)** Longitudinal extended field-of-view ultrasound image of the proximal biceps tendon, demonstrating the musculotendinous junction (arrowhead), beyond which the biceps brachii muscle belly is visualized (arrows).

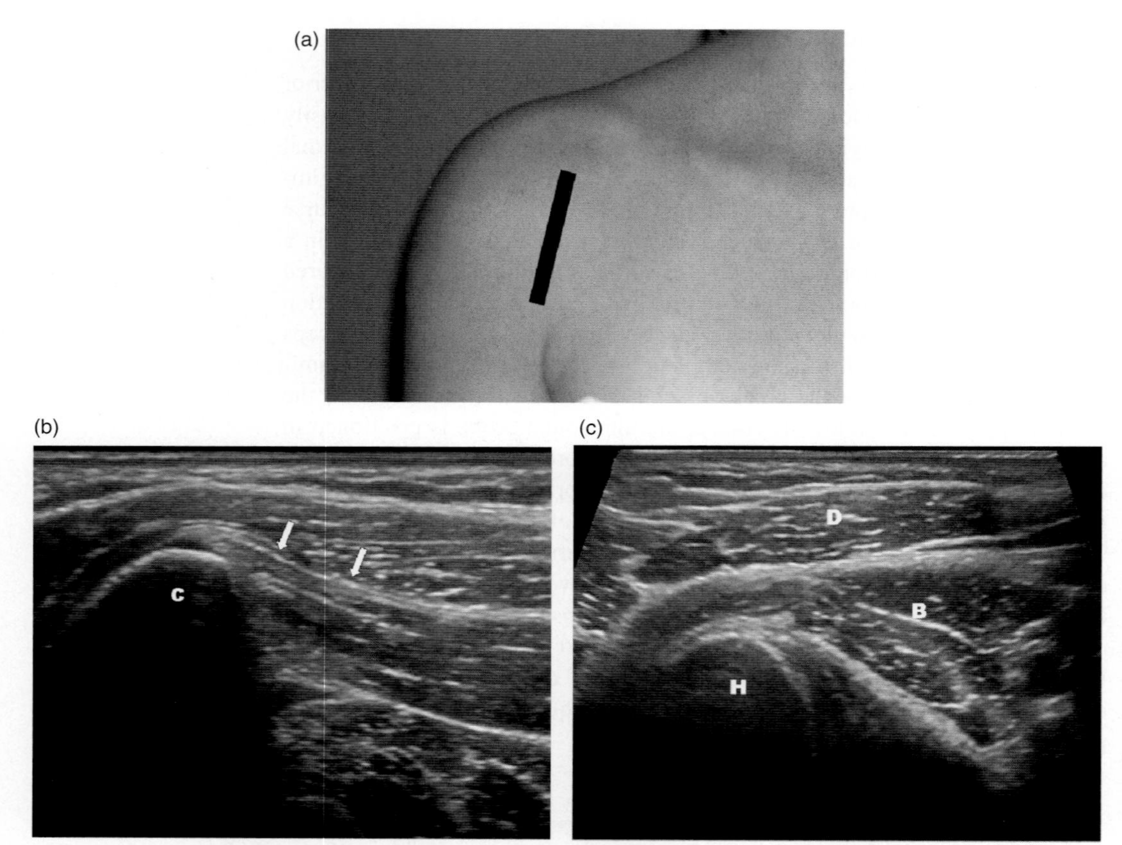

Figure 3.10. (**a**) The probe position for longitudinal evaluation of the short head of the biceps tendon, at its origin from the coracoid process. (**b**) Longitudinal ultrasound image at the level of the coracoid process (C), clearly demonstrates the short head of the biceps tendon (arrows). (**c**) Transverse ultrasound image of the anterior proximal arm demonstrating the biceps brachii (B), overlying anterior deltoid (D) fibers, and deeper humeral shaft (H).

The coracobrachialis and brachialis muscles can be evaluated in a similar fashion. The coracobrachialis is identified as the second tendon originating from the coracoid process (Figures 3.11 and 3.12a). From this position, the muscle has an inferolateral orientation, inserting over a 3- to 5-cm distance on the humeral shaft.[1] The brachialis arises from the lower half of the lateral humerus, arising from either side of the deltoid insertion. Distally, the fibers form a broad thick tendon that attaches to the ulnar tuberosity and a roughened area of the coronoid process of the ulna.[1] On transverse and longitudinal imaging, this muscle is identified lying deep to the biceps (Figure 3.12b and c). From this position of identification, the brachialis muscle and tendon can be followed proximally and distally. At the elbow joint, the joint capsule is immediately deep to the brachialis muscle (Chapter 4).

Insider Information 3.5
The brachialis muscle is the deepest muscle in the distal anterior arm. The biceps tendon is positioned anterior to this muscle; the humerus and elbow joint capsule are positioned immediately deep to it.

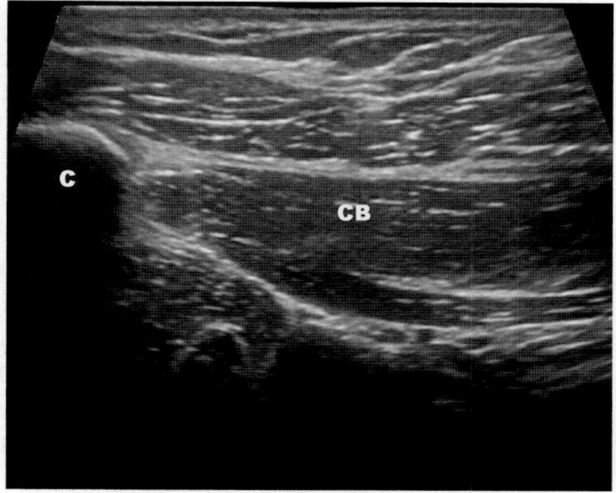

Figure 3.11. Longitudinal ultrasound image of the coracobrachialis muscle (CB) at its proximal origin from the coracoid process (C).

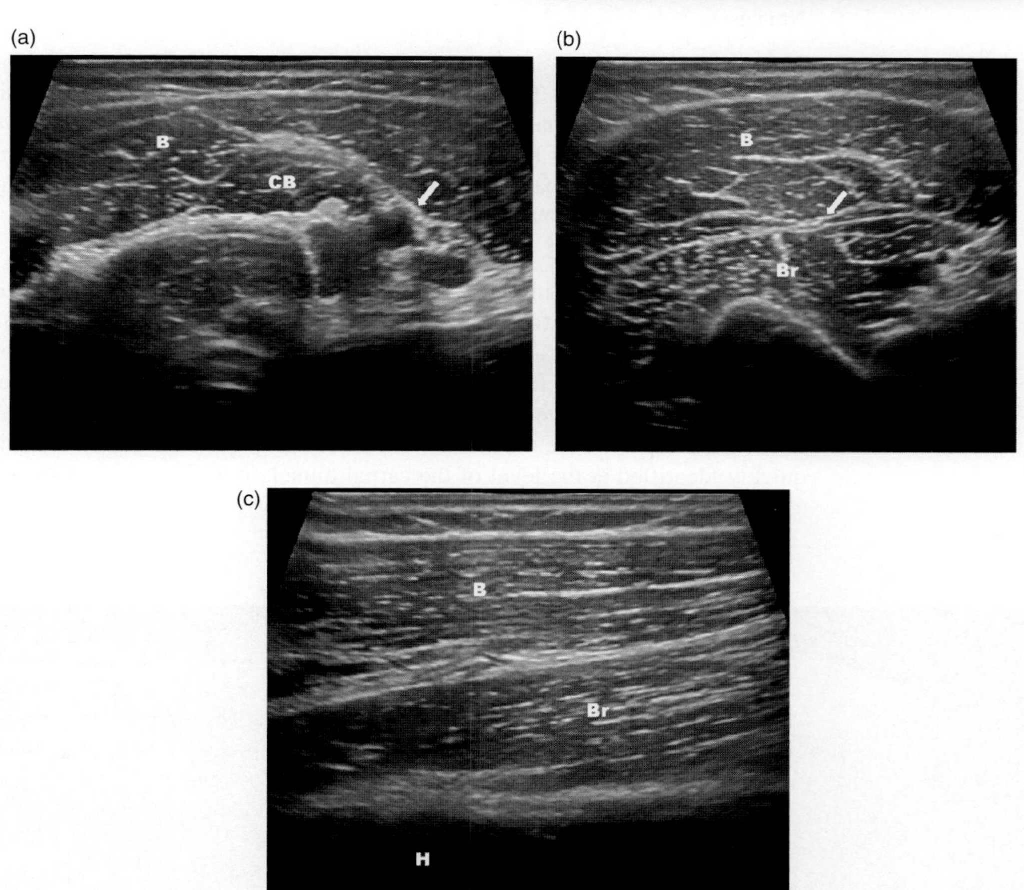

Figure 3.12. **(a)** Transverse ultrasound image of the proximal anterior arm demonstrating the coracobrachialis muscle (CB) lying deep and at the medial aspect of the biceps brachii (B). Note the brachial artery (arrow) at the medial aspect of the proximal coracobrachialis. **(b)** Transverse ultrasound image of the anterior mid arm identifies the biceps brachii (B) and deeper brachialis muscle (Br), with the intermuscular septum (arrow) identified as a hyperechoic structure separating the two muscle bellies. **(c)** Longitudinal ultrasound image of the anterior mid arm illustrates the brachialis muscle (Br) overlying the humeral shaft (H), with the biceps muscle (B) lying more superficially.

Posterior Compartment

Posteriorly, the triceps is easiest to evaluate from a distal to proximal orientation. It is useful to slightly abduct the arm in order to image both the medial and lateral aspects of this large muscle. This is easily accomplished with the patient placing their palm on the hip, or on the thigh, if in a seated position. The distal tendon is identified as a hyperechoic, compact linear structure, inserting onto the olecranon process. The tendon is evaluated in longitudinal (Figure 3.13) and transverse orientation and can also be assessed dynamically with flexion and extension of the forearm. This assists in evaluating the integrity of the distal tendon. From the olecranon process, the triceps tendon can be followed proximally, whereby the triceps muscle is easily identified and evaluated. The three heads of the triceps are recognized, and knowledge of this anatomy assists in better localizing any regional pathology (Figure 3.14).

Nerves

The median, ulnar, and radial nerves can be assessed along their proximal and distal course in the arm. There are important anatomical landmarks that assist in identifying the normal course and location of these nerves. The nerves should be evaluated in both longitudinal and transverse planes, observing echotexture, fascicular pattern, presence or absence of fusiform swelling, and relationship to any regional pathology.

Median Nerve

The median nerve lies in close approximation to the brachial artery, at the level of the antecubital fossa. For this reason, the brachial artery serves as a quick and easy anatomical landmark for the median nerve. From this position, the median nerve can be followed proximally into the arm. This is often easiest to perform in the transverse orientation (Figure 3.15a and b). If there is any doubt with respect to the median nerve position at the elbow, the nerve can be quickly identified at the level of the carpal tunnel, at the wrist, and followed

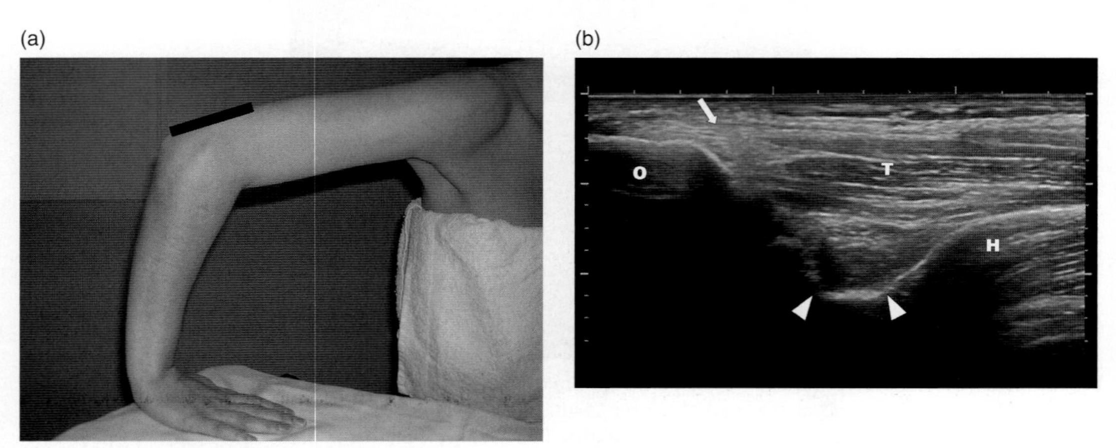

Figure 3.13. **(a)** The position of the ultrasound probe for longitudinal evaluation of distal triceps tendon and muscle. **(b)** Longitudinal extended field-of-view image illustrating the appearance of the distal triceps tendon (arrow) at its insertion onto the olecranon process of the ulna (O) and muscle (T). The olecranon fossa (arrowheads) and posterior humeral shaft (H) are visible.

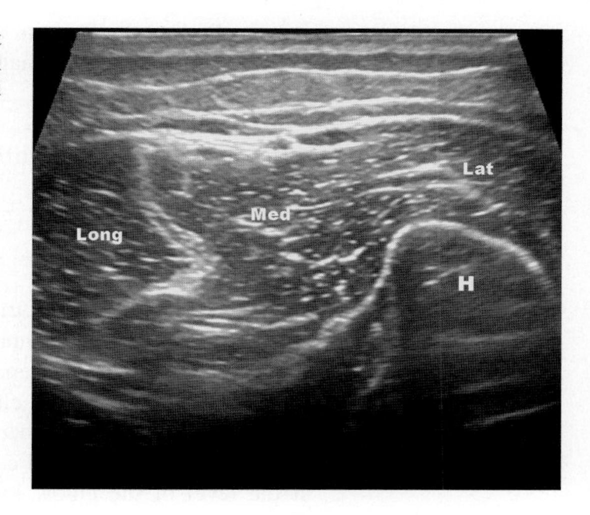

Figure 3.14. Transverse image of the posterior aspect of the mid arm demonstrating the long, medial, and lateral heads of the triceps muscle lying posterior and medial to the humeral shaft (H).

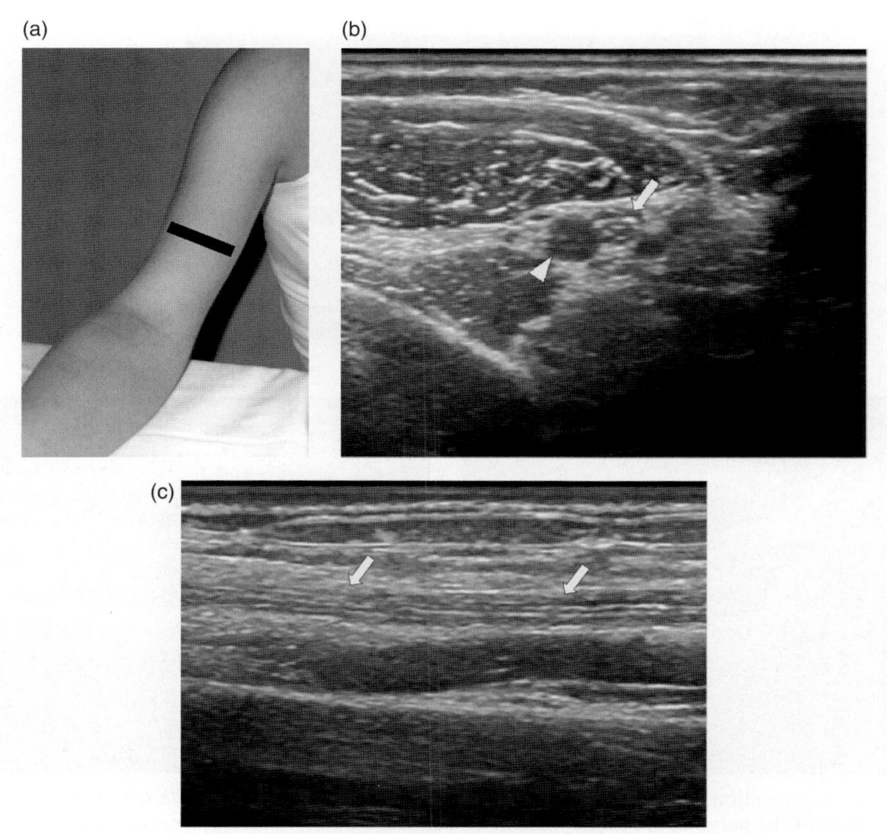

Figure 3.15. **(a)** The position of the ultrasound probe for identification of the median nerve, in transverse orientation. **(b)** Transverse ultrasound image at the medial aspect of the anterior arm demonstrates the oval-shaped appearance of the normal median nerve (arrow) positioned just medial to the brachial artery (arrowhead). **(c)** Longitudinal ultrasound image of the median nerve (arrows) at mid arm level. This image highlights the normal course, fascicular pattern of nerves observed on longitudinal imaging.

proximally into the forearm and arm. After being identified in the transverse orientation, the nerve is imaged along its longitudinal course (Figure 3.15c).

Insider Information 3.6
The median nerve is identified adjacent to the brachial artery in the antecubital fossa.

Ulnar Nerve

In the proximal half of the arm, the ulnar nerve is located medial, immediately adjacent to the brachial artery. At the mid arm, it pierces the intermuscular septum and continues descending along a medial course, anterior to the medial head of the triceps. At the elbow, it is identified lying adjacent to the medial epicondyle. As with the median nerve, the course and location of the ulnar nerve in the arm are often easiest to assess by first identifying this structure at the level of the elbow joint and following it proximally (Figure 3.16a). This is accomplished by bridging the ultrasound probe with one end on the

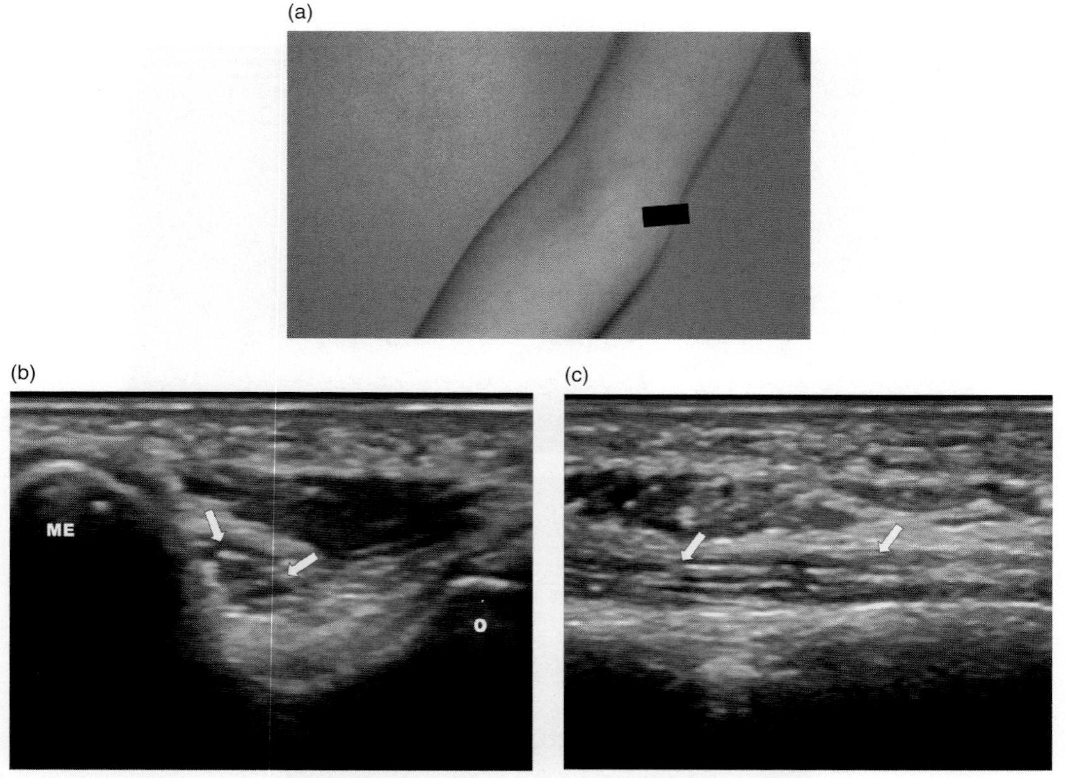

Figure 3.16. **(a)** The position of the ultrasound probe for evaluation of the ulnar nerve in the arm, commencing with identification of the nerve at the posteromedial aspect of the elbow joint. **(b)** Transverse ultrasound image of the ulnar nerve (arrows) at the level of the posteromedial elbow, with identification of the nerve immediately adjacent to the medial epicondyle (ME) of the humerus. The probe is placed, bridging between the medial epicondyle and the olecranon process (O) of the ulna. **(c)** Longitudinal ultrasound image of the ulnar nerve (arrows) at the level of the distal arm. After identifying this structure in the transverse plane **(b)**, the probe is turned longitudinally, with structure followed more proximally into the arm, in order to obtain this image.

olecranon process and the other on the medial epicondyle. In this position, the ulnar nerve is identified as a round to oval structure adjacent to the medial epicondyle, which is a key anatomical landmark for this nerve. In transverse and subsequently longitudinal orientation, the nerve can be followed proximally from this position, along its course in the arm (Figure 3.16b and c).

Radial Nerve

When imaging the radial nerve, the examiner may first identify the structure at the level of the deltoid tuberosity, from which point it can be followed proximally (posterior and superior) and distally (anterior and inferior).[10] This can be achieved with the ultrasound probe in the transverse position (Figure 3.17). At the level of the posterolateral humerus, the nerve runs alongside the brachial artery. Proximally, it can be identified between the coracobrachialis and inferior margin of the teres major muscles.[8] From this position, the nerve

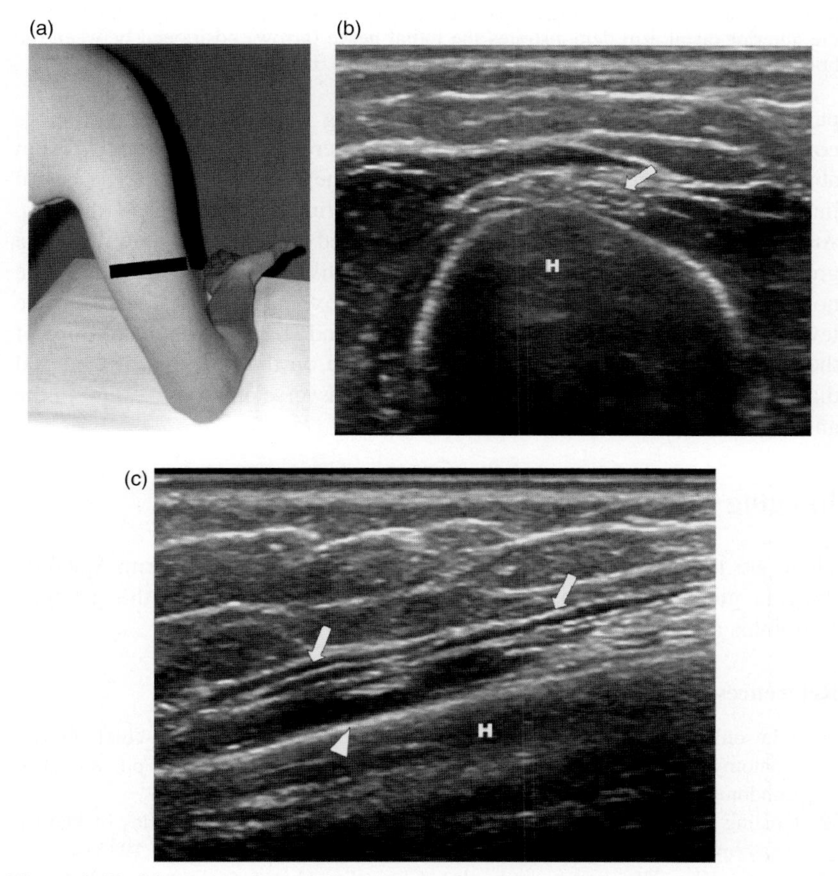

Figure 3.17. **(a)** Positioning of the ultrasound probe in the transverse plane, at the posterior aspect of the arm, for identification of the radial nerve. **(b)** Transverse image at the level of probe placement for **(a)** demonstrates the oval-shaped appearance of the radial nerve (arrow) lying immediately adjacent to the underlying humerus (H). **(c)** Longitudinal ultrasound image at the level of the posterior humerus (H) demonstrates the radial nerve (arrows), with typical fascicular ultrasound appearance, demonstrating its close proximity to the humeral cortex (arrowhead).

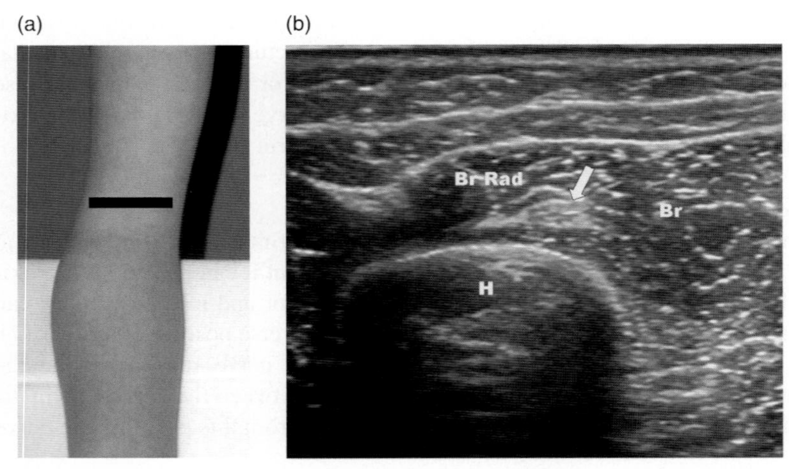

Figure 3.18. (**a**) The probe position for evaluation of the distal radial nerve that is now identified in the anterior compartment of the arm. (**b**) Transverse image at the level of the anterior distal arm demonstrates the radial nerve (arrow) positioned between the brachialis (Br) and brachioradialis (Br Rad) muscles. H, humerus.

passes inferiorly, between the lateral and long head of the triceps, before commencing its spiral course around the humerus.[10] Approximately 10 cm above the lateral epicondyle of the humerus, the nerve penetrates the lateral intermuscular septum and passes into the anterior compartment of the arm. At this point, the radial nerve can be identified anteriorly. It now lies in a groove between the brachialis and brachioradialis muscles (Figure 3.18). The normal radial nerve has a round appearance proximally, an oval shape at the level of the mid humerus, and returns to a round shape at the distal third of the humerus.[8] At the level of the spiral groove on the humerus, the normal diameter of this nerve is 4.0–4.2 mm in the transverse and 2.3–3.5 mm in the anteroposterior direction.[8]

Imaging Protocols

There are no set imaging protocols for the evaluation of the arm. Standard imaging guidelines are used. The examination is tailored to the patient's symptoms and the involved compartment.

References

1. Johnson D, Ellis H, eds. Upper arm. In: Standring S, editor-in-chief. Gray's Anatomy. The Anatomical Basis of Clinical Practice, 39th ed., pp. 851–858. London: Elsevier, 2005.
2. Gosling JA, Harris PF, Humpherson JR et al. Upper limb. In: Atlas of Human Anatomy, pp. 3.20–3.50. London: Gower Medical Publishing Ltd., 1985.
3. Moore KL. The upper limb. In: Clinically Oriented Anatomy, 2nd ed., pp. 626–793. Baltimore: Williams & Wilkins, 1985.
4. Silvestri E, Martinoli C, Derchi LE et al. Echotexture of peripheral nerves: Correlation between US and histologic findings and criteria to differentiate tendons. Radiology 1995;197: 291–296.
5. Fornage BD. Peripheral nerves of the extremities: Imaging with US. Radiology 1988;167:179–182.

6. Martinoli C, Bianchi S, Derchi L. Ultrasonography of peripheral nerves. Semin Ultrasound, CT MRI 2000;21(3):205–213.
7. Martinoli C, Bianchi S, Pugliese F et al. Sonography of entrapment neuropathies in the upper limb (wrist excluded). J Clin Ultrasound 2004;32:438–450.
8. Bodnar G, Buchberger W, Schocke M et al. Radial nerve palsy associated with humeral shaft fracture: Evaluation with US—initial experience. Radiology 2001;219:811–816.
9. Huang C, Ko S, Ko J et al. Contracture of the deltoid muscle: Sonographic evaluation with MRI correlation. AJR 205;185:364–370.
10. Loewy J. Sonoanatomy of the median, ulnar and radial nerves. Can Assoc Radiol J 2002;53(1):33–38.

4

The Elbow

Karen Finlay

The elbow is an important synovial hinge and pivot joint of the upper extremity. Given its superficial position, the elbow joint is easily evaluated by ultrasonography. This joint represents a common site of musculoskeletal complaints, which affect all age groups. Both joint and paraarticular structures are amenable to ultrasound evaluation. The elbow ultrasound examination lends itself to an organized anatomical approach: anterior, lateral medial, and posterior. Evaluation can be targeted to the area of the patient's symptoms or to a specific clinical question.

Imaging Indications

The indications for elbow joint evaluation by ultrasound are extensive and varied. The most common elbow soft tissue pathology is epicondylitis.[1] Regional tendon abnormalities are frequent and problematic. Ultrasound can evaluate these structures for the presence of tendinopathy, tears, and enthesiopathy. Soft tissue injuries, soft tissue masses, bursitis, ulnar nerve impingement, and entrapment abnormalities are also amenable to assessment. The scope of elbow sonographic evaluation also includes articular abnormalities, including joint effusions, assessment of complications from arthritis, presence of intraarticular bodies, and synovitis. Occasionally, incidental bone surface abnormalities can be appreciated, for example, an occult radial head fracture. Assistance with interventional procedures is a strong indication for elbow ultrasound. This includes ultrasound-guided joint aspiration and injections and synovial and soft tissue biopsies.

A successful approach to sonographic imaging of the elbow joint requires proper equipment and technique, a systematic approach to the examination, as well as a thorough understanding of the regional anatomy and function of the soft tissues and joints of the elbow. In addition, it is important to review available clinical information, and to elicit a brief history from the patient.

Technical Review

The elbow joint ultrasound is performed using high-resolution, multifrequency linear array transducers. Both large standard and smaller footprint probes are useful in evaluating the elbow. Smaller footprint probes often prove useful for evaluating smaller structures, for example, the collateral ligaments, as well as those positioned between and around prominent bony landmarks, such as the ulnar nerve. The choice of probes and ideal frequency is also affected by body habitus. In general, the highest frequency that permits adequate penetration of the structures of interest is recommended.

Color and power Doppler are useful for demonstrating hyperemia and the relation of regional structures and pathology to normal arteries and veins. Doppler is also useful for assisting in determining the cystic versus solid nature of any hypoechoic or anechoic abnormalities identified. For superficial structures, the use of a generous amount of gel is recommended. As an alternative, a standoff pad may be utilized but is usually not necessary. Tissue harmonics and compound imaging represent new technologies assisting in visualization and assessment of soft tissue structures. Extended field of view imaging further enhances the ability of ultrasound to image and document findings.[2] This technique is especially helpful for demonstrating findings for clinicians, as it assists in illustrating and measuring the finding, its relationship to adjacent structures, as well as the extent of pathology.

Anatomy

Surface Anatomy

The cubital fossa is a triangular space or depression at the anterior aspect of the elbow. The fossa is bounded by medial and lateral muscle groups that form the respective boundaries of the space. The medial elevation consists of the pronator teres muscle; the brachioradialis muscle forms the lateral elevation. Conventionally, an imaginary line traversing between the two humeral epicondyles defines the proximal boundary of the fossa. Distally, the medial and lateral muscle groups converge to create a triangular configuration. The brachialis and supinator muscles form the floor of the fossa. The deep fascia, strengthened by the bicipital aponeurosis, forms the roof of the fossa, which is covered by the superficial fascia and skin.[3]

With the elbow joint flexed, the tendon of the biceps brachii is visible as a cordlike structure crossing the front of the elbow crease. This structure can be palpated. In addition, the bicipital aponeurosis can be palpated proximally, where it passes on an oblique course over the median nerve and brachial artery.[3] With forearm flexion against resistance, the brachialis muscle can be palpated on either side of the distal biceps tendon (Chapter 5, Figure 5.1).

On a thinner patient, the lateral and medial epicondyles are visible as discrete bony prominences on the distal humerus and are important landmarks for ultrasound examination of the elbow. On the posterior aspect of the elbow, the triceps brachii is identified as a longitudinally oriented eminence with a flattened tendon extending to the visible bony prominence of the olecranon process. The anconeus is a triangular area lateral to the olecranon process, separated from the extensor muscle group by an obliquely oriented indentation.

Elbow Joint

The elbow joint is a complex hinge-pivot joint, with three discrete articular components: the ulnohumeral joint, between the ulnar trochlear notch and the trochlea of the humerus; the radiocapitellar joint, between the radial head and the capitellum of the humerus; and the proximal radioulnar joint. Four discrete movements are facilitated at the elbow joint: flexion, extension, supination, and pronation.

> **Insider Information 4.1**
> There are three discrete articulations at the elbow joint: the ulnohumeral joint, radiocapitellar joint, and proximal radioulnar joint.

There are many important bony landmarks on the distal humerus (Figure 4.1). These include the medial and lateral epicondyle, capitellum, and trochlea. The coronoid fossa is a small, hollow area on the anterior aspect of the distal humerus that is positioned immediately above the trochlea. This fossa provides room for the coronoid process of the ulna during flexion. The olecranon fossa is a larger hollow area on the posterior aspect of the distal humerus that accommodates the olecranon process during elbow extension. The capitellum is a rounded area at the anterior and inferior aspect of the lateral humeral condyle that articulates with the head of the radius. The radial head has a slightly convex disc-like shape; it articulates with the hemispherical capitellum. The radial fossa is a shallow depression above the capitellum that accommodates the radial head with full flexion of the elbow. The trochlea is present at the anterior, inferior, and posterior surfaces of the condyle of the humerus. It articulates with the trochlear notch on the ulna. The capitellum and trochlea are separated from one another by a shallow groove. There is an additional small fossa on the humerus, just above the lateral aspect of the

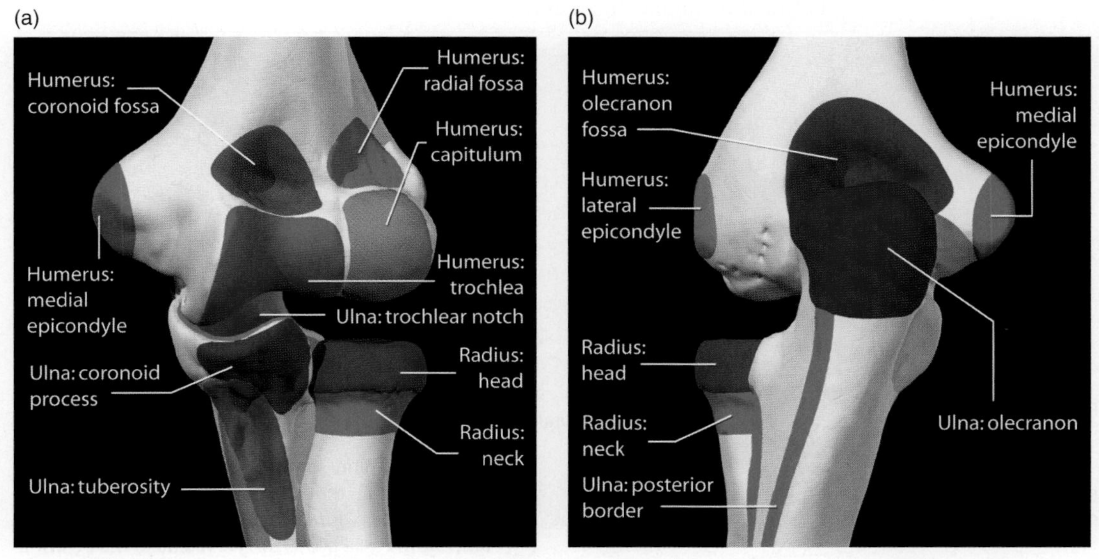

Figure 4.1. The important bony landmarks around the elbow joint: **(a)** anterior and **(b)** posterior views.

capitellum, termed the radial fossa, which accommodates the margin of the radial head on full elbow flexion.

The proximal radioulnar joint is a pivot type synovial joint that facilitates movement of the radius on the ulna. The radial head articulates with the adjacent radial notch of the ulna and is held in place by the annular ligament. The radioulnar joint is enclosed within the articular capsule of the elbow joint.[3]

The joint capsule and collateral ligaments provide joint stability. The synovial cavities of the elbow joint and proximal radioulnar joint are in free communication with each other.[3] The normal joint capsule investing the elbow joint consists of a thin, outer fibrous capsule and inner synovial lining. The synovial membrane descends distally—just below the lower border of the annular ligament around the radial neck.[4] This inferior extension of the synovial capsule creates a saclike structure at the level of the neck of the radius. This anatomical arrangement allows the radius to freely rotate within the annular ligament.[3] The anterior joint capsule inserts onto the anterior humerus, proximal to the coronoid and radial fossa and distal to the margin of the coronoid process of the ulna and annular ligament. Posteriorly, the joint capsule inserts into the humerus, just proximal to the olecranon fossa.[5] The normal elbow fat pads lie between these, with the posterior fat pad in the olecranon fossa larger than the anterior fat pad in the coronoid fossa (Figure 4.2).[4] The joint capsule is easily visualized posteriorly, lying in a position deep to the distal triceps tendon and superficial to the posterior fat pad. The normal joint capsule appears as a compact linear echogenic structure, with normal thickness in the adult population approaching 2 mm.[6] The fibrous joint capsule and synovial membrane around the proximal radioulnar joint are continuous with the other two elbow joints.

Insider Information 4.2
The joint capsule and synovial lining around the elbow are extensive, with the synovial membrane extending down the proximal neck of the radius, below the annular ligament.

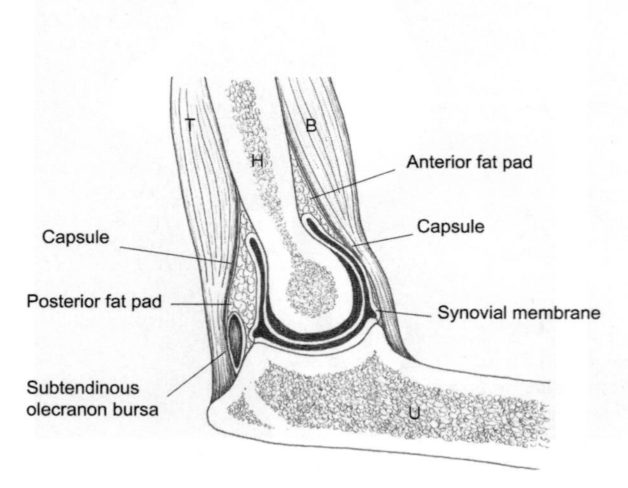

Figure 4.2. Mid-sagittal elbow joint capsule, demonstrating the joint capsule inserting above the coronoid fossa anteriorly and above the olecranon fossa posteriorly. Note also the position of the anterior and posterior fat pads.

Table 4.1. The Ligaments of the Elbow Joint.

Ulnar collateral ligament (medial collateral ligament)
Anterior bundle
Posterior bundle
Transverse bundle
Radial collateral ligament complex (lateral collateral ligament)
Radial collateral ligament
Lateral ulnar collateral ligament
Accessory collateral ligament
Annular ligament

Ligaments

The collateral ligaments reinforce the relatively weak or lax elbow joint capsule at its medial and lateral aspects (Table 4.1). The ulnar collateral ligament, also known as the medial collateral ligament, consists of three separate components: the anterior, posterior, and transverse bundles (Figure 4.3a). The anterior bundle is a strong structure that becomes taut with elbow extension, playing an important role in stabilizing against valgus stress. This anterior band is located between the anteroinferior aspect of

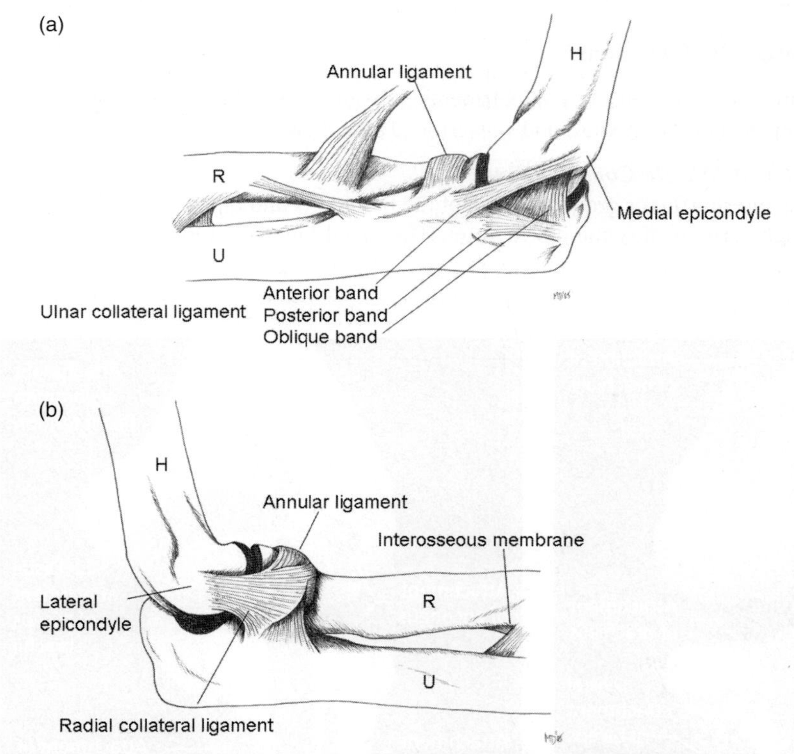

Figure 4.3. The elbow ligaments. **(a)** The ulnar (U) side of the elbow joint illustrates the components of the ulnar collateral ligament: the anterior, posterior, and transverse or oblique bundles. **(b)** The radial (R) side of the elbow joint, demonstrating the radial collateral ligament complex. The radial collateral ligament "proper" extends from the inferior aspect of the lateral epicondyle to merge with the annular ligament distally. H, humerus; R, radius; U, ulna.

the medial epicondyle and the medial margin of the coronoid process. In contrast, the posterior bundle is weak and fanlike, becoming taut with elbow flexion. It extends between the posteroinferior medial epicondyle and the medial olecranon margin. The transverse component serves to deepen the socket between the coronoid process and the olecranon and has little role in maintaining joint stability.[4] On ultrasound, the important anterior bundle has a hyperechoic, fibrillar appearance.[7] This ligament is usually symmetric in asymptomatic persons, when comparing right side to left, with a normal mean midpoint transverse thickness of 4 mm, obtained on a long axis view.[8]

The radial collateral ligament complex contains four components: the radial collateral ligament, lateral ulnar collateral ligament, accessory collateral ligament, and annular ligament (Figure 4.3b). The radial collateral ligament "proper" extends from the inferior aspect of the lateral epicondyle, deep to the common extensor tendon, merging at insertion with the fibers of the annular ligament. The lateral ulnar collateral ligament originates more posteriorly, extending to the supinator crest of the ulna, and has a major role in stabilizing against varus stress.[5] The accessory lateral collateral ligament is variably present.

The annular ligament encircles the radial head, attaching to the radial notch of the ulna. It serves to maintain radial head articulation with the ulna (Figure 4.3b).

Muscles and Tendons

Four important muscle compartments surround the elbow joint (Figure 4.4): anterior, lateral, medial, and posterior (Table 4.2).

Anterior Muscle Compartment

The anterior flexor group consists of the brachialis and biceps brachii muscles, which serve to flex the elbow joint. The distal biceps tendon is formed from

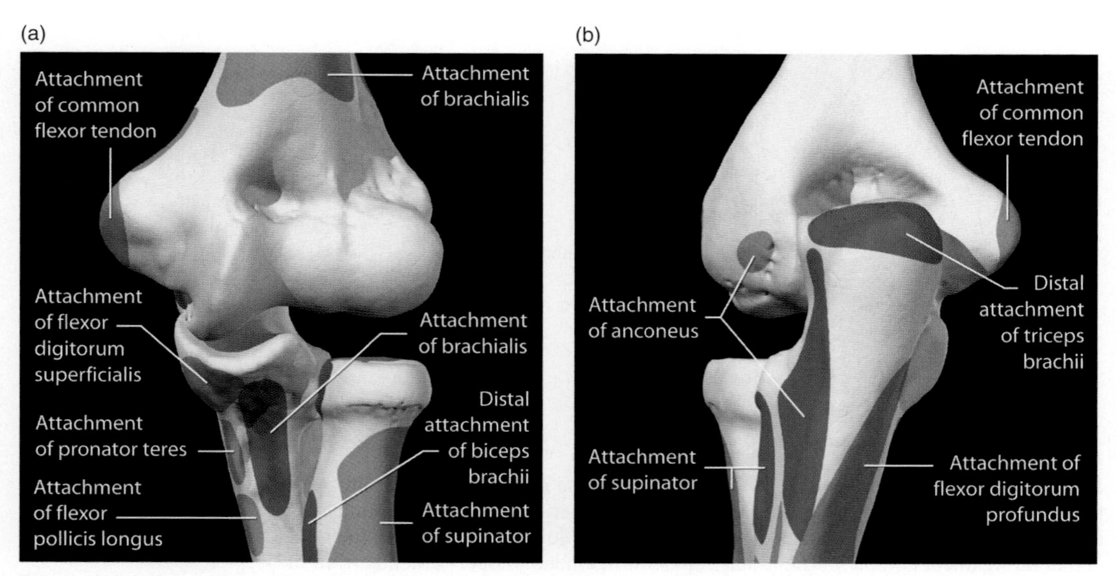

Figure 4.4. The muscle origin (red) and insertion (blue) points around the elbow joint: **(a)** anterior and **(b)** posterior views.

Table 4.2. Muscles and Tendons of the Elbow Joint: Origin Insertion, and Action.

Muscle	Origin	Insertion	Main action
Anterior			
Brachialis	Anterior surface lower one-half of humerus	Coronoid process of ulna	Forearm flexion
Biceps brachii—long head	Supraglenoid tubercle scapula	Radial tuberosity and bicipital aponeurosis	Forearm supination Elbow flexion
Biceps brachii—short head	Coracoid process of scapula	Joins with long head to insert onto the radial tuberosity and bicipital aponeurosis	Forearm supination Elbow flexion
Brachioradialis	Upper two-thirds of lateral supracondylar ridge of humerus	Styloid process of radius, distal one-half of radius, antebrachial fascia	Forearm flexion at elbow Forearm pronation and supination
Lateral			
Extensor carpi radialis longus	Lower one-third of lateral supracondylar ridge of humerus	Dorsum of second metacarpal at base	Extends wrist Abducts hand
Extensor carpi radialis brevis	Common extensor tendon, lateral supracondylar ridge of humerus	Dorsum of third metacarpal at base	Extends wrist Abducts hand
Extensor digitorum	Lateral epicondyle of humerus via common extensor tendon	Extensor expansion of digits 2–5	Extends digits 2–5 Extends wrist if fingers flexed Abducts digits
Extensor digiti minimi	Lateral epicondyle of humerus via common extensor tendon	Joins extensor digitorum tendon to fifth digit; inserts into extensor expansion	Extends and abducts fifth digit
Extensor carpi ulnaris	First head—lateral epicondyle of humerus via common extensor tendon Second head—posterior border of ulna	Medial side base of fifth metacarpal	Extends wrist Adducts hand
Supinator	Lateral epicondyle of humerus, supinator crest and fossa of ulna, radial collateral and annular ligaments	Lateral side, proximal one-third of radius	Supinator forearm
Medial			
Flexor carpi radialis	Medial epicondyle of humerus via common flexor tendon; antebrachial fascia and intermuscular septa	Base of second and third metacarpals	Flexes wrist Abducts hand
Flexor carpi ulnaris	Medial epicondyle of humerus via common flexor tendon, ulnar head from medial border of olecranon and upper two-thirds of posterior ulna	Pisiform, hook of hamate, base of fifth metacarpal	Flexes wrist Adducts hand

(Continued)

Table 4.2. *(Continued)*

Muscle	Origin	Insertion	Main action
Flexor digitorum superficialis	Common flexor tendon (humeroulnar head); middle one-third radius (radial head)	Shafts of middle phalanges digits 2–5	Flex the metacarpophalangeal and proximal interphalangeal joints
Palmaris longus	Medial epicondyle of humerus via common flexor tendon	Central portion of flexor retinaculum; superficial portion of palmar aponeurosis	Flexes wrist
Pronator teres	Medial epicondyle of humerus via common flexor tendon (humeral head); coronoid process of ulna (ulnar head)	Lateral aspect of radius at mid shaft	Pronates forearm Weakly flexes elbow
Posterior			
Triceps brachii—long head	Infraglenoid tubercle of scapula	Olecranon process of ulna	Adducts arm, extends shoulder
Triceps brachii—lateral head	Posterolateral aspect of humerus	Olecranon process of ulna	Extends forearm at elbow
Triceps brachii—Medial head	Lower one-half of posteromedial humerus	Olecranon process of ulna	Extends forearm at elbow
Anconeus	Posterior surface, lateral epicondyle of humerus	Lateral aspect of olecranon and upper one-quarter of ulna	Extends forearm at elbow; supports elbow when in full extension

the union of the long and short heads of the biceps brachii and commences approximately 7 cm above the elbow joint, forming into a flattened tendon. The tendon lies in a superficial position above the elbow joint, taking a steep and slightly oblique course between the medial and lateral muscle groups, to insert onto the radial tuberosity (Figures 4.5a and 4.6). It is important to recognize that the biceps brachii tendon has no tendon sheath. In addition to the biceps insertion onto the radial tuberosity, there is a biceps aponeurosis, which fuses with the deep fascia on the medial aspect of the forearm (Chapter 3, Figure 3.4a).[4] This triangular membrane runs from the margin of the distal biceps tendon, across the cubital fossa, and blends in with the deep fascia overlying the medial flexor muscle group.[3] This fascia serves to protect these medial structures of the forearm, as well as to decrease the pressure on the distal biceps tendon during forearm supination and pronation actions. In terms of muscle action at the elbow, the biceps serves as a strong supinator of the forearm, with the elbow joint flexed, particularly when power is required against resistance, for example, in screwdriver action.[3] The brachialis muscle, which lies posterior to the biceps brachii, is the main flexor of the forearm at the elbow joint. This muscle originates from the anterior surface of the distal humerus, as well as from the intermuscular septum. It inserts onto the coronoid process and the tuberosity of the ulna (Figures 4.5a and 4.6).

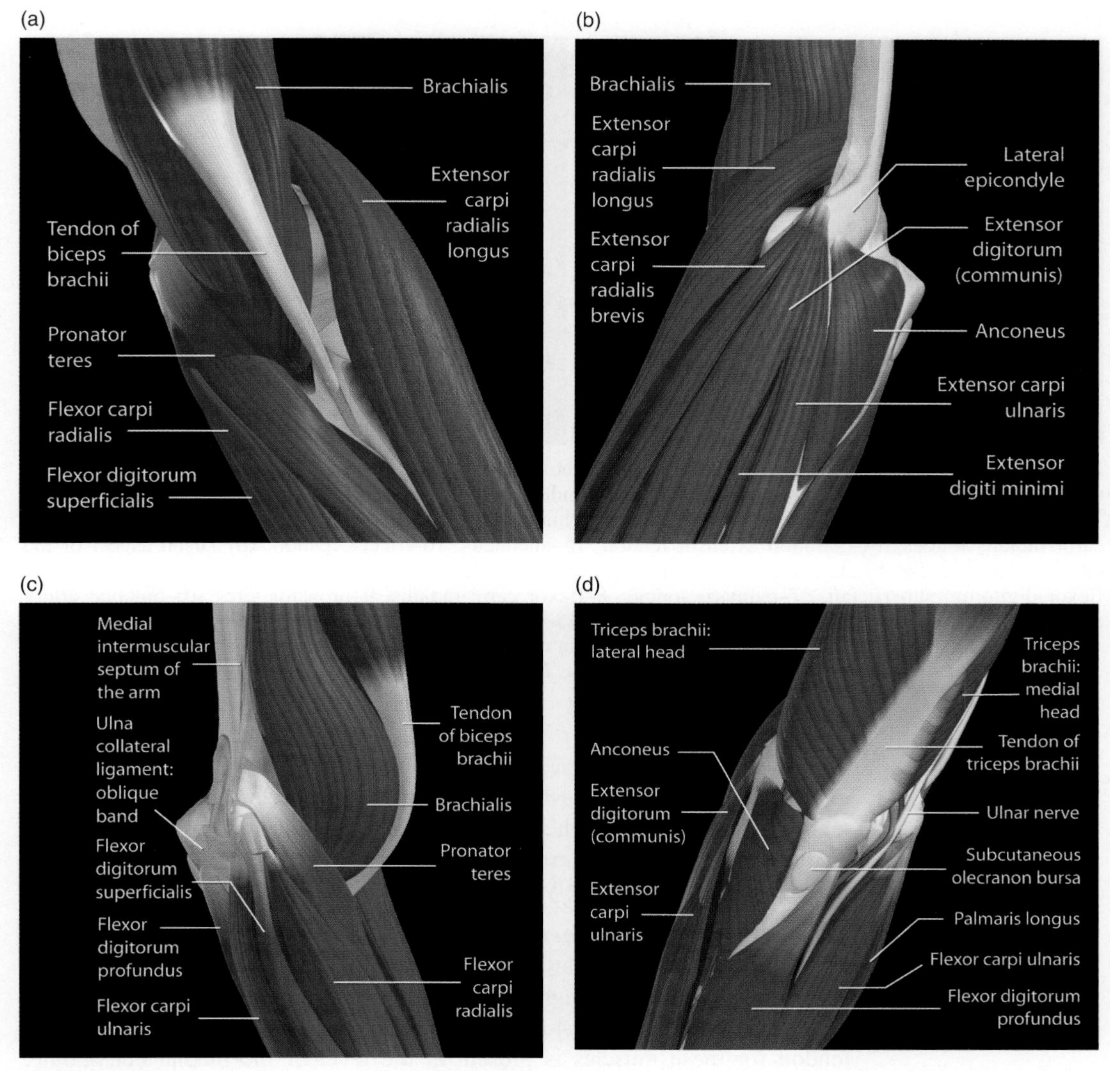

Figure 4.5. **(a)** An anterior view of the elbow, demonstrating the distal biceps tendon. **(b)** A lateral view of the elbow, demonstrating the components of the common extensor tendon and adjacent muscles at the lateral epicondyle. **(c)** A medial view of the elbow, demonstrating the common flexor tendon at the medial elbow. **(d)** A posterior view of the elbow demonstrating the large triceps muscle and tendon. The anconeus muscle is identified at the posterior and lateral aspect of the elbow. Note the superficial position of the ulnar nerve.

Lateral Muscle Compartment

The lateral muscle group includes the extensors of the wrist and hand, as well as the supinator and brachioradialis muscles. The tendons contributing to the common extensor tendon consist of tendon fibers from the extensor carpi radialis brevis, extensor digitorum, extensor digiti minimi, and extensor carpi ulnaris (Figures 4.4, and 4.5b and Table 4.3). The common tendon consists of both superficial and deep components. The superficial portion is largely made up of fibers from the extensor digitorum; the deep fibers are predominantly formed by the extensor radialis brevis. The extensor digiti

(a)

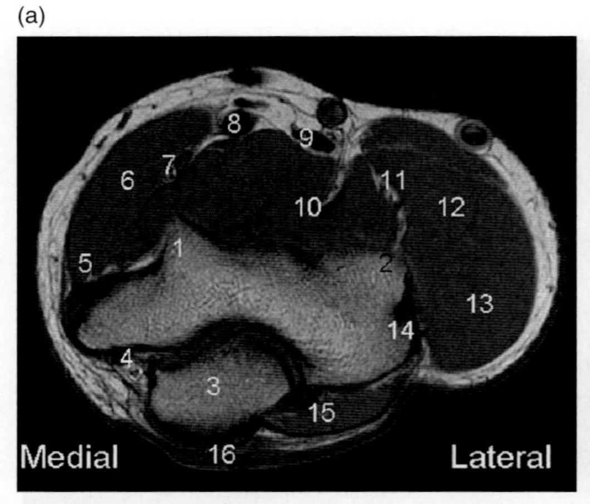

(b)

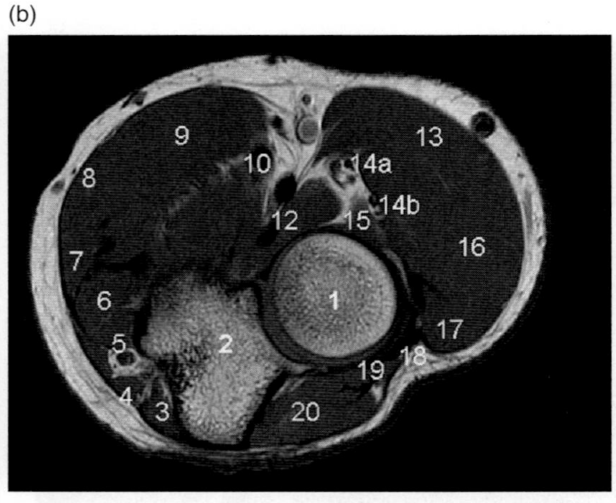

Figure 4.6. Axial T1-weighted MRI anatomy of the elbow. (**a**) Proximal aspect of the elbow joint: 1–humerus, trochlea, 2–humerus, capitellum, 3–ulna, olecranon, 4–ulnar nerve, 5–common flexor tendon, 6–pronator teres, 7–median nerve, 8–brachial artery, 9–biceps, 10–brachialis, 11–radial nerve, 12–brachioradialis, 13–extensor carpi radialis longus, 14–common extensor tendon, 15–anconeus, 16–triceps tendon. (**b**) Distal aspect of the elbow joint: 1–radial head, 2–ulna, 3–flexor digitorum profundus, 4–flexor carpi ulnaris, 5–ulnar nerve, 6–flexor digitorum superficialis, 7–palmaris longus, 8–flexor carpi radialis, 9–pronator teres, 10–brachial artery and median nerve, 11–biceps tendon, 12–brachialis, 13–brachioradialis, 14a–radial nerve, superficial branch, 14b–radial nerve, deep branch, 15–supinator, 16–extensor carpi radialis longus and brevis, 17–extensor digitorum, 18–common extensor tendon, 19–extensor carpi ulnaris, 20–anconeus.

minimi and extensor carpi ulnaris are minor contributors to the common extensor tendon. At the level of the lateral epicondyle, all the contributing tendon fibers blend together to form the common extensor tendon origin. At the epicondyle, the intertwined tendon fibers of each of the contributing tendons cannot be discretely separated.

Medial Muscle Compartment

Medially, the flexor muscles group consists of the flexor carpi radialis, flexor carpi ulnaris, palmaris longus, flexor digitorum superficialis, and pronator teres muscles (Figures 4.4 and 4.5c and Table 4.4). The common flexor tendon for these muscles is present at the level of the medial epicondyle. The exception is the pronator teres. This muscle has two separate heads. The larger attachment is present above the medial epicondyle, just proximal to the common tendon. The smaller attachment arises from the coronoid process of the ulna. The flexor carpi ulnaris, which is the most medial and superficial of the forearm flexors, also has two heads: the humeral and the ulnar. The humeral head is the smaller one and contributes to the common flexor tendon. The larger ulnar head has a more extensive relationship to the medial aspect of

Table 4.3. The Common Extensor Tendon.

Extensor carpi radialis brevis
Extensor digitorum
Extensor digiti minimi
Extensor carpi ulnaris

Table 4.4. The Common Flexor Tendon.

Flexor carpi radialis
Flexor carpi ulnaris
Palmaris longus
Flexor digitorum superficialis
Pronator teres

the olecranon, the proximal two-thirds of the posterior ulna, and the adjacent intermuscular septum. The two separate heads are connected to each other by a tendinous arch.[4] The ulnar nerve and posterior ulnar recurrent artery pass under this arch.

Posterior Muscle Compartment

The posterior extensor muscle group consists of the triceps and anconeus muscles (Figures 4.5d and 4.6). The powerful triceps extensor muscle is formed from the three heads of the triceps muscle, which merge to form a common tendon, inserting onto the olecranon process of the ulna. The anconeus muscle arises from the posterior aspect of the lateral epicondyle and covers the lateral portion of the annular ligament and radial head, inserting onto the lateral olecranon process and superior part of posterior surface of the ulna.[3] This muscle is morphologically and functionally closely related to the triceps muscle.[3] The anconeus abducts the ulna during forearm pronation and contracts when the joint needs stabilization against flexion. In addition, it assists the triceps in extension of the forearm. In a small percentage of individuals, an anomalous muscle called the anconeus epitrochlearis is present arising from the medial border of olecranon and adjacent triceps and inserting into the medial epicondyle.

Nerves

At the elbow joint, the main nerve trunks, namely the ulnar, median, and radial nerves, are visible on ultrasound, which permits evaluation of their caliber, echotexture, course, and relationship to adjacent structures and pathology (Figures 4.5d and 4.6, and Chapter 12, Figures 12.3 and 12.10). The normal ulnar nerve traverses along a groove on the posteromedial aspect of the humerus, at the level of the medial epicondyle. On ultrasound, the normal ulnar nerve appears as a round or oval structure on short axis view, with multiple discrete slightly echogenic foci dispersed within.[9–11] These echogenic foci represent the normal nerve fascicles in cross section. The ulnar nerve is usually of uniform thickness, typically measuring 2–3 mm at the posterior aspect of the olecranon fossa.[12] Longitudinally, the ulnar nerve appears as a cordlike hypoechoic structure, with parallel hyperechoic linear structures throughout, again illustrating the fascicular pattern of nerves.[10,12,13]

The median nerve is identified anteriorly in the antecubital fossa, medial to the brachial artery. The nerve is positioned beneath the bicipital aponeurosis, prior to its distal course between the heads of the pronator teres muscle. At the elbow, the radial nerve lies in a groove between the brachialis and brachioradialis muscles proximally and extensor carpi radialis distally.

Table 4.5. Bursae of the Elbow.

Subcutaneous olecranon bursa
Subtendinous olecranon bursa
Cubital or bicipitoradial bursa
Radioulnar bursa

Bursae

There are several bursae present at the elbow joint (Table 4.5). The olecranon bursa is a flattened potential space positioned between the surface of the olecranon process and the subcutaneous tissues (Figure 4.5d). This bursa is more correctly referred to as the subcutaneous olecranon bursa.[3] Its normal appearance on ultrasound consists of a very thin hypoechoic cleft in the soft tissues with a subtle hyperechoic outline. Less recognized, there is a bursa deep to the triceps tendon that helps it slide over the olecranon process. This deeper structure is called the subtendinous olecranon bursa and is present just proximal to the tendon insertion.[3] Distention and pathology of this deeper bursa are much less common than its superficial counterpart.

The cubital bursa or bicipitoradial bursa is located at the distal biceps insertion onto the radial tuberosity. This bursa is subtendinous in position, lying between the biceps insertion and the underlying radius and serving to reduce the friction between these two structures.

The less well-known radioulnar bursa is identified between the extensor digitorum, the radiohumeral joint, and the supinator muscle. It lies posterior to the supinator muscle, lateral to the distal biceps tendon and medial in relation to the ulna.[3]

Deep Fascia

The deep brachial fascia of the arm continues into the forearm as the antebrachial fascia. The fascia is attached to the humerus at the epicondyles of the humerus and the olecranon process of the ulna. There are two intermuscular septa of the fascia, which extend from the brachial fascia to attach to the medial and lateral supracondylar ridges of the humerus.

Technique

For the evaluation of the elbow joint, the patient is seated facing the examiner, with the arm extended comfortably on a bedside table or stretcher.[14–16] Techniques have been described for evaluating the patient in a supine position.[17] It is helpful to divide the examination into four parts: anterior, lateral, medial, and posterior (Table 4.6). Once skilled in the complete elbow examination, it is possible to tailor the examination to assess the patient's specific site of complaints or a targeted clinical question.

Different positions of the elbow joint redistribute joint fluid. The presence of a joint effusion is better recognized at the posterior elbow, rather than the anterior elbow, with the elbow in a flexed position.[18] When examining the joint, it is important to distinguish articular cartilage from joint fluid and hypoechoic synovium. Graded compression of the joint space can assist in

Table 4.6. Muscles and Tendons of the Elbow Joint: Position for Ultrasound Examined.

Muscle	Position examined
Anterior	
Brachialis	Anterior approach Elbow mildly flexed, forearm neutral
Biceps brachii—Long head	Elbow flexed
Short head	Forearm supinated
Lateral	
Brachioradialis	Lateral approach
Extensor carpi radialis longus	Elbow mildly flexed, forearm neutral
Extensor carpi radialis brevis	Elbow mildly flexed, forearm neutral
Extensor digitorum	Elbow mildly flexed, forearm neutral
Extensor digiti minimi	Elbow mildly flexed, forearm neutral
Extensor carpi ulnaris	Elbow mildly flexed, forearm neutral
Supinator	Anterior approach Elbow mildly flexed, forearm supinated
Medial	
Flexor carpi radialis	Medial approach
Flexor carpi ulnaris	Elbow extended, forearm fully supinated
Flexor digitorum superficialis	Elbow extended, forearm fully supinated
Palmaris longus	Elbow extended, forearm fully supinated
Pronator teres	Elbow extended, forearm fully supinated
Posterior	
Triceps brachii—Long head	
Lateral head	Posterior approach, elbow flexed, arm abducted
Medial head	
Anconeus	Posterior approach, elbow flexed or extended

differentiating joint fluid from thickened synovium. If any synovial abnormality is observed, it can be assessed with power Doppler.[19,20]

Anterior Approach

With the arm in the supinated position, the examination begins in the transverse plane, placing the transducer parallel to the elbow crease (Figure 4.7a). In this position, the distal humeral cartilage, cortical surface, and subchondral bone are evaluated, while moving the transducer proximally and distally. The normal cartilage appears as a hypoechoic layer of uniform thickness, parallel to the hyperechoic underlying subcortical bone (Figure 4.7b). Once at the distal aspect of the humerus, the transducer is rotated to the longitudinal plane and moved from the medial to lateral aspect of the joint, evaluating in turn the medial trochlear ulnar joint space (Figure 4.8) and the lateral radiocapitellar joint space (Figure 4.9). Assessment includes evaluation of the synovial lining and the presence of any joint fluid. The normal anterior joint fat pad appears as a hyperechoic structure that in the setting of a joint effusion is displaced

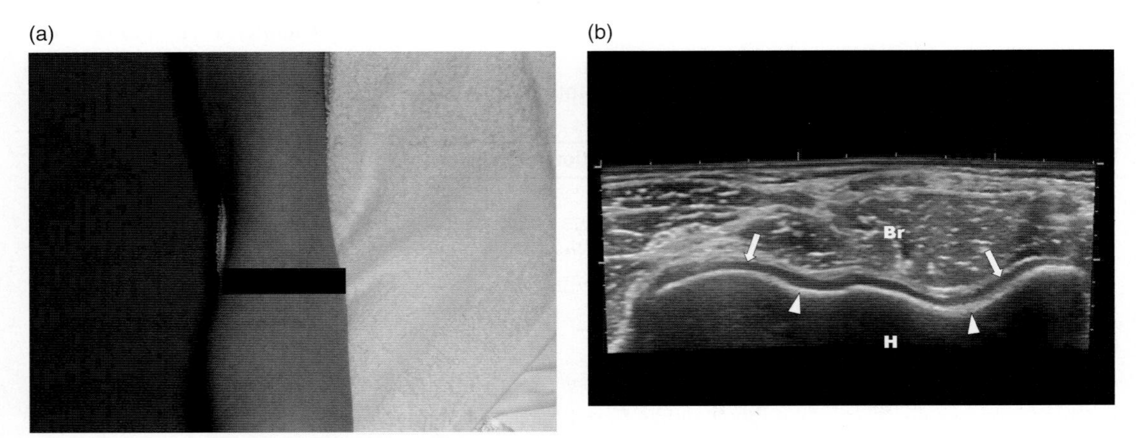

Figure 4.7. (a) The position of the ultrasound probe for transverse assessment of the anterior elbow joint. **(b)** Transverse image of the distal humerus, demonstrating the thin, uniform, hypoechoic cartilage (arrows) overlying the hyperechoic parallel surface of the subchondral bone (arrowheads). Note the brachialis muscle (Br) overlying the anterior elbow at this level.

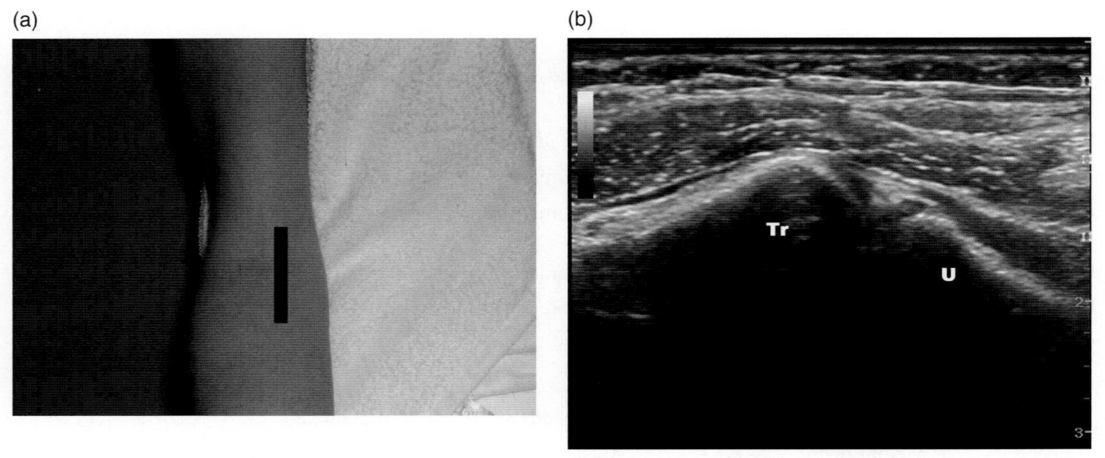

Figure 4.8. (a) The probe placement, sagittal orientation, for evaluation of the medial joint space and trochlear ulnar joint. **(b)** Corresponding longitudinal image of the trochlear ulnar joint. Tr, trochlea; U, ulna.

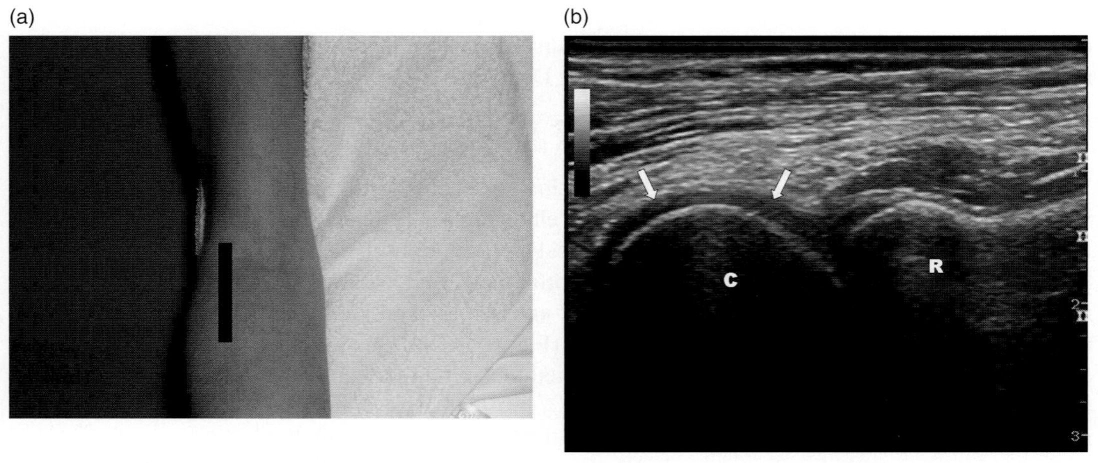

Figure 4.9. (a) Probe placement, sagittal orientation, for evaluation of lateral joint space and radiocapitellar joint. **(b)** Corresponding longitudinal ultrasound image of the radiocapitellar joint. The hyaline cartilage over the surface of the capitellum appears smooth and uniform (arrows). C, capitellum; R, radius.

anteriorly.[21] The opposing articular margins and cortical surfaces of the radius and ulna are assessed. It is necessary to carefully evaluate the contour and appearances of the cartilaginous and articular bone surfaces, being alert to any cartilaginous defects, thinning, osteophytes, erosions, or disruptions that would suggest trauma. Normal hypoechoic cartilage should be observed over the articular surfaces. The normal joint space contains a thin layer of joint fluid.[6] The brachialis muscle is identified lying immediately anterior to the joint capsule medially. The brachioradialis muscle is radial or lateral to the brachialis muscle.

It is useful to dynamically assess the joint space with supination and pronation so as to assist in the detection of loose bodies.[22] Evaluation of the anterior joint space includes interrogation of the coronoid fossa (Figure 4.10a), radial fossa (Figure 4.10b), and radial neck recess (Figure 4.10c). For evaluation of the radial neck recess, the radial head is identified at the anterior joint space where it articulates with the capitellum. From this location, the

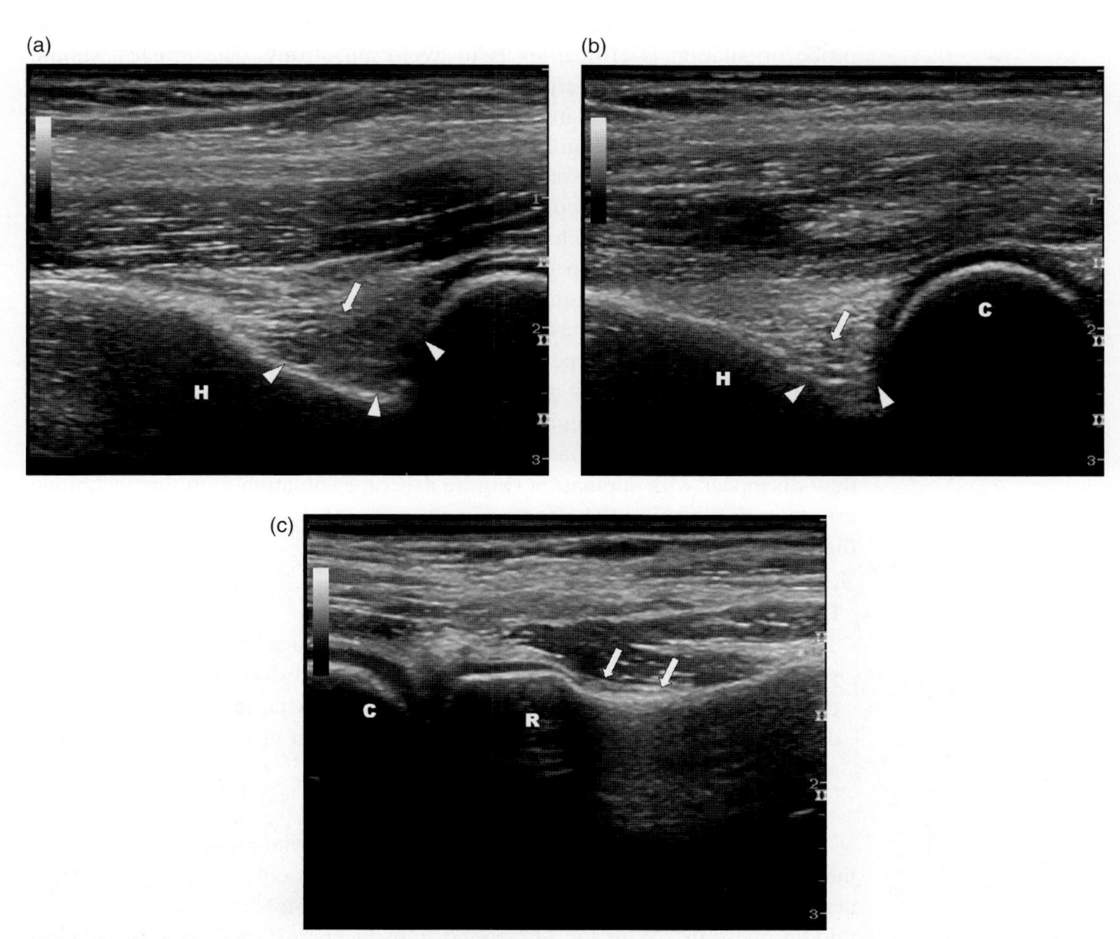

Figure 4.10. (**a**) Longitudinal image of the coronoid fossa (arrowheads) of the humerus (H). Note the hyperechoic fat (arrow) filling the space. In the setting of an effusion, this fat pat is displaced anterior. (**b**) Longitudinal image of the radial fossa (arrowheads) of the humerus (H). Note this fossa has a similar appearance to the coronoid fossa illustrated in (**a**) and is also normally filled with fat (arrow). C, capitellum. (**c**) Longitudinal image of the radial neck recess (arrows). C, capitellum; R, radius.

transducer is moved distally to identify the radial neck. The transducer is then fanned in a medial and lateral longitudinal fashion around the visible circumference of the anterior radius. Assessment of the radial neck recess is enhanced by rotating the proximal radius, achieved by supination and pronation of the forearm.

Insider Information 4.3
The brachialis muscle is identified immediately anterior to the joint capsule. The distal biceps tendon is positioned superficial to this muscle and lateral to the brachial artery.

The distal biceps tendon is assessed in both planes. This structure is positioned superficial to the brachialis muscle and lateral to the brachial artery. This tendon is challenging to evaluate, given its deep oblique course toward its insertion onto the radial tuberosity. In cases in which it is difficult to identify the tendon, the examination can begin more proximally at the musculotendinous junction and then follow the tendon distally. The ultrasound probe orientation is critical so as to avoid anisotropy. The forearm should be placed in maximal external rotation, with the probe in a sagittal oblique orientation (Figure 4.11a and b). The biceps tendon is also evaluated in the transverse orientation (Figure 4.11c). The radial tuberosity and the bicipitoradial bursa should be assessed. An alternate technique has been reported that utilizes a posterior approach for evaluating the distal biceps tendon at its insertion.[23] For this technique, the transducer is placed in the transverse plane on the posterior aspect of the proximal forearm with the forearm in the pronated position (Figure 4.12a). In this orientation, the radial tuberosity is identified as a broad-based bony prominence. The distal biceps tendon appears as a tapering hyperechoic structure, inserting onto the tuberosity (Figure 4.12b). The fibers are oriented parallel to the skin surface, directly overlying the curvilinear contour of the radius. Dynamically evaluating with forearm supination and pronation also assists in identifying the distal fibers, as they disappear with supination (Figure 4.12c). Evaluation with this technique assists in diminishing the effects of anisotropy of the last few centimeters of the tendon insertion.

Insider Information 4.4
To image the distal biceps tendon anteriorly, place the forearm in full supination. Remember: the tendon takes a deep and slightly oblique course toward insertion onto the radial tuberosity. If the distal few centimeters are difficult to image, the posterior technique assists in visualizing the tendon at insertion.

The median nerve is amenable to ultrasound evaluation at the level of the cubital fossa. If the fossa is divided into three equal parts, the median nerve is typically found at the junction between the medial one-third and the middle one-third. With the ultrasound transducer in a transverse orientation (Figure 4.7a), the median nerve is identified just medial to the brachial artery. The nerve is assessed in both a transverse (Figure 4.13a) and longitudinal (Figure 4.13b) orientation, assessing caliber, course, and echotexture.

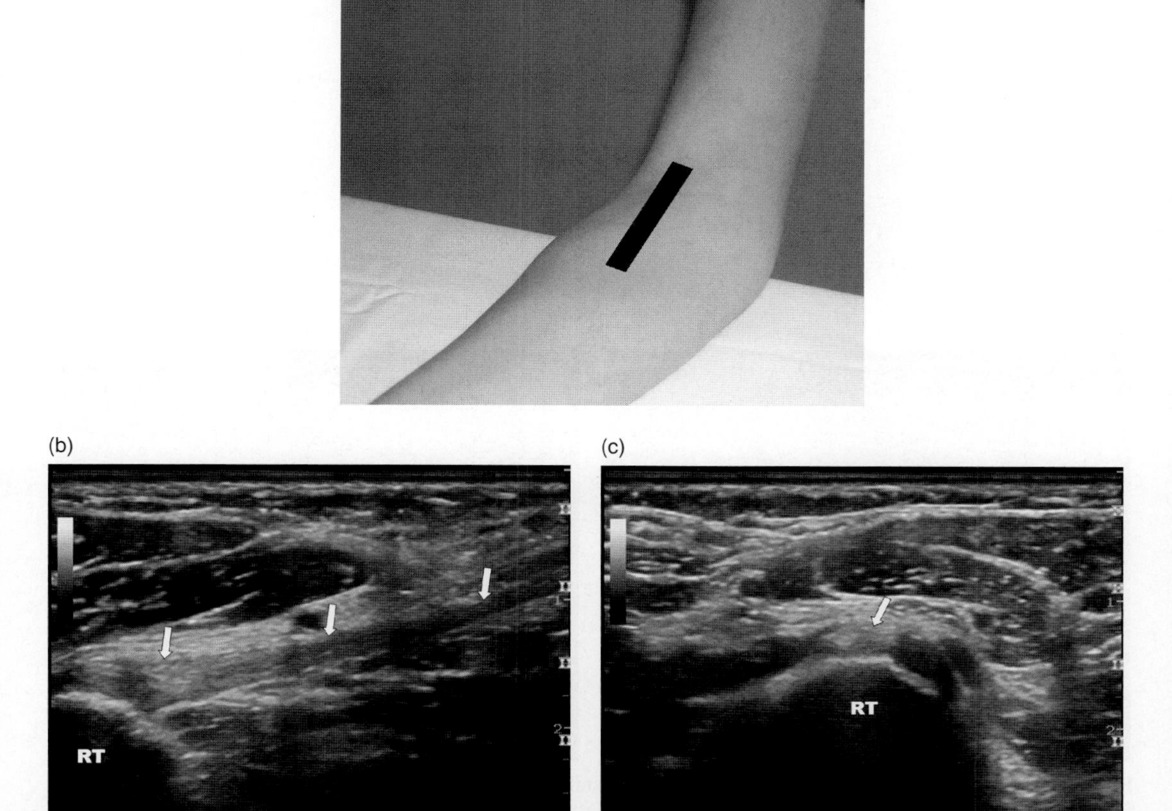

Figure 4.11. (**a**) Probe placement for assessment of the distal biceps tendon. (**b**) Longitudinal image of the distal biceps tendon (arrows), following the tendon to insertion on the radial tuberosity (RT). (**c**) Transverse ultrasound of the distal biceps tendon (arrow) at the level of the radial tuberosity (RT).

The radial nerve is easiest to identify as it courses in a fixed position around the humerus, at its midpoint (Chapter 3). From this position, the nerve can be followed to its position just proximal to the elbow joint. It is often easiest to identify and follow the nerve with the ultrasound probe in a transverse orientation (Figure 4.14). At the level of the lateral epicondyle, it may be appreciated that the nerve splits into superficial and deep terminal rami. Again, this division is easier to appreciate in the transverse orientation.

Lateral Approach

To examine the lateral aspect of the elbow joint, the patient is positioned with the elbow flexed, forearm extended, with both palms together (praying position) (Figure 4.15a). The lateral epicondyle is assessed for the presence of any surface irregularities, or enthesiopathy. The attachment of the common extensor tendon has a uniform hyperechoic triangular configuration that can be identified traversing the lateral aspect of the radiocapitellar joint

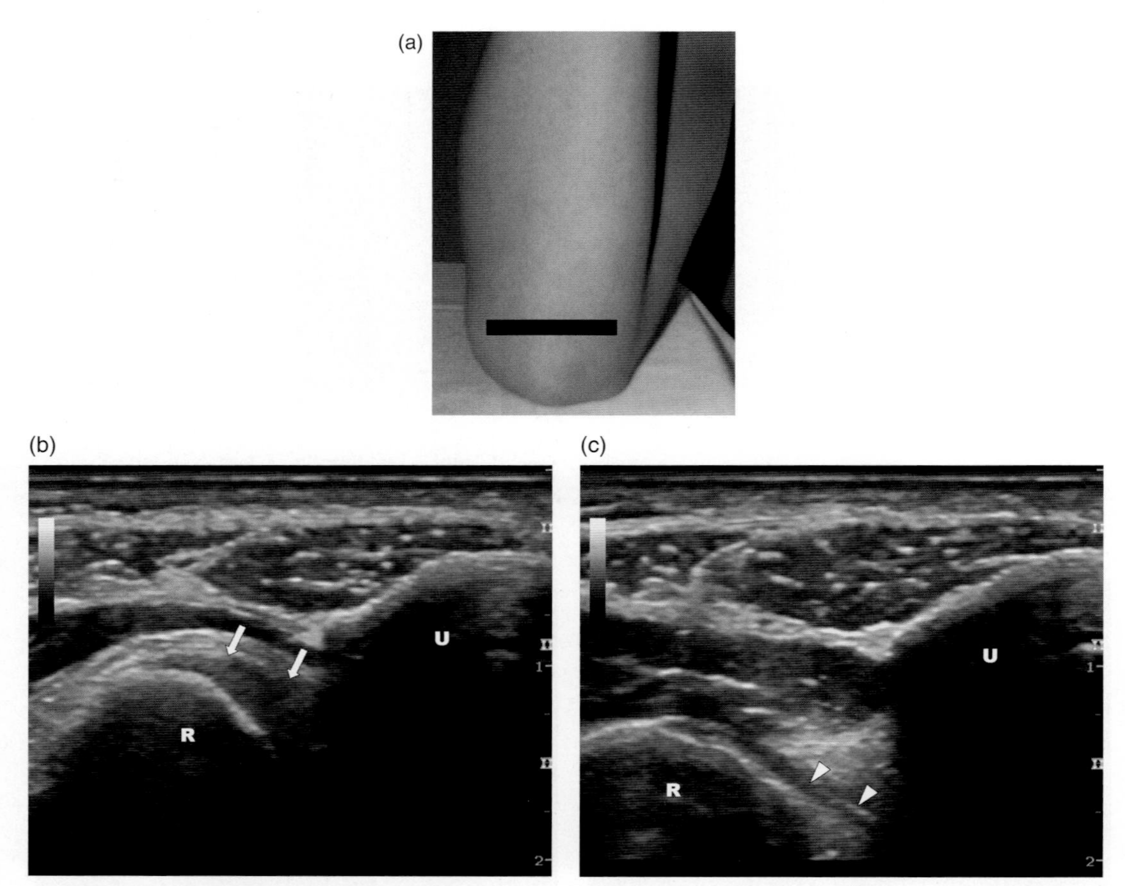

Figure 4.12. **(a)** Probe position for evaluation of the distal biceps tendon insertion on the radial tuberosity, with a posterior scanning technique. **(b)** Transverse image at the level of probe placement illustrated in **(a)**, with the forearm in pronation, identifies the distal biceps tendon insertion (arrows) as a tapering structure over the radial surface (R). U, ulna. **(c)** Transverse image at the same level as **(a)** and **(b)** with the forearm in supination illustrates the disappearance of the normal BT insertion (arrowheads). U, ulna.

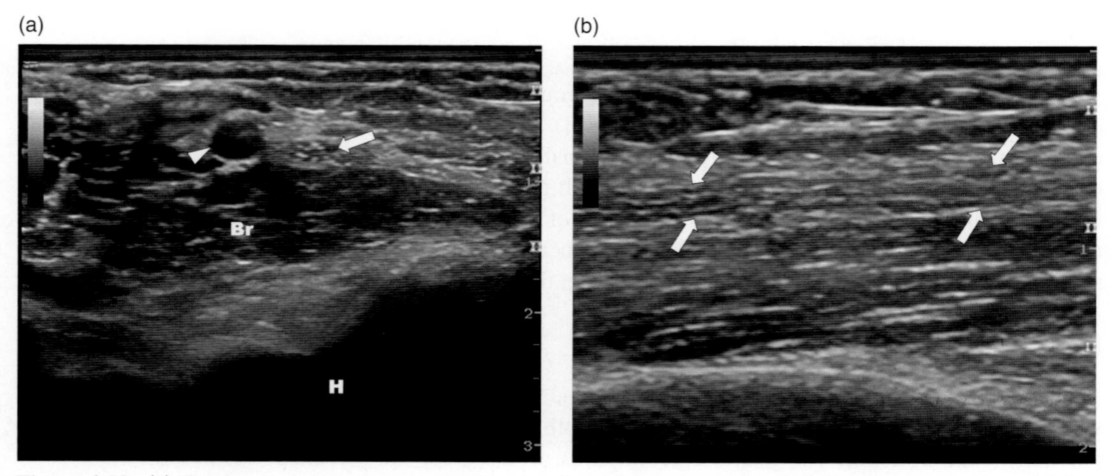

Figure 4.13. **(a)** Transverse image just proximal to the elbow joint demonstrates the median nerve (arrow) lying at the medial aspect of the brachial artery (arrowhead). Br, brachialis; H, humerus. **(b)** Longitudinal image at the same level as **(a)** identifies the course fascicular echotexture of the median nerve (arrows).

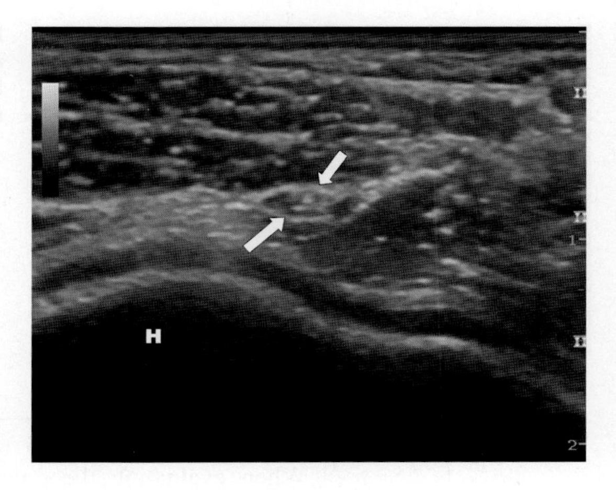

Figure 4.14. Transverse image at the level of the distal humerus identifies the radial nerve in cross section (arrow). H, humerus.

(Figure 4.15b). Both the superficial and deep components of this common tendon are evaluated. The contributing tendons that make up the superficial component of this tendon cannot be discretely identified. The extensor carpi radialis longus and brachioradialis tendons are identified in a more proximal position separate from the common extensor tendon. Next, with the hand pronated, extend the elbow, in order to evaluate the radial collateral ligament. With the ultrasound transducer in a longitudinal orientation at the level of the lateral epicondyle, the radial collateral ligament is identified immediately deep to the common extensor tendon, blending distally with the annular ligament fibers. It appears as a thin, linear structure, with a compact fibrillar appearance (Figure 4.16). It has a slightly different course from the overlying common extensor tendon.

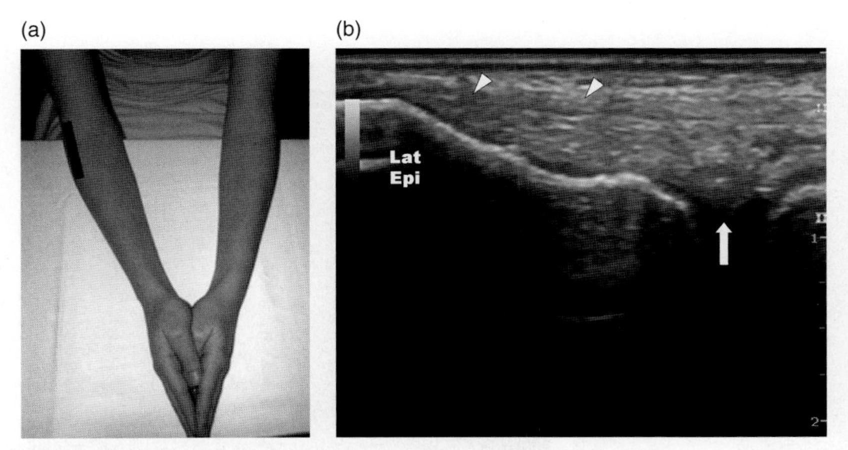

Figure 4.15. **(a)** Proper probe placement and patient positioning for assessment of the lateral elbow and common extensor tendon. **(b)** Longitudinal image at the level of the lateral epicondyle (Lat Epi) demonstrates the hyperechoic triangular appearance of the common extensor tendon (arrowheads). The tendon is observed traversing over the lateral joint space (arrow).

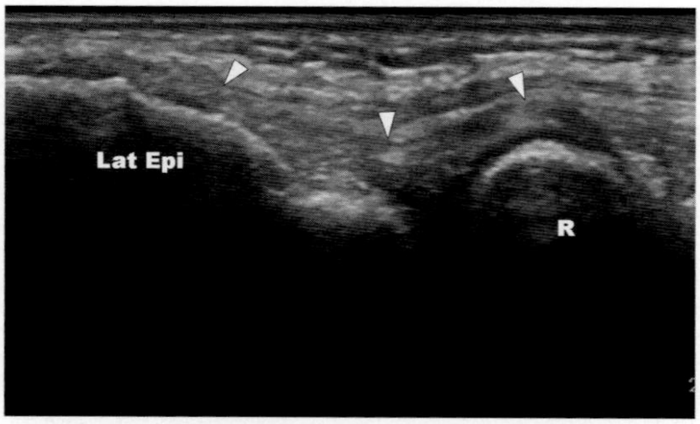

Figure 4.16. Longitudinal image of the radial collateral ligament (arrowheads) identified extending between the lateral humeral epicondyle (Lat Epi) and the radius (R).

Insider Information 4.5

When evaluating the epicondyles and common tendons, remember to evaluate the bone surface of the epicondyles, observing surface irregularities and enthesophytes, as well as observing the status of the overlying common tendon.

Medial Approach

To evaluate the medial aspect of the elbow joint, the patient is positioned with the elbow extended and the forearm fully supinated (Figure 4.17a). The medial epicondyle surface and appearance are evaluated, as well as the common flexor tendon attachment. The normal common flexor tendon appears as a hyperechoic "beak" or triangular structure, with a compact fibrillar appearance (Figure 4.17b). The medial common flexor origin has a broader appearance than the more cordlike lateral common extensor origin. Comparison with the opposite elbow is frequently warranted in order to appreciate subtle changes.

As described previously, the ulnar collateral ligament is composed of three components; the anterior band is the most important functionally and the most readily visible with ultrasound. This compact hyperechoic fibrillar structure is

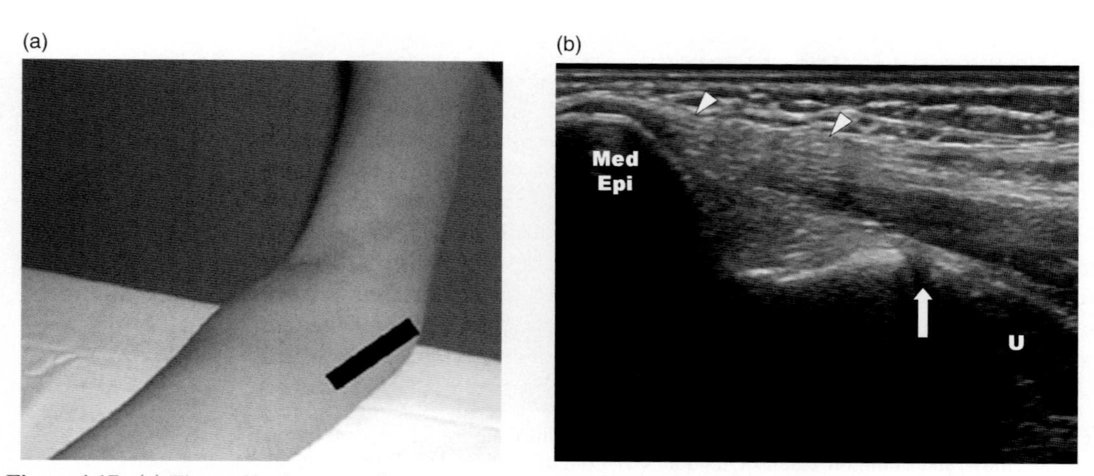

Figure 4.17. (**a**) The probe placement for assessment of the medial elbow and common flexor tendon. (**b**) Longitudinal image at the level of the medial epicondyle (Med Epi) demonstrating the compact fibrillar appearance of the common flexor tendon (arrowheads). The medial joint space is visible (arrow). U, ulna.

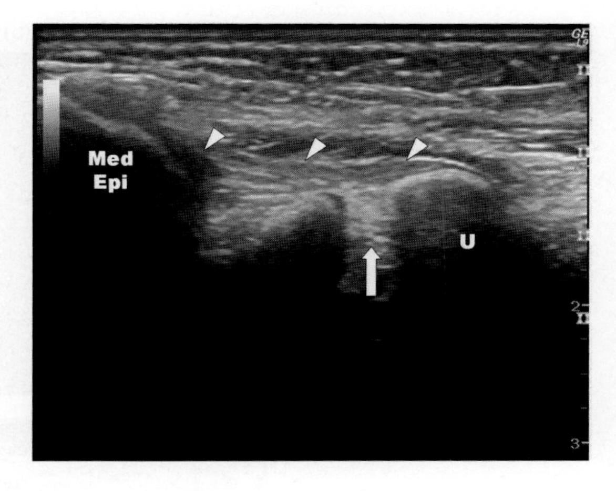

Figure 4.18. Longitudinal image of the medial elbow demonstrates the anterior band of the ulnar collateral ligament (arrowheads), identified as extending from the medial epicondyle of the humerus (Med Epi) to the ulna (U). The medial joint space is visible (arrow).

identified arising from the proximal ulna, inserting onto the medial epicondyle (Figure 4.18). If the patient has prominent bony landmarks, the generous use of ultrasound gel or a smaller compact probe can assist in better visualizing and assessing this structure. To evaluate this structure, place the ultrasound transducer along the course of the common flexor tendon, at the level of the medial epicondyle. At this position, the ulnar collateral ligament lies deep to the tendon. To visualize the ligament, the ultrasound probe often needs to be oriented slightly off the plane of the common flexor tendon in order to trace the ligament from the humerus to its attachment on the ulna. Dynamic techniques for evaluating this ligament for injury have been reported.[24]

Insider Information 4.6
The most important component of the ulnar collateral ligament is the anterior bundle. Once you identify the medial epicondyle, remember the oblique anatomical orientation of this ligament, as it traverses to the proximal ulna. Remembering this anatomy will assist in finding this small but important structure on ultrasound.

Posterior Approach

For evaluation of the posterior elbow, the patient is positioned with the palm down on a table and the elbow is flexed to 90° (Figure 4.19a). Alternatively, the patient can be imaged with their hand on their hip, in the sitting position. In longitudinal (Figure 4.19b) and short axis (Figure 4.19c) planes, the posterior joint space, olecranon fossa, triceps tendon, and olecranon process are evaluated. The distal triceps tendon is easily identified inserting onto the olecranon process. Tendon evaluation is enhanced with flexion and extension, as dynamic scanning assists in evaluating the integrity of the tendon fibers and any focal areas of altered echogenicity. The olecranon fossa is identified as a shallow, convex area in the distal humerus, normally filled with the posterior hyperechoic fat pad (Figure 4.19c). Gel and light touch technique are required to evaluate the olecranon bursa because this structure, when distended with some bursal fluid, is easily compressed. When

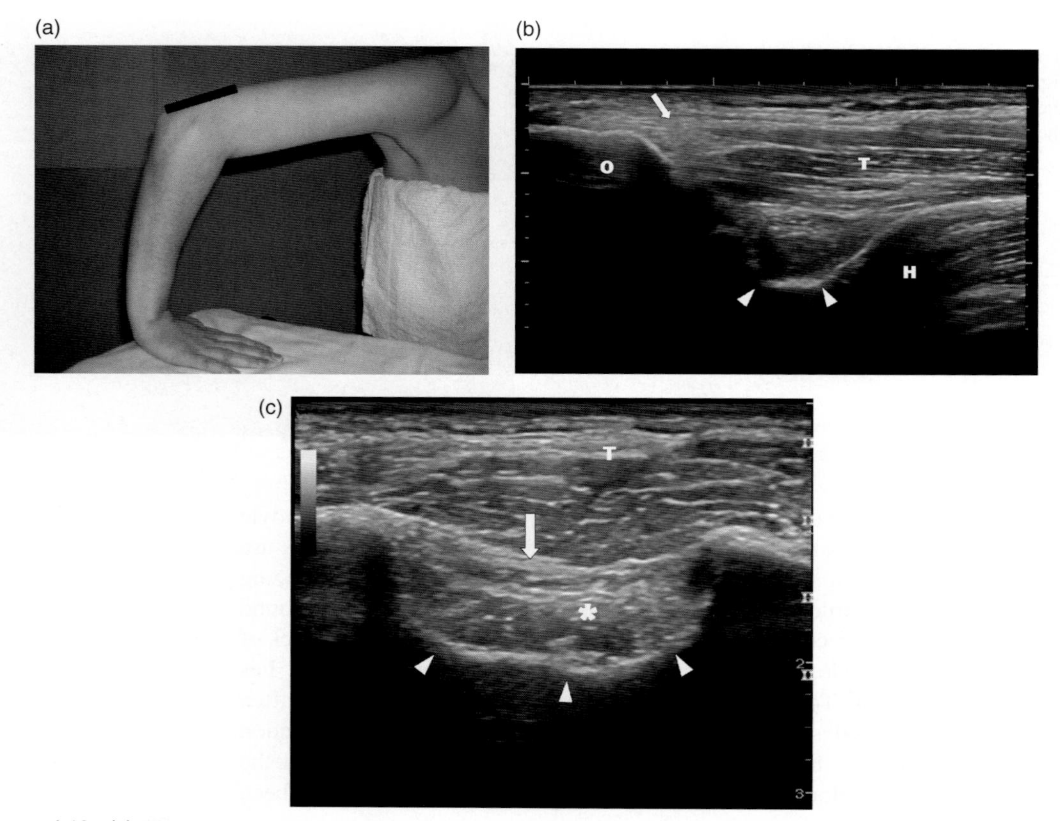

Figure 4.19. (**a**) The probe position for assessment of the posterior elbow joint and triceps tendon. (**b**) Longitudinal extended field of view imaging of the distal triceps muscle (T) and tendon (arrow) demonstrating insertion onto the olecranon process (O). The olecranon fossa (arrowheads) is identified as a deep groove on the posterior aspect of the humerus (H). (**c**) Transverse image at the level of the posterior humerus. The triceps muscle and tendon (T) are illustrated. Deep to this, the posterior joint capsule is visualized (arrow), with fat (asterisk) filling the olecranon fossa (arrowheads).

scanning the elbow, or viewing static images, the anconeus muscle serves as a useful landmark for the lateral elbow.

Insider Information 4.7
Remember to use a very light touch technique when evaluating the subcutaneous olecranon bursa in order to avoid compressing the bursa.

To evaluate the ulnar nerve within the medial olecranon groove, the transducer is bridged between the medial epicondyle and the olecranon process (Figure 4.20a). The nerve is identified in close proximity to the medial epicondyle, appearing as a hypoechoic, oval structure (Figure 4.20b). Once identified, the nerve is evaluated in the longitudinal plane (Figure 4.20c). Comparison with the opposite side is often useful. Dynamic assessment with flexion and extension of the elbow, with the transducer in the transverse plane, is useful to assess both the distal triceps tendon and ulnar nerve to determine if there is any subluxation, dislocation, or snapping sensation. For this evaluation, it is important to perform this technique with only gentle

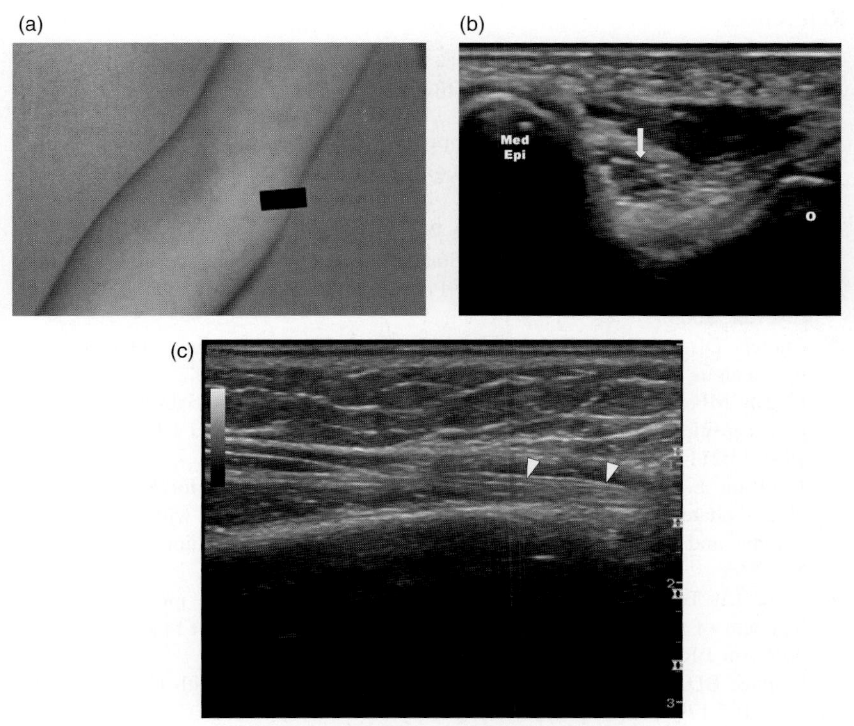

Figure 4.20. (**a**) The probe position for evaluation of the ulnar nerve. The probe is bridged between the olecranon process and the medial epicondyle. (**b**) Corresponding transverse image of the ulnar nerve (arrow) positioned adjacent to the medial epicondyle (Med Epi). O, olecranon process. (**c**) Longitudinal image of the ulnar nerve (arrowheads) at the posterior elbow.

pressure on the transducer, as firm pressure may prevent displacement on dynamic evaluation. In these different positions, the location of the ulnar nerve relative to the medial epicondyle can be assessed. The examiner should also be alert to the presence of any bone spurs or space-occupying lesions that may compress or compromise the ulnar nerve. Using the same technique, the position of the muscle belly of the medial head of the triceps can also be evaluated. Occasionally, this muscle may dislocate over the apex of the medial epicondyle, causing a snapping sensation that mimics ulnar nerve pathology.[25] The normal medial head of the triceps stays positioned posterior to the medial epicondyle during flexion and extension movements.

Imaging Protocols

The elbow joint examination may include a comprehensive joint assessment, or targeted evaluation. For the assessment of nonspecific or nonlocalized elbow joint pain, the examiner may follow a standard approach, including an evaluation of the anterior, posterior, medial, and lateral structures (see the Appendix). More commonly, the study is tailored to the site of patient symptoms or to specified clinical questions.

References

1. van Holsbeeck MT. Sonography of the elbow, wrist, and hand. In: van Holsbeeck M, Introcaso JH, eds., pp. 517–571. Musculoskeletal Ultrasound. St. Louis: Mosby, 2001.
2. Barbarie JE, Wong AD, Cooperberg PL et al. Extended field-of-view sonography in musculoskeletal disorders. AJR 1998;171:751–757.
3. Moore KL. The upper limb. In: Clinically Oriented Anatomy, 2nd ed., pp. 626–793. Baltimore: Williams & Wilkins, 1985.
4. Johnson D, Ellis H, eds. Elbow. In: Standring S, editor-in-chief. Gray's Anatomy. The Anatomical Basis of Clinical Practice, 39th ed., pp. 859–866. London: Elsevier, 2005.
5. Daniels DL, Mallisee TA, Erickson SJ et al. The elbow joint: Osseous and ligamentous structures. Radiographics 1998;18:229–236.
6. Hogan MF, Rupich RC, Bruder JB et al. Age-related variability in elbow joint capsule thickness in asymptomatic children and adults. J Ultrasound Med 1994;13:211–213.
7. Jacobson J, Propeck P, Jamadar DA et al. US of the anterior bundle of the ulnar collateral ligament: Findings in five cadaver elbows with MR arthrographic and anatomic comparison—initial observations. Radiology 2003;227: 561–566.
8. Ward LI, Teefey SA, Paletta GA et al. Sonography of the medial collateral ligament of the elbow: A study of cadavers and healthy adult male volunteers. AJR Am J Roentgen 2003;180:389–394.
9. Fornage BD. Peripheral nerves of the extremities: Imaging with US. Radiology 1988;167:179–182.
10. Silvestri E, Martinoli C, Derchi LE et al. Echotexture of peripheral nerves: Correlation between US and histologic findings and criteria to differentiate tendons. Radiology 1995;197:291–296.
11. Martinoli C, Bianchi S, Derchi L. Ultrasonography of peripheral nerves. Semin Ultrasound, CT MRI 2000;21(3):205–213.
12. Okamoto M, Abe M, Shirai, H et al. Morphology and dynamics of the ulnar nerve in the cubital tunnel: Observation by ultrasonography. J Hand Surg (Br) 2000;25:85–89.
13. Loewy J. Sonoanatomy of the median, ulnar and radial nerves. Can Assoc Radiol J 2002;53:33–38.
14. Martinoli C, Bianchi S, Giovagnorio F, Pugliese F. Ultrasound of the elbow. Skeletal Radiol 2001;30:605–614.
15. Martinoli C, Bianchi S, Zamorani MP, Sunsunequi JL, Derchi LD. Ultrasound of the elbow. Eur J Ultrasound 2001;14:21–27.
16. Finlay K, Ferri M, Friedman L. Ultrasound of the elbow. Skeletal Radiol 2004;33:63–79.
17. Barr LL, Babcock DS. Sonography of the normal elbow. AJR Am J Roentgenol 1991;157:793–798.
18. De Maeseneer M, Jacobson JA, Jaovisidha S et al. Elbow effusions: Distribution of joint fluid with flexion and extension and imaging implications. Invest Radiol 1998;33:117–125.
19. Breidahl WH, Newman JS, Taljanovic MS, Adler RJ. Power Doppler sonography in the assessment of musculoskeletal fluid collections. AJR 1996;166:1443–1446.
20. Newman JS, Aderl RS, Bude RO, Rubin JM. Detection of soft-tissue hyperemia: Value of power Doppler sonography. AJR Am J Roentgenol 1994;163:385–389.
21. Miles KA, Lamont AC. Ultrasonic demonstration of the elbow fat pads. Clin Radiol 1989;40:602–604.
22. Bianchi S, Martinoli, D. Detection of loose bodies in joints. Radiol Clin North Am 1999;37:679–690.

23. Giuffre BM, Lisle DA. Tear of the distal biceps branchii tendon: A new method of ultrasound evaluation. Australasian Radiol 2005;49:404–406.
24. Nazarian LN, McShane JM, Cicotti MG et al. Dynamic US of the anterior band of the ulnar collateral ligament of the elbow in asymptomatic major league baseball pitchers. Radiology 2003;227:149–154.
25. Jacobson JA, Jebson PJ, Jeffers A et al. Ulnar nerve dislocation and snapping triceps syndrome: Diagnosis with dynamic sonography—report of three cases. Radiology 2001;220:601–605.

5

The Forearm

Karen Finlay and Lawrence Friedman

The forearm is identified as the portion of the upper extremity positioned between the elbow and wrist joints. Many important anatomical structures are present within the forearm, several of which can be followed from the elbow joint proximally to the wrist joint distally. These include the main nerves of the forearm, as well as the important flexor and extensor muscle groups.

Ultrasonography can be an extremely useful imaging tool for localizing the specific area of patient concern in the forearm, as well as for assessing local pathology. Dynamic assessment during the flexion, extension, supination, and pronation actions of the forearm musculature assists in evaluating local pathology.

Imaging Indications

Indications for ultrasound examination of the forearm include investigation of forearm muscle injuries or tears and tendon degeneration. Occasionally, underlying bony pathology may be recognized, such as occult fractures, although this is not a primary role for ultrasound. With increasing recognition of the value of ultrasound in assessing nerves and regional structures, ultrasonography can be utilized to assess the caliber and course of forearm nerves in the setting of suspected compression syndromes, nerve sheath tumors, or surrounding soft tissue pathology.

Knowledge of the course of nerves and anatomical compartments is important when ultrasound is utilized to perform interventional procedures, such as biopsy. As a general rule, it is useful to note that nerves are usually identified adjacent to regional vessels; hence, power Doppler is very useful. Ultrasound can also be used to assist with interventional procedures, including biopsies, targeted injections, or aspirations.

Technical Review

Both large standard and smaller footprint multifrequency linear array probes may be utilized. Smaller footprint probes often prove useful for evaluating smaller structures, such as the forearm nerves, as their course on transverse imaging can be specifically targeted with the smaller field of view. The type of pathology being evaluated, as well as the patient's body habitus, affects the choice of probes and ideal frequency. Generally, the forearm can be evaluated with higher frequencies, given the superficial nature of most of the anatomical structures. In general, the ultrasound examination of the forearm is usually undertaken with multifrequency high-resolution linear array 7- to 15-MHz transducers.

Anatomy

Surface Anatomy

On the dorsal surface of the mid forearm, two discrete muscle bundles are visible (Figures 5.1). The lateral longitudinal eminence consists of the brachio-radialis and extensor carpi radialis longus and brevis. The medial group consists of the extensor digitorum and minimi, as well as the extensor carpi ulnaris.

The brachioradialis is a dominant muscle, which is initially identified as a rounded soft tissue structure above the lateral epicondyle that extends inferiorly to form a prominent visible mass on the radial side of the proximal forearm. Its tendon can be followed to the radial styloid.

There are several important palpable bony landmarks around the elbow joint that are utilized in the examination of the forearm (Figure 5.2). These include the medial and lateral epicondyles of the humerus and the olecranon process of the proximal ulna proximally. The anterior cubital fossa and distal biceps tendon are additional important proximal landmarks; these are on the volar aspect of the forearm. These structures can be palpated in most individuals, guiding evaluation of the proximal forearm at its junction with the elbow joint. Distally, a useful visible landmark at the wrist is the transverse crease,

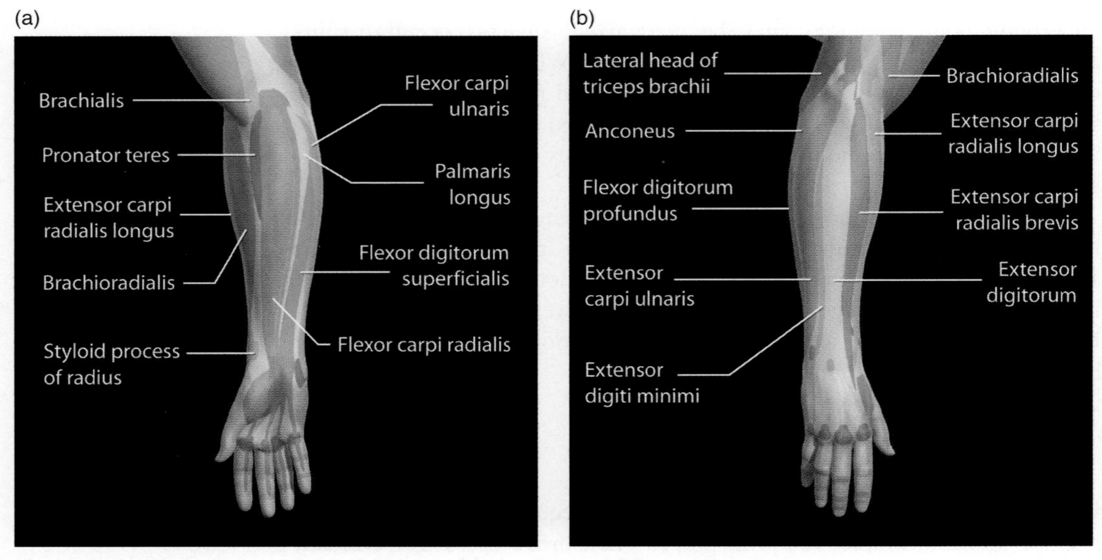

Figure 5.1. The surface anatomy of the arm: **(a)** anterior and **(b)** posterior views.

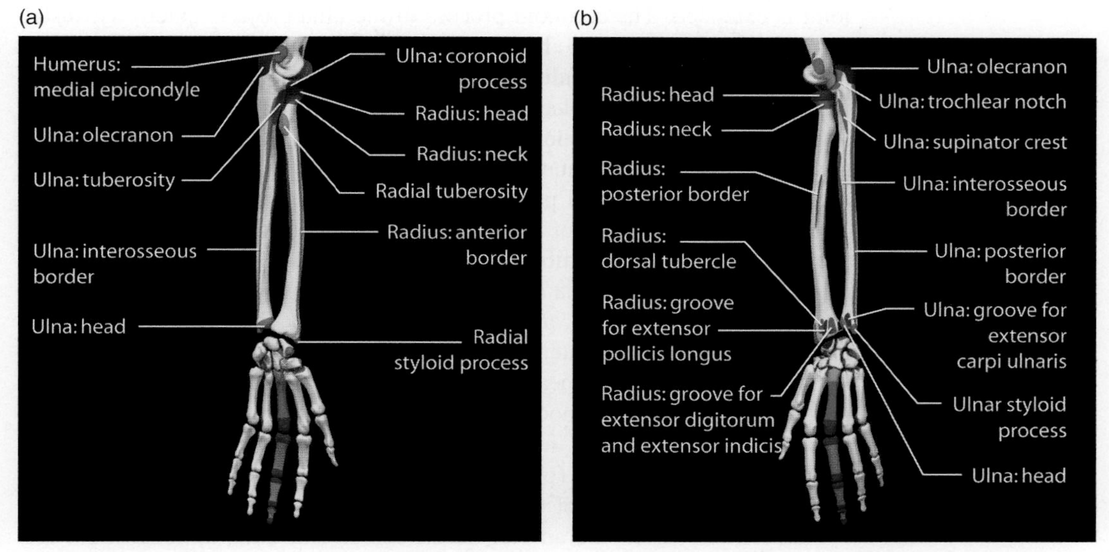

Figure 5.2. The important bony landmarks of the forearm and hand: (**a**) anterior and (**b**) posterior views.

on the volar aspect, corresponding to the level of the flexor retinaculum. Distal palpable bony landmarks include the pisiform, at the volar and ulnar aspect of the wrist, and the radial styloid, at the lateral or radial aspect of the wrist.

Bones

The forearm extends from the elbow joint to the wrist and contains two long bones: the radius and the ulna. These have a parallel relationship in supination (palm facing up), with the radius crossing the ulna in pronation (palm facing down). The proximal radius has a disc-shaped head, a cylindrical neck, and a prominent tuberosity on its anteromedial surface for attachment of the distal biceps tendon. The radius has three surfaces and three borders. The anterior surface has a slightly concave contour for its proximal three-fourths and a flattened contour in its distal one-fourth.[1] The posterior surface is generally flat. There is a gentle, convex configuration to the lateral surface. The anterior border is clearly discriminated proximally and distally; in between it is less distinct, due to the rounded configuration of the bone. The posterior border is well defined only at the midpoint of the radius. The interosseous border is sharp, except at the level of the radial tuberosity proximally and near the level of the ulnar notch distally. The distal radius expands to represent the widest portion of this bone. The ulnar notch at the distal end of the radius articulates with the distal ulna at the distal radioulnar joint.

The ulna is the longer and more medially positioned bone of the forearm. It has important regional landmarks proximally and distally. Proximally at the elbow joint the ulna has two processes: the olecranon and coronoid processes. The large posterior olecranon process has a concave anterior surface and anterior-oriented tip, creating a large hook-like appearance. The beak-shaped tip of this process enters the olecranon fossa of the humerus when the elbow joint is extended. The coronoid process of the ulna projects anteriorly, distal to the olecranon process. This structure enters the coronoid fossa of the humerus, with the elbow fully flexed. The trochlear notch is a convex surface positioned between the olecranon and coronoid processes, which form an articulation with the trochlear process of the humerus. It has a constricted area in its mid-portion, at the junction of these two processes. There are distinct medial and lateral parts of this process, separated by a small ridge. The thick proximal shaft of the ulna has a triangular configuration from the proximal to distal midportion. Distally, the ulna has a more slender, cylindrical appearance. The ulna has an anterior, posterior, and medial surface, as well as anterior, posterior, and interosseous borders. The anterior surface is positioned between the anterior and interosseous borders. This surface has a longitudinally grooved appearance. The medial surface, between the anterior and posterior borders, is smooth and convex. The posterior surface is identified between the posterior and interosseous borders. The distal aspect of the ulna is referred to as the head (opposite to the radius), which is palpable on the dorsal and medial aspect of the wrist.

An interosseous membrane unites the radius and ulna; although thin, the membrane is very strong. It extends between the respective interosseous ridges obliquely downward and inward. In addition to connecting the two forearm bones, this membrane serves as an attachment for some of the forearm muscles (Figure 5.3). This membrane commences 2–3 cm distal to the radial tuberosity.[2]

Muscles and Tendons

The muscles of the forearm act on the elbow joint and the wrist joint, as well as some of the joints of the digits (Table 5.1). The bulk of the muscles are present at the medial and lateral aspect of the proximal forearm, with

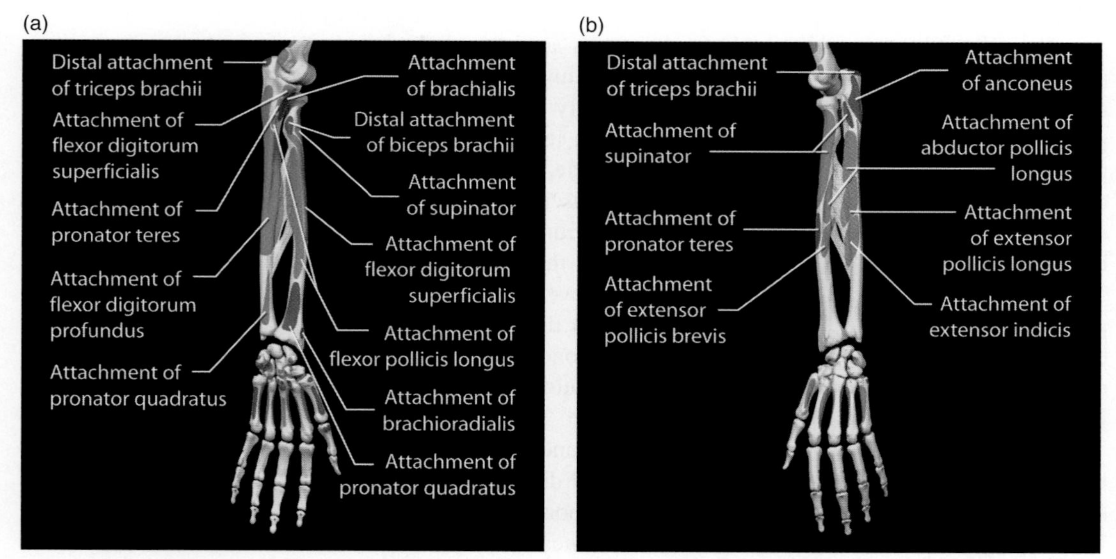

Figure 5.3. The muscle origin (red) and insertion (blue) of the forearm and hand: **(a)** anterior and **(b)** posterior views. Note the longitudinal extent of the interosseous membrane between the radius and ulna.

Table 5.1. Forearm Muscles: Origin, Insertion, and Action[a].

Muscle	Origin	Insertion	Main action
Brachioradialis	Upper two-thirds of lateral supracondylar ridge of humerus	Styloid process of radius, distal one-half of radius, antebrachial fascia	Forearm flexion at elbow Forearm pronation and supination
Extensor carpi radialis longus	Lower one-third of lateral supracondylar ridge of humerus	Dorsum of second metacarpal at base	Extends wrist Abducts hand
Extensor carpi radialis brevis	Common extensor tendon, lateral supracondylar ridge of humerus	Dorsum of third metacarpal at base	Extends wrist Abducts hand
Extensor digitorum	Lateral epicondyle of humerus via common extensor tendon	Extensor expansion of digits 2–5	Extends the digits 2–5 Extends wrist if fingers flexed Abducts digits
Extensor digiti minimi	Lateral epicondyle of humerus via common extensor tendon	Joins extensor digitorum tendon to fifth digit; inserts into extensor expansion	Extends and abducts fifth digit
Extensor carpi ulnaris	First head—lateral epicondyle of humerus via common extensor tendonSecond head— posterior border of ulna	Medial side base of fifth metacarpal	Extends wrist Adducts hand
Supinator	Lateral epicondyle of humerus, supinator crest, and fossa of ulna, radial collateral and annular ligaments	Lateral side, proximal one-third radius	Supinates forearm

(*Continued*)

Table 5.1. (*Continued*)

Muscle	Origin	Insertion	Main action
Flexor carpi radialis	Medial epicondyle of humerus via common flexor tendon	Base of second and third metacarpals	Flexes wrist Abducts hand
Flexor carpi ulnaris	Medial epicondyle of humerus via common flexor tendon, ulnar head from medial border of olecranon and upper two-thirds of posterior ulna	Pisiform, hook of hamate, base of fifth metacarpal	Flexes wrist Adducts hand
Flexor digitorum superficialis	Common flexor tendon (humeroulnar head); middle one-third of radius (radial head)	Shafts of middle phalanges digits 2–5	Flex the MCP and PIP joints
Flexor digitorum profundus	Posterior border of ulna; proximal two-thirds of medial border of the ulna; interosseous membrane	Base of distal phalanx digits 2–5	Flexes MCP, PIP, and DIP joints
Palmaris longus	Medial epicondyle of humerus via common flexor tendon	Central portion of flexor retinaculum; superficial portion of palmar aponeurosis	Flexes wrist
Flexor pollicis longus	Anterior surface of radius and interosseous membrane	Base of distal phalanx of thumb	Flexes MCP and IP joints of thumb
Pronator teres	Medial epicondyle of humerus via common flexor tendon (humeral head); coronoid process of ulna (ulnar head)	Lateral aspect of radius at mid shaft	Pronates forearm Weakly flexes elbow

[a]MCP, metacarpophalangeal; PIP, proximal interphalangeal; DIP, distal interphalangeal; IP, interphalangeal.

the tendons of these muscles passing into the region of the distal forearm and wrist. The flexor-pronator group arises from a common flexor tendon on the medial epicondyle of the humerus, frequently referred to as the common flexor origin (Figure 5.4a). Distal to the elbow joint, deeper muscle groups arise from the anterior or dorsal surface of the ulna and radius (Figure 5.4b). The extensor-supinator group arises from a common extensor tendon from the lateral epicondyle, known as the common extensor origin (Figures 5.4c and d).

The muscles of the forearm are separated by the radius and ulna, as well as the interosseous membrane (Table 5.2), into anterior (flexor) and posterior (extensor) compartments (Figure 5.5). It is important for imagers to be aware of the forearm compartments, particularly when considering potential interventional procedures. The antebrachial fascia, or deep fascia of the forearm, surrounds the forearm musculature and divides it into three compartments: the mobile wad, volar, and dorsal compartments.[2,3] Septae arise from the deep surface of this fascia, passing between the forearm muscles. These provide anchoring for muscle attachments to the underlying radius and ulna, as well as the interosseous membrane.[2] The volar or anterior compartment contains the flexor muscles of the forearm, which are arranged in superficial and deep groups. The superficial muscles include the flexor carpi radialis and ulnaris, flexor digitorum superficialis and palmaris longus, flexor pollicis longus, and pronator teres. These tendons arise from the medial epicondyle by a common tendon, excluding the pronator teres (Figure 5.4a).

The dorsal compartment contains the extensor muscles. In the deepest position, the supinator muscle is identified. More superficially, the dorsal compartment muscles include the extensor digitorum, extensor digiti minimi, and extensor carpi ulnaris, from radial to ulnar position, respectively (Figures 5.4c and d). The proximal and lateral compartment, also known as the mobile wad, includes the brachioradialis and extensors carpi radialis longus

Table 5.2. Forearm Muscles: Position for Ultrasound Evaluation.

Muscle	Position examined
Brachioradialis	Lateral approach
Extensor carpi radialis longus	Elbow mildly flexed, forearm neutral
Extensor carpi radialis brevis	Elbow mildly flexed, forearm neutral
Extensor digitorum	Elbow mildly flexed, forearm neutral
Extensor digiti minimi	Elbow mildly flexed, forearm neutral
Extensor carpi ulnaris	Elbow mildly flexed, forearm neutral
Supinator	Anterior approach
	Elbow mildly flexed, forearm supinated
Flexor carpi radialis	Medial approach
Flexor carpi ulnaris	Elbow extended, forearm fully supinated
Flexor digitorum superficialis	Elbow extended, forearm fully supinated
Flexor digitorum profundus	Elbow extended, forearm fully supinated
Palmaris longus	Elbow extended, forearm fully supinated
Flexor pollicis longus	Anterior approach, forearm supinated
Pronator teres	Anteromedial approach, forearm supinated

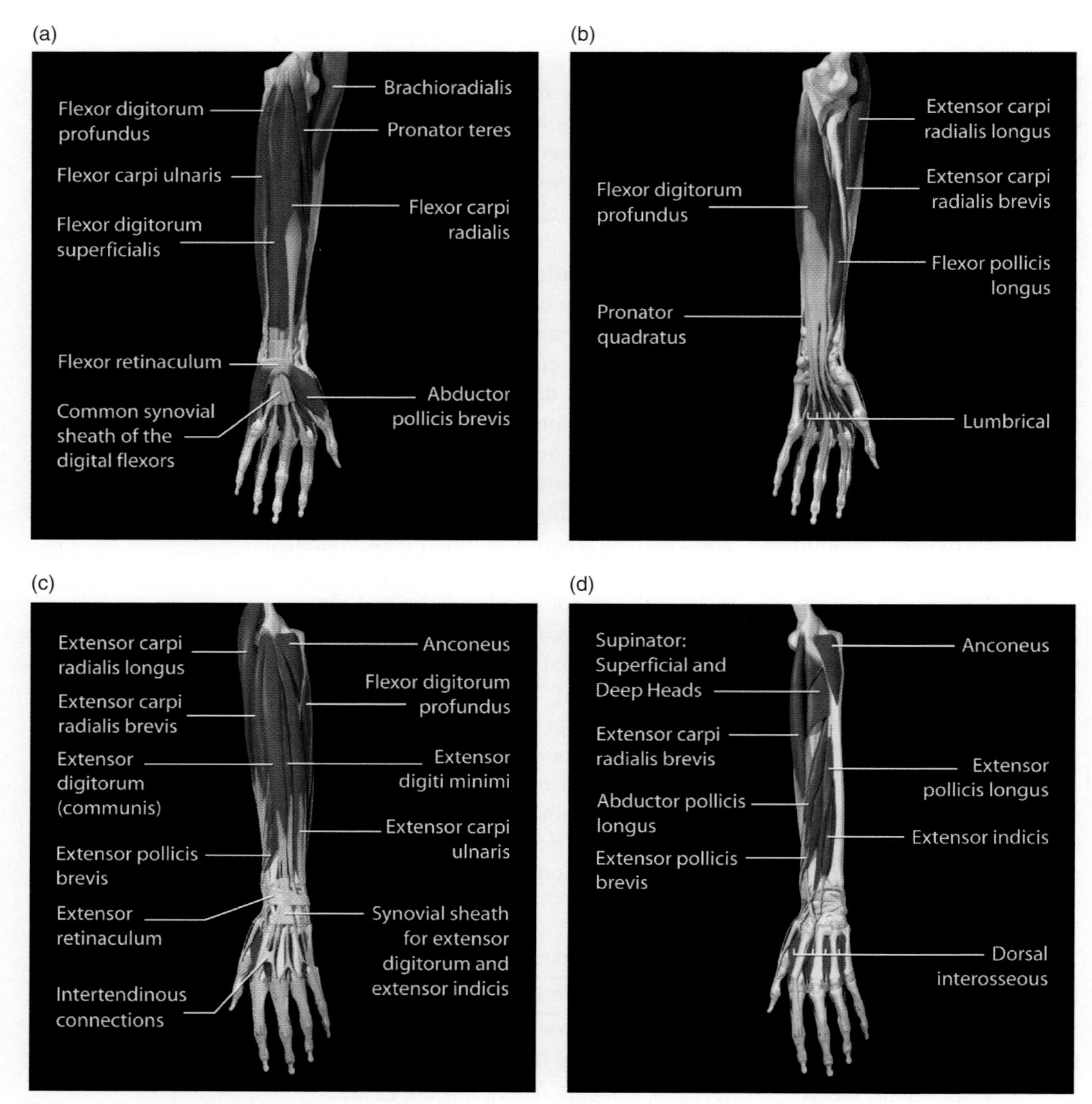

Figure 5.4. The muscles of the arm. **(a)** Oblique view of the medial forearm, demonstrating the flexor muscles at the medial epicondyle and forearm, and **(b)** post removal flexor digitorum superficialis. **(c)** Oblique view of the lateral forearm, demonstrating the extensor muscles at the lateral epicondyle and forearm, and **(d)** post removal extensor digitorum and indicis.

and brevis.[2,3] The brachioradialis is identified as the most superficial muscle along the radial aspect of the forearm. There are no major neurovascular structures located in the mobile wad.

Insider Information 5.1

Mobile wad: two wrist extensors and one forearm flexor.

Volar compartment: muscles that flex the wrist and digits and pronate the forearm.

Dorsal compartment: muscles that extend the wrist and digits.

(a)

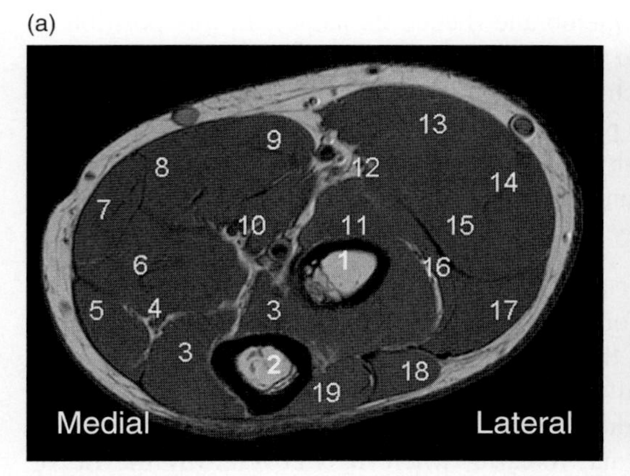

(b)

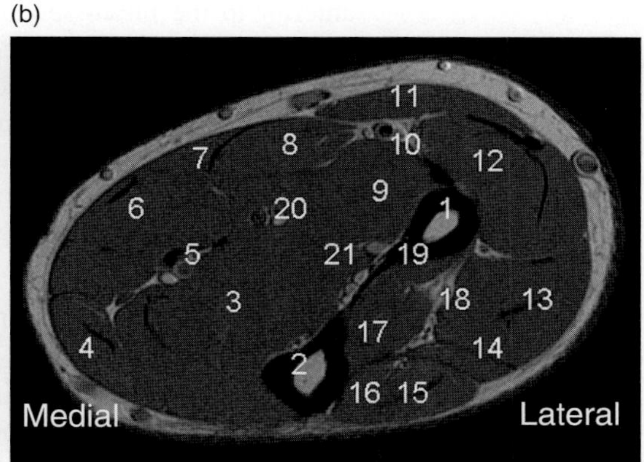

Figure 5.5. Axial T1-weighted MRI anatomy of the arm. **(a)** Proximal forearm: 1–radius, 2–ulna, 3–flexor digitorum profundus, 4–ulnar nerve, 5–flexor carpi ulnaris, 6–flexor digitorum superficialis, 7–palmaris longus, 8–flexor carpi radialis, 9–pronator teres, 10–median nerve, 11–supinator, 12–radial nerve, superficial branch, 13–brachioradialis, 14–extensor carpi radialis longus, 15–extensor carpi radialis brevis, 16–radial nerve, deep branch, 17–extensor digitorum, 18–extensor carpi ulnaris, 19–anconeus. **(b)** Mid forearm: 1–radius, 2–ulna, 3–flexor digitorum profundus, 4–flexor carpi ulnaris, 5–ulnar nerve and artery, 6–flexor digitorum superficialis, 7–palmaris longus, 8–flexor carpi radialis, 9–flexor pollicis longus, 10–radial nerve and artery, 11–brachioradialis, 12–extensor carpi radialis longus, 13–extensor carpi radialis brevis, 14–extensor digitorum and extensor digiti minimi, 15–extensor carpi ulnaris, 16–extensor indicis, 17–extensor pollicis longus, 18–posterior interosseous nerve and artery, 19–abductor pollicis longus, 20–median nerve, 21–anterior interosseous nerve and artery.

Nerves

Important nerves course through the forearm, including the median and ulnar nerves, as well as branches of the radial nerve (Chapter 12, Figure 12.10a and b). Ultrasound can confidently evaluate the main nerve trunks.[4,5] Nerves demonstrate a characteristic ultrasound appearance, with small echogenic foci identified on transverse images, as well as prominent hyperechoic linear structures, interspersed through a hypoechoic background on longitudinal imaging.[6,7] This appearance is secondary to the fascicular microanatomy of nerves.

Median Nerve

The median nerve enters the forearm from the cubital fossa where it lies deep to the bicipital aponeurosis and traverses between the two heads of the pronator teres muscle (Chapter 12, Figure 12.10c). It crosses anterior to the ulnar artery and passes deep into the forearm to supply muscles in the anterior forearm muscles. In the forearm, it descends posterior and adherent to the flexor digitorum superficialis and anterior to the flexor digitorum profundus (Figure 5.5b).[2] Approximately 5 cm proximal to the flexor retinaculum, this nerve returns to a more superficial position, passing at the lateral edge of flexor digitorum superficialis, just prior to entering the carpal tunnel.[2] At this level, the median nerve lies between the tendons of the flexor digitorum superficialis and flexor carpi radialis and is deep to the palmaris longus.

The anterior interosseous nerve is an important branch of the median nerve in the forearm. This branch arises from the posterior aspect of the median nerve between the two heads of pronator teres, just distal to the elbow joint.[1,2] The anterior interosseous nerve is positioned beside the adjacent artery, just anterior to the interosseous membrane (hence its name). In this position, it courses between and deep to the flexor pollicis longus and flexor digitorum profundus. This motor branch supplies the pronator quadratus, flexor pollicis longus, and flexor digitorum profundus muscles. Because of its small size, the nerve branch itself is difficult to visualize; however, it is important to assess the muscle bulk and appearance of those nerves it innervates, particularly in situations in which pathology of the nerve is suspected.[8]

Ulnar Nerve

The ulnar nerve enters the forearm by passing behind the medial epicondyle of the humerus and entering the forearm between the two heads of the flexor carpi ulnaris. It descends in the medial aspect of the forearm and lies on the flexor digitorum profundus (Chapter 12, Figure 12.10a). It is positioned slightly deeper in the proximal forearm, where it is covered by the flexor carpi ulnaris (Figure 5.5). In the distal half of the forearm, the ulnar nerve is superficially located, just below skin and fascia, and is accompanied by the ulnar artery.

Radial Nerve

At the elbow, the radial nerve splits into deep (motor) and superficial (sensory) branches. This occurs at the level of the lateral epicondyle, although there is some anatomical variation of level for these branches. The branches include the superficial terminal branch; the posterior interosseous nerve; and the medial, lateral, and posterior cutaneous nerves of the forearm. The posterior interosseous nerve represents an important branch. In most individuals, it reaches the posterior aspect of the forearm by traversing around the lateral aspect of the radius and piercing the supinator muscle between its superficial and deep components (Chapter 12, Figure 12.10c). The arcade of Frohse is a strong fibrous arch, identified at the proximal margin of the supinator muscle, that bridges the nerve. The anatomical course and adjacent structures make the posterior interosseous nerve branch vulnerable to compression and entrapment at this level.[2,9] The radial nerve supplies no muscles in the hand.[1] Branches of the superficial branch of the radial nerve reach the distal forearm, traversing along its anterolateral (radial) aspect.

Technique

The forearm is positioned according to the compartment that needs to be investigated. The patient is seated opposite the examiner, with the elbow in varying degrees of extension. The degree of supination or pronation also depends on the area of interest. Evaluation of regional pathology is enhanced by knowledge of regional anatomy, particularly of the elbow joint and wrist joint. Frequently, it is easier to identify discrete muscles and nerves by following them proximally or distally from the elbow or wrist joints.

Muscles

For evaluation of all muscles and muscle compartments, careful and meticulous comparison with the opposite normal side should be employed, to exclude subtle pathology (Table 5.3).[10] This includes evaluation of muscle

Table 5.3. Muscle Compartments of the Forearm.

Flexor/volar compartment	Extensor/dorsal compartment	Mobile wad
Deep volar	Extensor digitorum	Brachioradialis
Flexor digitorum profundus	Extensor digiti mimimi	Extensor carpi radialis brevis
Flexor pollicis longus	Extensor carpi ulnaris	Extensor carpi radialis longus
Pronator quadratus		
	Supinator	
Superficial		
Flexor carpi radialis		
Flexor carpi ulnaris		
Flexor digitorum superficialis		
Palmaris longus		
Flexor pollicis longus		
Pronator teres		

bulk, echotexture, and musculotendinous junctions. Muscles can be examined in relaxation and with active contraction. Active contraction can often trigger the symptom or clinical finding of interest.[11] In addition, it assists in identifying the muscle of interest.

Flexor Muscles/Volar Compartment

To examine the flexor muscles, located in the volar compartment, the elbow is flexed approximately 90° and the forearm is positioned in supination (Figure 5.6). The superficial and deep flexors can be traced from the common flexor tendon at the medial epicondyle (Figure 5.7). The conjoint tendon is located slightly more dorsal along the medial epicondyle than might be expected. The probe is then maneuvered distally, in a medial to lateral orientation, in both the sagittal and transverse planes (Figures 5.8 and 5.9).

Extensor Muscles/Dorsal Compartment

The extensor compartment is best assessed with the forearm in pronation (Figure 5.10). The muscles can be visualized from their common origin at the lateral epicondyle (Figure 5.11), sweeping distally from medial to lateral in both planes (Figures 5.12 and 5.13). Again it should be noted that the conjoint extensor tendon is located in a deep position.

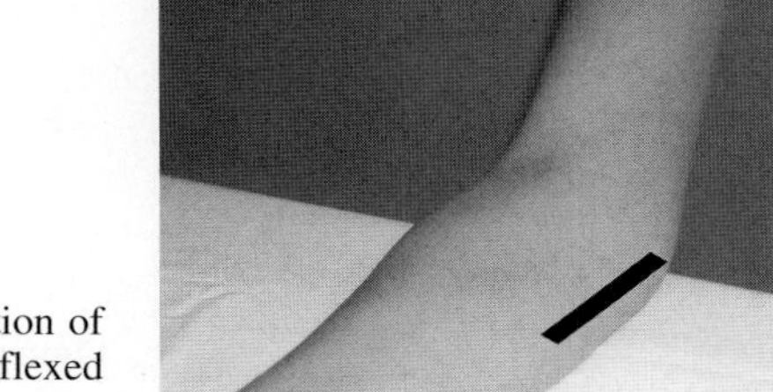

Figure 5.6. Image demonstrating patient positioning for examination of the flexor muscles, located in the volar compartment. The elbow is flexed and the forearm is positioned in supination.

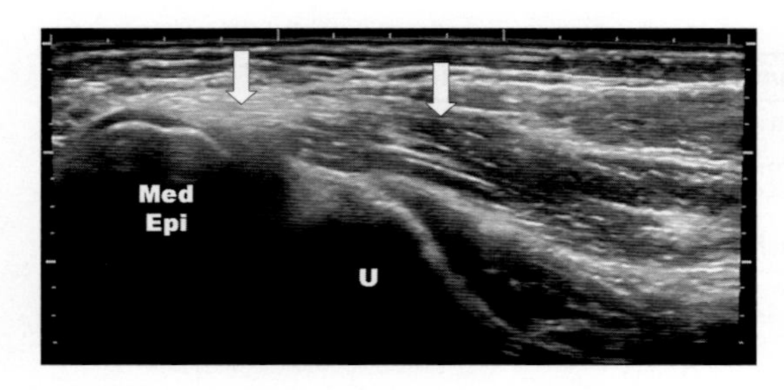

Figure 5.7. Longitudinal extended field of view image demonstrating the common flexor tendon extending to the level of the proximal forearm muscles (arrows). Ulna (U), medial epicondyle (Med Epi).

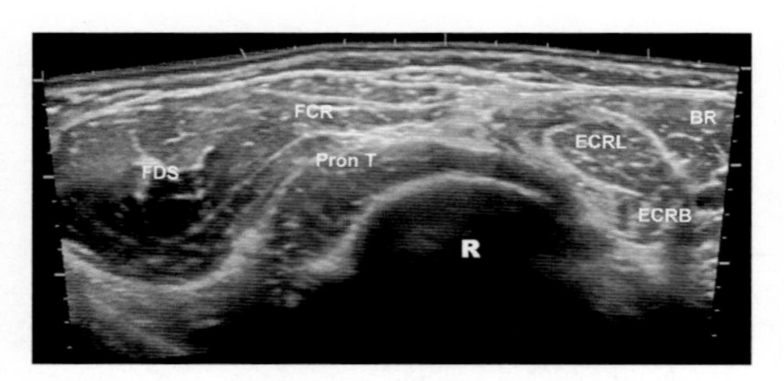

Figure 5.8. Transverse image of proximal forearm volar compartment muscles. Flexor digitorum superficialis (FDS), flexor carpi radialis (FCR), pronator teres (Pron T), extensor carpi radialis longus (ECRL), extensor carpi radialis brevis (ECRB), brachioradialis (BR), radius (R).

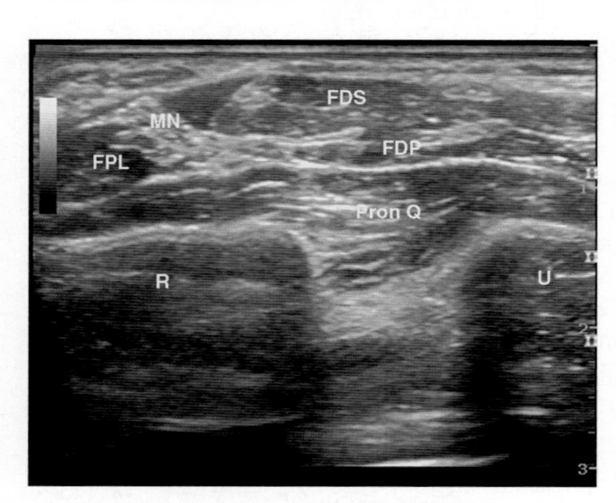

Figure 5.9. Transverse image of distal forearm volar compartment muscles. Flexor pollicis longus (FPL), median nerve (MN), flexor digitorum superficialis (FDS), flexor digitorum profundus (FDP), pronator quadratus (Pron Q), radius (R), ulna (U).

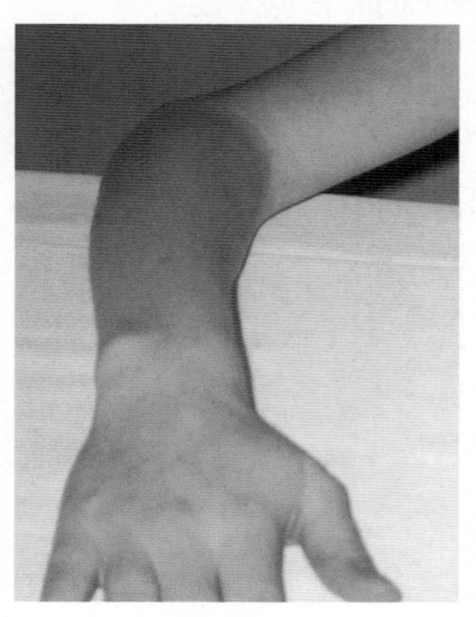

Figure 5.10. Image demonstrating patient position for evaluation of the extensor compartment. The patient is positioned with elbow flexed and forearm pronated.

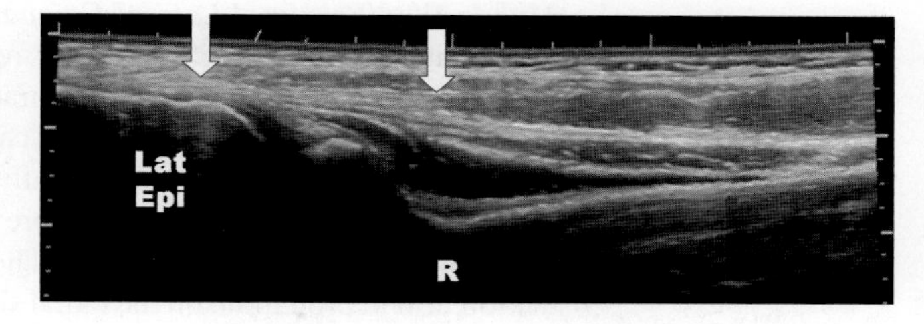

Figure 5.11. Longitudinal image demonstrating the common extensor tendon (arrows) extending from the lateral epicondyle of the humerus (Lat Epi) to the level of the proximal forearm muscles. Radius (R).

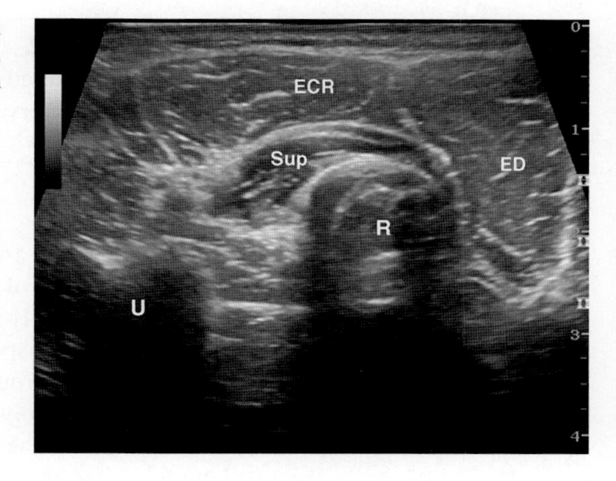

Figure 5.12. Transverse image of the proximal forearm dorsal compartment muscles. Supinator (Sup), extensor carpi radialis (ECR), extensor digitorum (ED), radius (R), ulna (U).

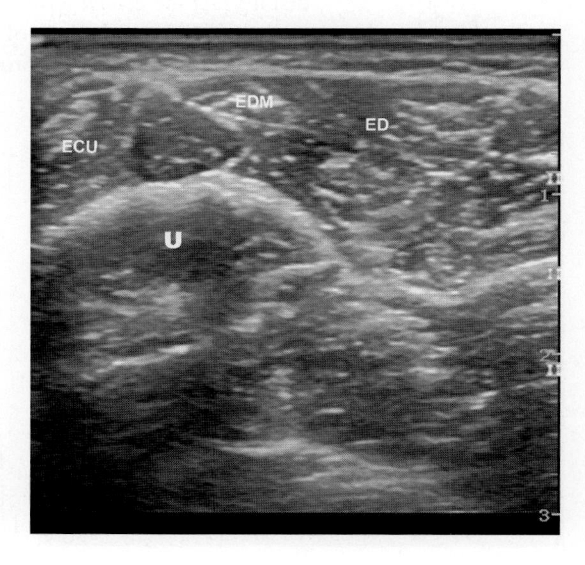

Figure 5.13. Transverse image of the distal forearm dorsal compartment muscles. Extensor carpi ulnaris (ECU), extensor digiti minimi (EDM), extensor digitorum (ED), ulna (U).

Mobile Wad/Proximal Lateral Compartment
Examination of the mobile wad may require moving the arm to best assess a particular muscle group. The brachioradialis is best examined with the elbow joint in partial extension. The muscle can then be traced from above the elbow, as it extends superficially and distally into the forearm (Figure 5.14). The extensor carpi radialis longus and brevis, on the other hand, may be easier to trace proximally from the wrist. They are located in compartment 2, with the forearm in pronation, on the radial side of Lister's tubercle (see Chapter 6).

Nerves

For evaluation of the forearm nerves, it is important to be aware of the normal ultrasound appearance of nerves, as well as their anatomical location (see Chapters 1 and 13).

> **Insider Information 5.2**
> If difficulty is encountered in identifying nerves versus tendons, dynamic evaluation can assist. Nerves demonstrate far less movement with muscle action than tendons do.

Median Nerve
The median nerve in the forearm can be identified at the junction of the medial and middle third of the antecubital fossa at the elbow, medial to the brachial artery. Distally it can be followed through the forearm to the decussation at the volar aspect of the wrist. It is often easiest to trace the median nerve proximally from the carpal tunnel, where it is located superficial to the common flexor tendons, on the radial side of the wrist. With the forearm positioned in supination, the median nerve can be easily traced, either in the short or long axis, into the cubital fossa region (Figure 5.15).

Ulnar Nerve
To assess the ulnar nerve, it is easiest to first identify it either proximally or distally. At the elbow joint, the ulnar nerve is identified immediately adjacent to the medial epicondyle of the humerus, in the cubital tunnel, and can be easily followed into the proximal forearm (Figure 5.16). In the distal half

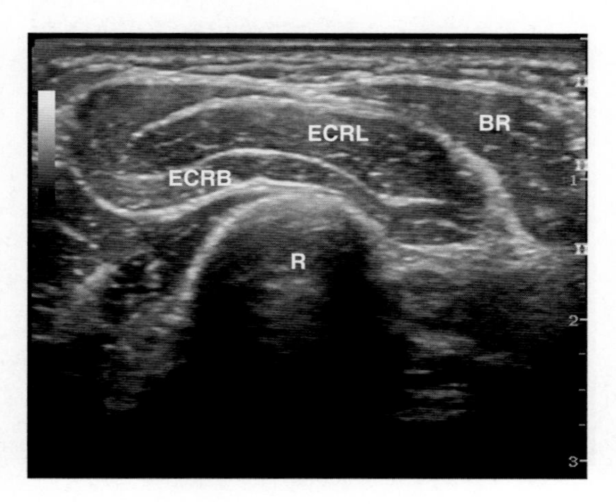

Figure 5.14. Transverse ultrasound image of the mobile wad muscles. Extensor carpi radialis longus (ECRL), extensor carpi radialis brevis (ECRB), brachioradialis (BR), radius (R).

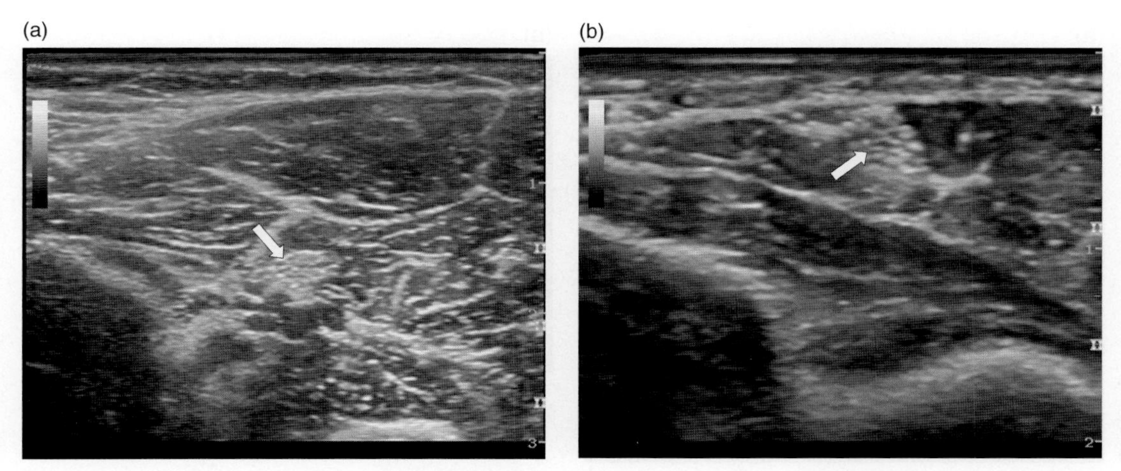

Figure 5.15. (**a**) Transverse ultrasound image of the median nerve (arrow) at the level of the proximal forearm. (**b**) Transverse ultrasound image of the median nerve distally (arrow), where the nerve is identified in a more superficial location.

of the forearm, the ulnar nerve is superficially located, just below skin and fascia, and is accompanied by the ulnar artery. It is easily identified at the wrist, adjacent to the ulnar artery, in Guyon's canal. From this position it can also be followed proximally into the forearm.

Radial Nerve

The radial nerve is identified at the level of the lateral epicondyle, on the radial aspect of the elbow. It lies in a groove between the brachialis and brachioradialis muscles. From this position, its branches can be followed into the proximal forearm. The important posterior interosseous nerve has a vulnerable course in the proximal forearm, as was previously described. The supinator muscle is easily identified in the proximal forearm as a roundly contoured muscle that covers the volar surface of the radius. Although challenging to image, the position and appearance of the normal and abnormal posterior interosseous nerve have been described (Figure 5.17).[9,12]

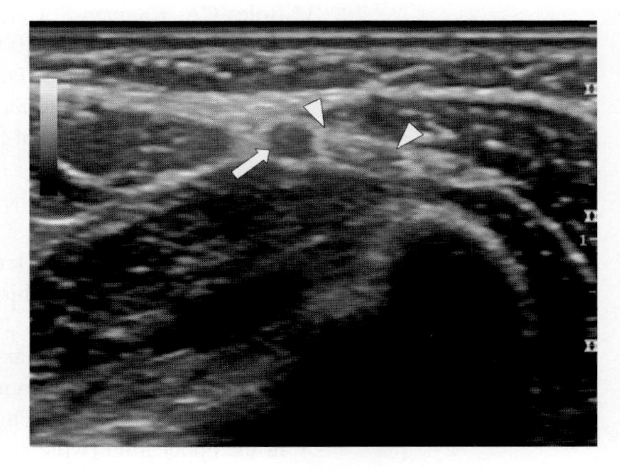

Figure 5.16. Transverse ultrasound image of the ulnar nerve (arrowheads) at the level of the proximal forearm, positioned adjacent to the ulnar artery (arrow).

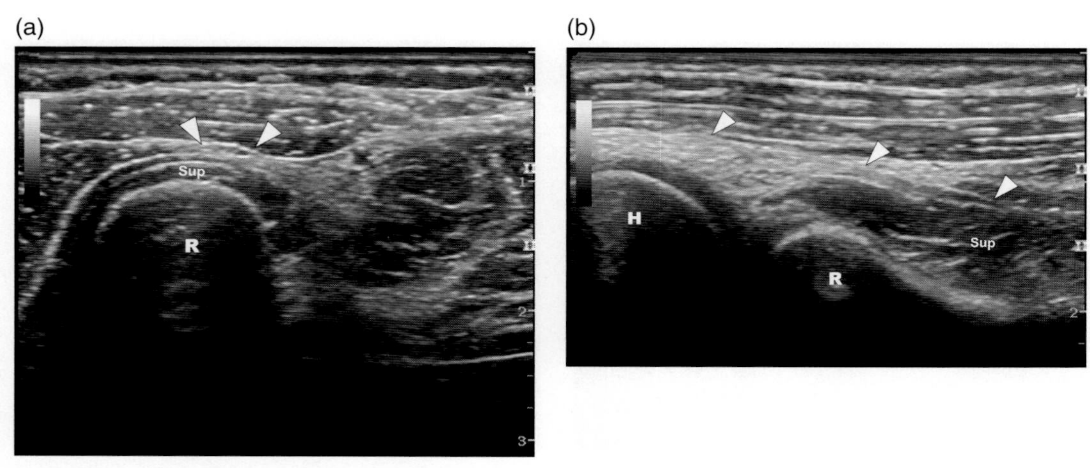

Figure 5.17. **(a)** Transverse ultrasound image of the proximal forearm at the level of the proximal radius (R) demonstrates the posterior interosseous nerve (arrowheads) lying just superficial to the supinator muscle (Sup). **(b)** Longitudinal ultrasound image of the posterior interosseous nerve (arrowheads) demonstrates the distal portion of this nerve piercing the supinator muscle (Sup). Humerus (H), radius (R).

Imaging Protocols

There are no set imaging protocols for ultrasound evaluation of the forearm. Standard imaging guidelines are used. The examination is typically targeted to the specific area of concern or clinical question, rather than a comprehensive examination. Often the forearm examination is an extension of the wrist or elbow study.

References

1. Moore KL. The upper limb. In: Clinically Oriented Anatomy, 2nd ed., pp. 626–793. Baltimore: Williams & Wilkins, 1985.
2. Johnson D, Ellis H, eds. Forearm. In: Standring S, editor-in-chief. Gray's Anatomy. The Anatomical Basis of Clinical Practice, 39th ed., pp. 867–887. London: Elsevier, 2005.
3. Boles CA, Kannam S, Cardwell AB. The forearm: Anatomy of muscle compartments and nerves. AJR 2000;174:151–159.
4. Martinoli C, Bianchi S, Derchi L. Ultrasonography of peripheral nerves. Semin Ultrasound, CT MRI 2000;21(3):205–213.
5. Loewy J. Sonoanatomy of the median, ulnar and radial nerves. Can Assoc Radiol J 2002;53:33–38.
6. Fornage BD. Peripheral nerves of the extremities: Imaging with US. Radiology 1988;167:179–182.
7. Silvestri E, Marinoli C, Derchi LE et al. Echotexture of peripheral nerves: Correlation between US and histologic findings and criteria to differentiate tendons. Radiology 1995;197:291–296.
8. Hide I, Grainger A, Naisby G et al. Sonographic findings in the anterior interosseous nerve syndrome. J Clin Ultrasound 1999;27:459–464.
9. Martinoli C, Bianchi S, Pugliese F et al. Sonography of entrapment neuropathies in the upper limb (wrist excluded). J Clin Ultrasound 2004;32:438–450.

10. van Holsbeeck MT. Sonography of muscle. In: van Holsbeeck M, Introcaso JH, eds. Musculoskeletal Ultrasound, pp. 23–75. St. Louis: Mosby, 2001.
11. Fornage BD. The case for ultrasound of muscles and tendons. Semin Musculoskeletal Radiol 2000;4:375–391.
12. Bodnar, G, Harpf C, Meirer R et al. Ultrasonographic appearance of the supinator syndrome. J Ultrasound Med 2002;21:2189.

6

The Wrist and Hand

Lawrence Friedman

The development of high-resolution multifrequency linear probes has allowed ultrasound to accurately depict the normal anatomy and pathology of the wrist. The superficial nature of the anatomical structures of the wrist and hand is ideally suited to ultrasound, which offers high resolution and dynamic capabilities. The wrist is now the second commonest joint evaluated by ultrasound at our center. This is due to increasing rheumatology referral for the assessment of active inflammatory changes, synovitis and joint effusion, as well as the detection of early erosive changes. Ultrasound is inexpensive, portable, and equally effective in both the hospital and outpatient facility.

Clinical Indications

Common indications for ultrasound of the wrist include tendon assessment for tendinosis, tears and rupture, subluxation, and dislocation, as well as for tenosynovitis, including de Quervain's and intersection syndrome. Muscles are evaluated for posttraumatic tears, rupture, and hematomas, intramuscular masses, and hernias. It is important to recognize normal anatomical accessory muscles. The intrinsic scapholunate and lunotriquetral ligaments and triangular fibrocartilage complex can be initially screened by ultrasound for injury. The median nerve and other nerves are readily and accurately evaluated for entrapment syndromes and neuropathy, neuromas, and fibrolipomatous hamartoma.

The joints are gaining increasing prominence in the assessment of synovitis and joint effusions in rheumatology patients as well as patients with suspected infections. The bones of the wrist and hand are superficial and are amenable to assessment of cortical surfaces for erosions and occult fractures. Vascular structures are easily assessed for aneurysms. Ultrasound is often used as the initial investigation to assess soft tissue masses such as ganglia, giant cell tumors, hemangiomas, and nerve sheath tumors and in the assessment of internal structures: solid, cystic, with calcification or ossification, internal flow, and vascularity. Aspects of foreign body assessment include localization, number, depth, and inflammatory response.

Technical Equipment

The wrist and hand are best assessed using a high-resolution multifrequency linear 9- to 15-MHz transducer. We prefer to use the small, linear hockey stick probe, which is excellent for assessing superficial small structures. The use of new high-frequency probes and a liberal amount of gel has eliminated the need for a stand-off pad in most patients. The probe should always be positioned perpendicular to the anatomy being evaluated, particularly structures prone to anisotropy.

Anatomy

The surface anatomy will initially be reviewed followed by a comprehensive discussion with respect to the following:

- Osseous structures
- Compartments including muscles, tendons, fascia, and retinacula
- Pulleys
- The triangular fibrocartilage complex
- Ligaments

Surface Anatomy

Important palpable bony landmarks include the distal radial styloid and ulna styloid processes. The rounded head of the ulna lies proximal to the styloid process and is felt as a rounded prominence dorsally. Lister's tubercle, also known as the dorsal tubercle of the radius, is easily palpable as a small, bony prominence on the dorsal surface of the radius just proximal to the radiocarpal joint space, junction radial, and middle third of the wrist. This is a very useful starting point in the evaluation of the extensor compartments. The lunate bone lies just distal to the tubercle in the midline. The extensor pollicis longus tendon lies either within a groove on Lister's tubercle or on its ulnar aspect and can be felt moving on extension of the thumb. The anatomical snuff box is easily palpable as a depression on the lateral aspect of the wrist, with the radial styloid process and scaphoid forming the floor, and the extensor pollicis longus medially, and extensor pollicis brevis and abductor pollicis longus laterally. Pain in this location may be associated with a fracture involving the scaphoid bone. The first dorsal web space is an important landmark in the assessment of the ulnar collateral ligament of the thumb and Stener's lesion.

The pisiform bone lies between the two transverse creases on the volar and medial aspect of the wrist. Along the volar aspect of the wrist, one or two prominent creases are identified that are exaggerated with flexion. The proximal transverse crease on the volar wrist lies at the level of the wrist joint, and the distal crease lies at the proximal aspect of the flexor retinaculum (Figure 6.1). Apposition of the thumb and fifth finger will accentuate a plane between the thenar and hypothenar muscles. The median nerve is usually located between this plane and the wrist crease.

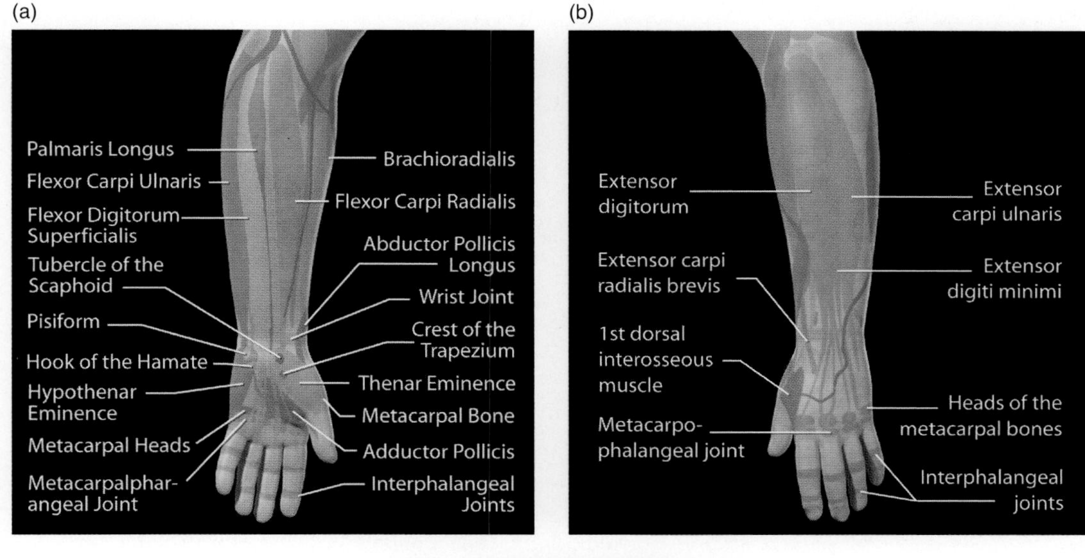

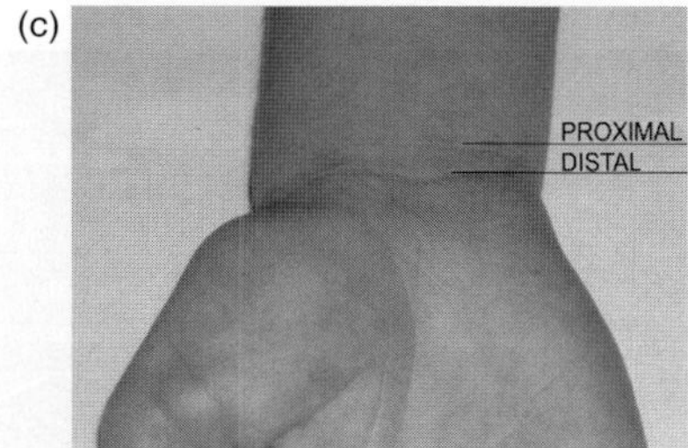

Figure 6.1. Surface anatomy of the arm and hand: **(a)** anterior, **(b)** posterior, and **(c)** lateral views. **(c)** The wrist in flexion shows proximal and distal creases.

The dorsal hoods are easily visible over the dorsal "knuckles," and a hood injury is usually clinically evident as the tendon subluxes or dislocates during flexion of the fingers. The proximal and distal interphalangeal joints are clearly visible as creases on the palmar aspect of the hand.

Bones

The bones of the wrist consist of the distal radius and ulna, the proximal carpal row (comprising the scaphoid, lunate, and triquetrum with pisiform), the distal carpal row (comprising the trapezium, trapezoid, capitate, and hamate), and the bases of the metacarpals. The osseous structures are divided into three major compartments as defined by arthrographic studies: the distal radioulnar (DRU) and the radiocarpal (RC) and mid-carpal (MC) (Figure 6.2).[1]

Lister's tubercle, located on the dorsal aspect of the distal radius, can be felt as a small bony protuberance and represents an important bony landmark in the evaluation of the extensor tendons and intrinsic ligaments of the wrist. The pisiform located proximally, the hook of hamate located distally on the volar and ulnar aspect of the wrist, the scaphoid tubercle located proximally, and the trapezium located distally on the volar and radial aspect of the wrist are important bony landmarks for locating the flexor retinaculum.[2]

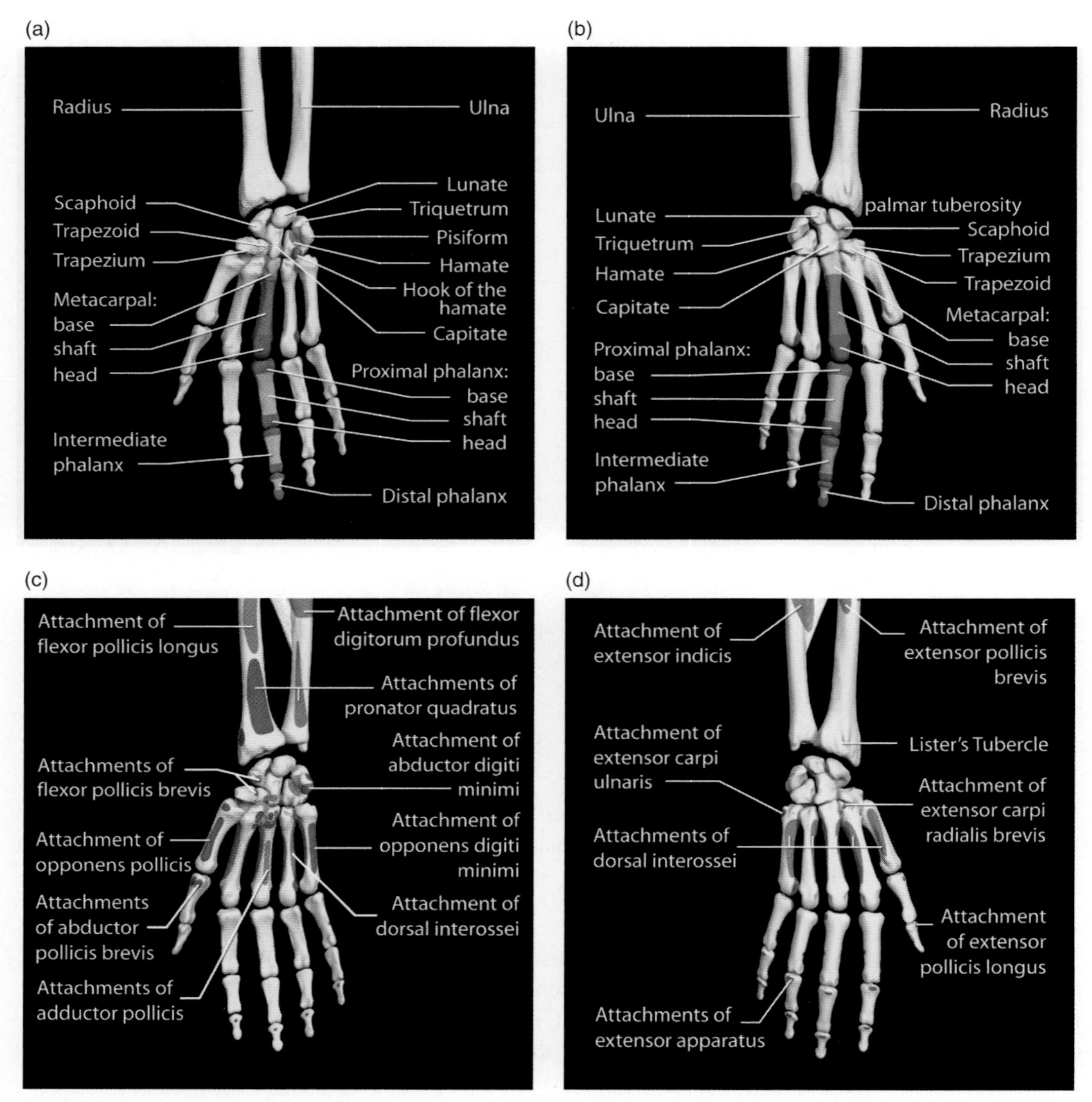

Figure 6.2. The important bony landmarks of the hand: (**a**) volar and (**b**) dorsal views; and muscle origin (red) and insertion (blue) points of the hand: (**c**) volar and (**d**) dorsal views.

Extensor Compartment Wrist

The extensor retinaculum is a broad, thickened band contained in the deep fascia of the forearm that runs obliquely across the extensor surface of the wrist joint, attaching proximally to the anterolateral border of the radius above the styloid process and lateral border of the pronator quadratus. It attaches to the pisiform and triquetral bones, but not to the ulna. The retinaculum functions as an anchor, restraining the extensor tendons of the forearm in all positions (Figure 6.3).

More distally, the extensor retinaculum divides into fibrous septa that pass to the bones of the forearm, dividing the extensor tunnel into six compart-

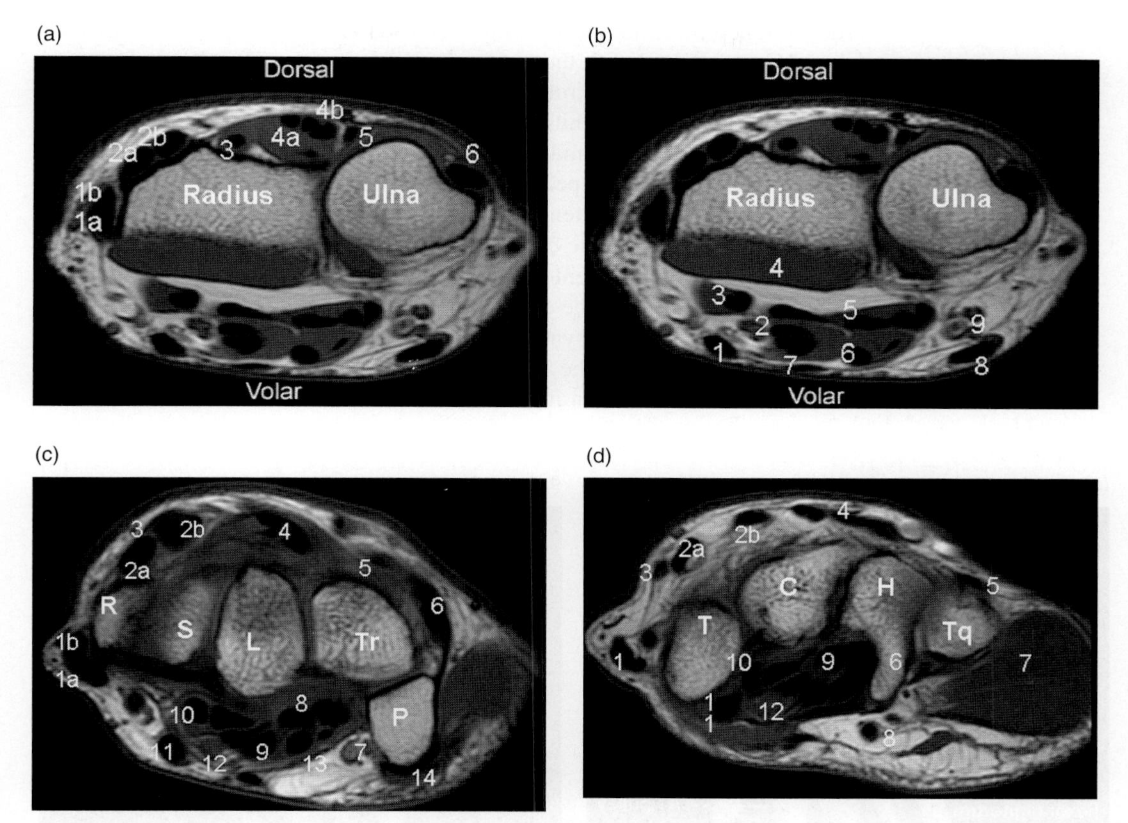

Figure 6.3. Axial T1-weighted MRI anatomy of the wrist. **(a)** Axial wrist extensor compartment tendons at the level of Lister's tubercle (LT): 1a–abductor pollicis longus, 1b–extensor pollicis brevis, 2a–extensor carpi radialis longus, 2b–extensor carpi radialis brevis, 3–extensor pollicis longus, 4a–extensor indicis, 4b–extensor digitorum, 5–extensor digiti minimi, 6–extensor carpi ulnaris. **(b)** Axial wrist flexor compartment tendons at the level of Lister's tubercle: 1–flexor carpi radialis, 2–median nerve, 3–flexor pollicis longus, 4–pronator quadratus muscle, 5–flexor digitorum profundus, 6–flexor digitorum superficialis, 7–palmaris longus, 8–flexor carpi ulnaris, 9–ulnar nerve. **(c)** Axial wrist at the level of the proximal carpal row: R, radius; S, scaphoid; L, lunate; Tr, triquetrum; P, pisiform. 1a–abductor pollicis longus, 1b–extensor pollicis brevis, 2a–extensor carpi radialis longus, 2b–extensor carpi radialis brevis, 3–extensor pollicis longus, 4–extensor indicis and digitorum, 5–extensor digiti minimi, 6–extensor carpi ulnaris, 7–ulnar nerve, 8–flexor digitorum profundus, 9–flexor digitorum superficialis, 10–flexor pollicis longus, 11–flexor carpi radialis, 12–median nerve, 13–flexor retinaculum, 14–flexor carpi ulnaris. **(d)** Axial wrist at the level of the hamate hook. T, trapezium; C, capitate; H, hamate; Tq, triquetrum. 1–abductor pollicis longus and extensor pollicis brevis, 2a–extensor carpi radialis longus, 2b–extensor carpi radialis brevis, 3–extensor pollicis longus, 4–extensor indicis and digitorum, 5–extensor digiti minimi, 6–hook of hamate, 7–hypothenar muscles, 8–ulnar nerve, 9–flexor digitorum superficialis and profundus, 10–flexor pollicis longus, 11–flexor carpi radialis, 12–median nerve.

ments (Figures 6.3a, 6.4e).[2–4] Compartment 1 is the most radial or lateral compartment. It lies over the lateral surface of the distal radius tip and contains the abductor pollicis longus and extensor pollicis brevis tendons, usually lying in separate synovial sheaths. The groove on the ulnar side of the radial tubercle (Lister's tubercle) contains the extensor pollicis longus tendon, compartment 3, invested with its own synovial sheath. Compartment 2 harbors the tendons on the radial aspect of Lister's tubercle, the extensor pollicis longus and brevis, with brevis closest to the tubercle. Each tendon is usually contained in its own synovial sheath. An easy way to remember the order of tendons within these compartments is to first recognize that Lister's tubercle is associated with the extensor pollicis longus. Then heading toward compartment 1, the order rotates between brevis and longus. On the radial side of the tubercle, we initially encounter the radial extensors and as we approach the line of the thumb, the pollicis tendons. Compartment 4 is located on the medial or ulnar aspect of the extensor pollicis longus in a shallow groove in which all four tendons of the common extensor tendon lie. The four tendons are in intimate contact over the extensor indicis tendon; all five tendons in this compartment are surrounded by a common synovial sheath. Compartment 5 lies over the distal radioulnar joint and is host to the extensor digiti minimi in its own synovial sheath. Compartment 6 is located in the groove near the base of the ulnar styloid through which the extensor carpi ulnaris passes, contained in its own synovial sheath.

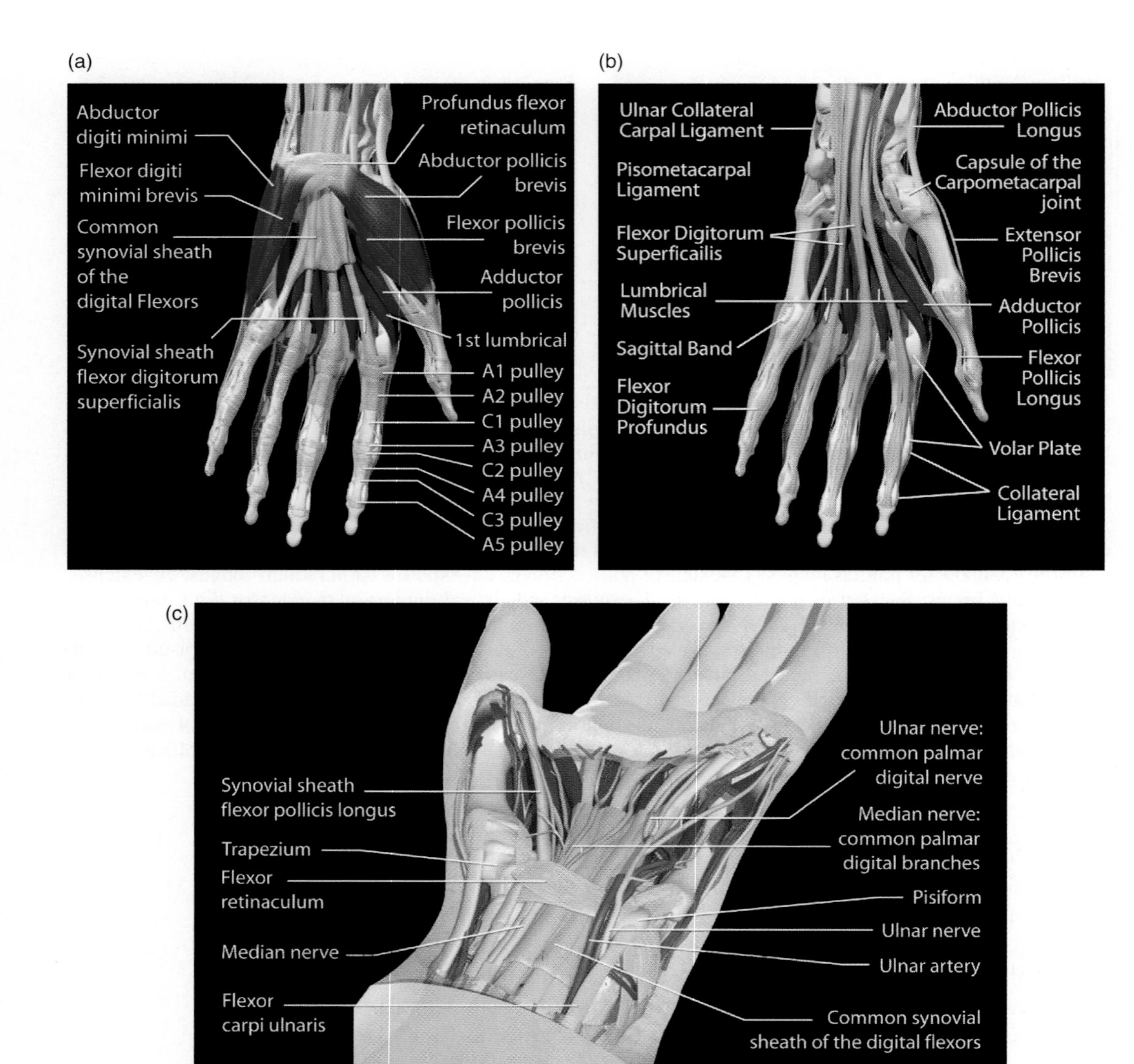

Figure 6.4. The muscles of the hand: **(a)** volar compartment demonstrating flexor sheaths, **(b)** volar compartment with retinaculum, thenar and hypothenar muscles, flexor retinaculum removed, **(c)** carpal tunnel,

(d)

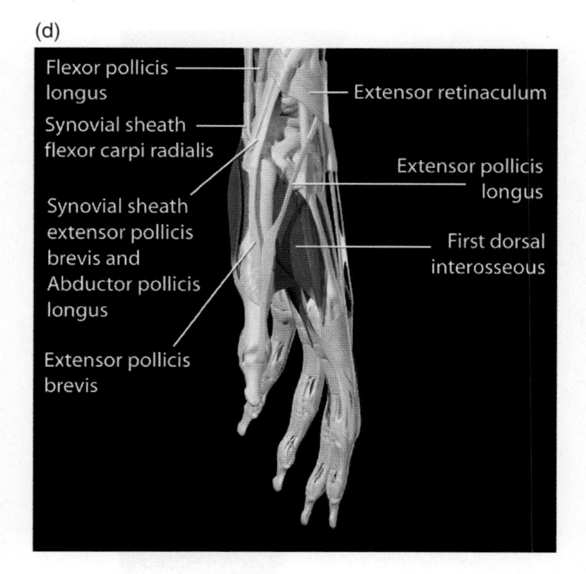

(e)

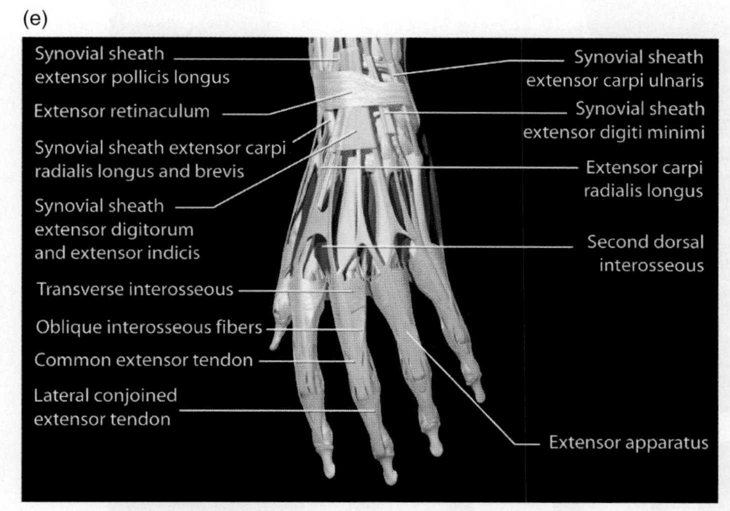

Figure 6.4. (*Continued*) **(d)** lateral demonstrating extensor compartment 1, and **(e)** dorsal view.

> **Insider Information 6.1**
> Lister's tubercle serves as the most useful bony landmark in assessing the extensor tendons (compartments 1–6) and dorsal instrinsic ligaments of the wrist.

Hands and Fingers

Distal to the extensor retinaculum, the extensors of the hand insert at the bases of their respective metacarpal bones. The superficial extensor tendons of the fingers extend over the dorsum of the hand to attach to the deep fascia and interconnect near the metacarpal heads by oblique fibrous bands (Figures 6.4e and 6.5c).

(a)

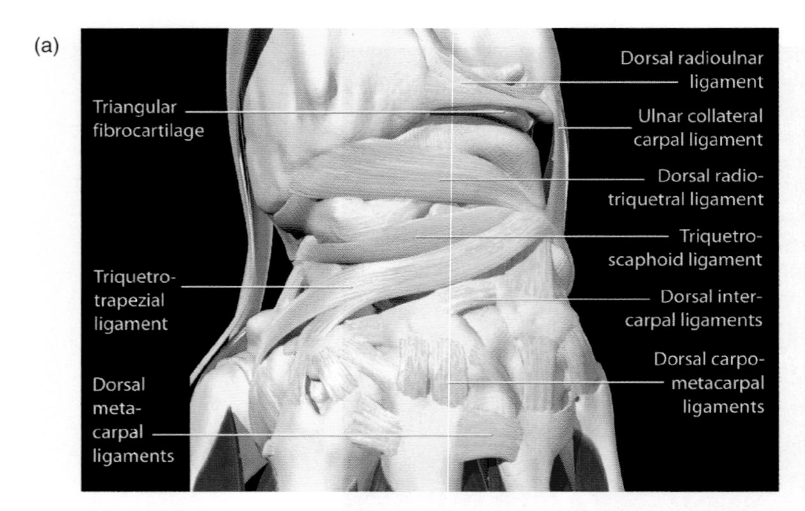

(b)

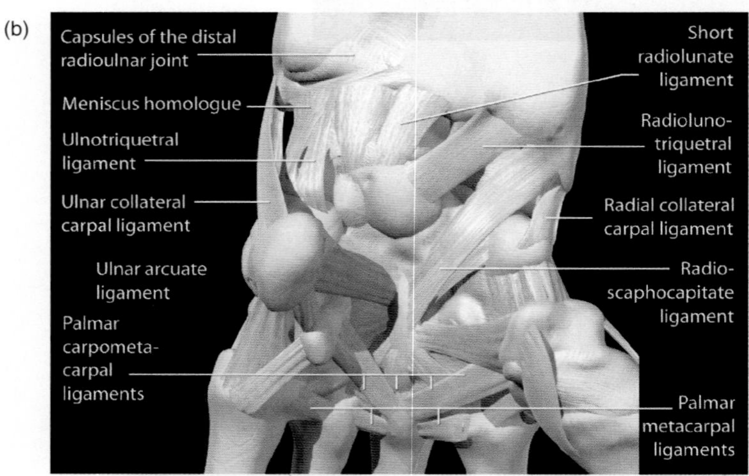

(c)

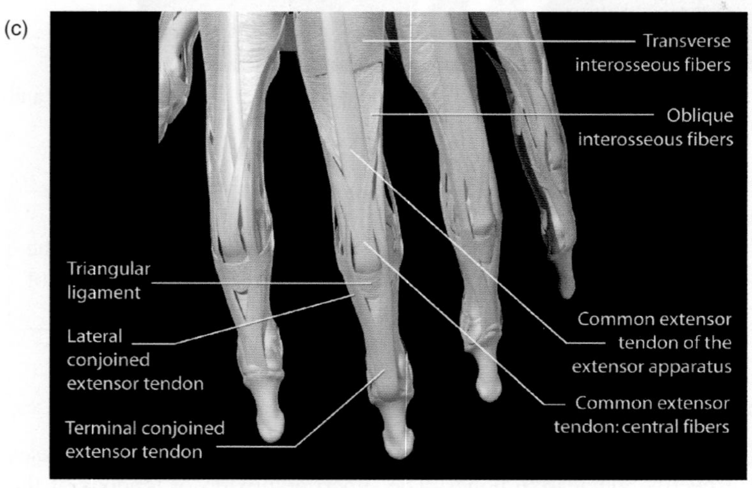

Figure 6.5. (**a**) Dorsal and (**b**) volar extrinsic ligaments of the hand and (**c**) the extensor hood.

The extensor tendons, excluding the thumb, have a characteristic insertion pattern.[2,3,5] Beyond the metacarpophalangeal joint most of the tendon is free and broadens out on the dorsal surface of the proximal phalanx and then divides into three slips. The central slip extends onto the base of the middle phalanx, while the two lateral slips pass around the middle slip (Figure 6.6a). Each receives a strong attachment from the tendons of the lumbrical and interosseous muscles, forming a broad extensor expansion. More proximally, the fibers from the interossei and lumbricals extend across the dorsum of the proximal phalanges to complete the extensor expansion. The connected interosseous tendons and slips of the common extensor expansion pass distally across the middle phalanx, join, and then insert together into the base of the distal phalanx.

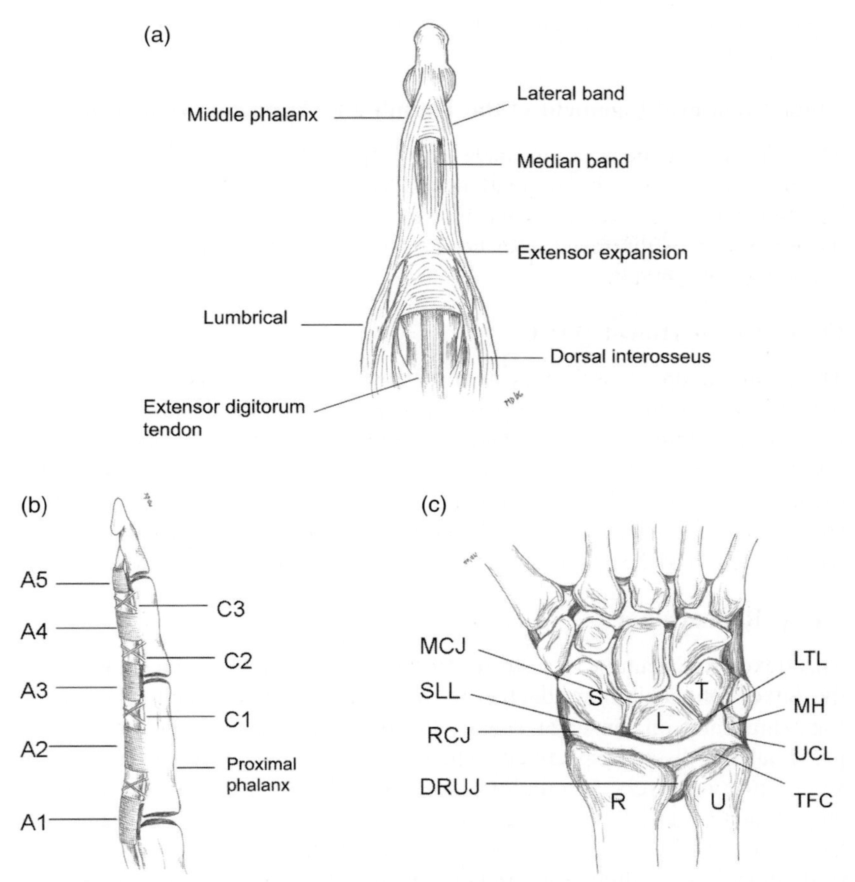

Figure 6.6. (**a**) Extensor expansion, (**b**) flexor tendon pulley system—-anular (A) and cruciate (C), and (**c**) coronal wrist joint compartments. DRUJ, distal radioulnar joint; RCJ, radiocarpal joint space; MCJ, midcarpal joint space; SLL, scapholunate ligament; LTL, lunotriquetral ligament; TFC, triangular fibrocartilage; UCL, ulnar collateral ligament; MH, meniscal homologue; S, scaphoid; L, lunate; T, triquetrum; R, radius; U, ulna.

Extensor Hood

The extensor hood is a triangular fibrous expansion on the dorsum of the proximal phalanx of each digit, with the base of the triangle wrapped around the dorsal and collateral aspects of the metacarpophalangeal joint.[4,5] A tendon of extensor digitorum (or extensor pollicis longus in the case of the thumb) joins with the central aspect of the expansion and is separated from the metacarpophalangeal joint by a small bursa. The interossei and lumbrical muscles attach to this expansion. This is further stabilized by links to the deep transverse metacarpal ligament. The end result is a movable hood that passes distally during dynamic flexion of the metacarpophalangeal joint.

Thumb

The extensor pollicis brevis and longus tendons insert separately into the proximal and distal phalanges. There is no extensor hood, but the extensor pollicis longus receives a fibrous expansion from both the abductor pollicis brevis and adductor pollicis to form the adductor aponeurosis.[2,3,5] This expansion functions as an anchor for the long extensor tendon on the dorsum of the thumb.

Ulnar Collateral Ligament of the Thumb and Adductor Aponeurosis

The adductor aponeurosis is made up of fibers from the adductor pollicis and abductor pollicis brevis tendons of the thumb.[2,3,5] The ulnar collateral ligament takes an oblique course inferior to the adductor aponeurosis from the ulnar side of the metacarpal head to the radial tubercle of the proximal phalanx of the thumb.

Flexor Compartment Wrist

The palmar aponeurosis is part of an extension of the degenerated tendon of palmaris longus and extends as part of the tendon from the distal border of the flexor retinaculum where it expands toward the bases of the fingers.[2–4] It then divides into four separate slips going to each finger. Each slip subsequently divides into two bands, inserting into the proximal phalanges, the flexor sheaths, and the deep transverse ligament. Dupuytren's contracture involves the contraction of the aponeurosis or slip resulting in a fixed flexion deformity.

Flexor Retinaculum

The flexor retinaculum is a strong fibrous flexor band. On the radial side, the flexor retinaculum is attached to the scaphoid tubercle and ridge of the trapezium, and on the ulnar side to the pisiform and hook of the hamate, proximal and distal, respectively. The radial aspect of the flexor retinaculum splits into two layers, forming a tunnel through which the tendon of flexor carpi radialis and its synovial sheath pass.[2,3] The muscles of the thenar and hypothenar eminences arise from the retinaculum. Several structures pass through the retinaculum. Superficially, the tendon of palmoris longus is fused to the midline of the retinaculum as it passes distally before expanding into the palmar aponeurosis. The ulnar aspect of the retinaculum joins the pisiform-hamate ligament. The flexor carpi ulnaris tendon lies separately within Guyon's canal adjacent to the ulnar nerve and medial to the ulnar artery (Figure 6.4c).

Carpal Flexor Tunnel

The deep bony concave surface of the wrist posteriorly and the flexor retinaculum anteriorly create a large passageway, through which the flexor tendons and median nerve traverse (Figures 6.2, 6.3, 6.4a–c).[2,6] The four superficial flexor tendons pass through in two rows with the middle and ring finger tendons lying anterior to the index and little finger tendons. The tendons of the flexor digitorum profundus, however, all lie in the same plane. The tendon to the index finger is separate, while the other three tendons are joined and split free only when they reach the palm.[2] All the superficial and deep flexor tendons are encased in a common synovial sheath. The median nerve enters the carpal tunnel intimately related to and deep to the flexor retinaculum and then runs alongside and anterior to the flexor tendons, covered by a fibrofatty layer. An important normal variant to be aware of is the presence of a persistent prominent median artery that is often accompanied by a bifid median nerve. It is essential to be aware of this anomaly if surgery is contemplated. The palmaris longus tendon lies just superficial to the median nerve outside the carpal tunnel. The tendon of flexor pollicis longus is surrounded by its own synovial sheath and passes through the radial side of the carpal tunnel.

Insider Information 6.2
The median nerve resembles an "ovary" closer to the radial aspect of the carpal tunnel and can be seen bouncing superficial to the flexor tendons during dynamic flexion and extension of the fingers.

Thenar Eminence

The thenar eminence is composed of three muscles that originate from the flexor retinaculum (Figure 6.4a).[2,3] The most radial, the abductor pollicis brevis, arises from the radial tubercle and flexor retinaculum and inserts into the radial side of the base and tendon of the extensor pollicis longus. Its main actions include abduction of the thumb, abduction of the proximal phalanx at the metacarpal phalangeal joint, and rotation of the proximal phalanx. The flexor pollicis brevis arises from the flexor retinaculum along the ulnar side of the abductor pollicis brevis and inserts into the radial sesamoid of the thumb and radial border of the proximal phalanx. Its action is to flex the proximal phalanx and draw the thumb across the palm. The opponens pollicis deep to the above two muscles also arises from the flexor retinaculum and inserts along the whole radial border of the first metacarpal (thumb). Its action is to oppose the thumb. All three muscles are supplied by the median nerve.

Hypothenar Eminence

The hypothenar eminence is also composed of three muscles (Figure 6.3a).[2,3] The abductor digiti minimi is the most ulnar of the group and arises from the pisiform bone and flexor retinaculum inserting into the ulnar side of the base of the proximal phalanx and extensor expansion. Its action is to abduct the little finger toward the ulnar side away from the midline of the palmar surface. The flexor digiti minimi arises from the flexor retinaculum and inserts into the base of the proximal phalanx. The opponens digiti minimi arises from the flexor retinaculum and hook of the hamate and inserts into the ulnar border of the fifth metacarpal bone. All three muscles help to cup the palm and are supplied by the ulnar nerve.

Long Flexor Tendons and Lumbrical Muscles

In the palm the flexor tendons are superficial to the flexor profundus digitorum.[2,3] The four lumbricals arise from each of the four profundus tendons. They then proceed along the radial side of the metacarpophalangeal joint. On the palmar surface of the deep transverse ligament of the palm, each develops a tendon that runs in a fibrous canal to reach the extensor expansion on the dorsum of the first phalanx. Usually the ulnar lumbricals are supplied by the ulnar nerve and the two radial lumbricles by the median nerve.

Adductor Pollicis Muscle

The adductor pollicis muscle lies deep in the palm in contact with the metacarpals and interossei (Figure 6.4a).[2,3] The transverse head arises from the whole length of the palmar border of the third metacarpal and then extends, fan shaped, to the ulnar sesamoid of the thumb as well as the ulnar side of the base of the proximal phalanx and tendons of the extensor pollicis longus. The oblique head originates from the bases of the second and third metacarpals, the trapezoid and capitate, by a crescentic origin that includes the insertion of the flexor carpi radialis. This muscle is supplied by the ulnar nerve, and its action is to approximate the thumb to the index finger.

Interosseous Muscles

Interosseous muscles include two groups: the palmar and dorsal interossei.[2,3] The palmar interosseous muscles are smaller and arise from only one metacarpal, while the dorsal muscles are larger and arise from both metacarpals in the space in which they lie. The palmar adduct and dorsal abduct the fingers. The thumb and middle fingers have no palmar interossei, and the thumb and little finger have no dorsal interossei.

Flexor Fibrous Sheaths

From the metacarpal heads to the distal phalanges, all five digits are provided with a strong unyielding fibrous sheath in which the flexor tendons lie.[2,3] In the thumb, the fibrous sheath is occupied only by the flexor pollicis longus tendon, whereas in the other four fingers the sheaths are occupied by the tendons of the superficial and deep flexors. The superficial flexors split to spiral around the deep flexors within the sheath. The proximal ends of the fibrous sheaths of the fingers receive the insertions of the four slips of the palmar aponeurosis. The sheaths are strong and dense over the phalanges and are weak and lax over the joints.

Synovial Flexor Sheaths

The flexor sheath surrounding the flexor pollicis longus extends from above the flexor retinaculum to the insertion of the tendon into the terminal phalanx of the thumb. The common sheath surrounding the superficial and deep flexors starts a short distance proximal to the wrist and extends down into the palm. In the little finger it extends the whole length to the insertion at the terminal phalanx. In the remaining three fingers, which include the index, middle, and ring fingers, the common flexor sheath ends just distal to the flexor retinaculum. At this point, a separate synovial sheath lines the fibrous flexor sheath over the phalanges.[2,3] As a result, an area of bare tendon exists for these three fingers where the lumbrical muscles arise. The fourth lumbrical obliterates the synovial sheath along its origin from the tendon to little finger.

Digital Attachments of Flexor Tendons

In the palm, the superficialis tendon remains superficial to the profundus tendon until it divides at the level of the proximal third of the proximal phalanx.[2,3,5] Here the two slips of the superficialis tendon pass around the profundus tendon, reunite deep to the profundus tendon, and then attach at a site in the proximal half of the middle phalanx. The profundus tendon passes through the divided superficialis tendon to insert at the base of the distal phalanx (Figure 6.4b).

Finger Flexor Tendon Pulley System

The flexor synovial sheath extends from the neck of the metacarpal to the distal interphalangeal joint. A series of retinacular structures, which thicken the sheath at five specific points, form the annular pulley system (pulleys A1-A5) (Figures 6.4a, 6.6b).[5,7] Additional fibers that crisscross between the annular pulleys create the cruciate pulley system (pulleys C1-C3). These pulleys combine to prevent excursion of the flexor tendons from the metacarpophalangeal and interphalangeal joints during finger flexion.

The A1 pulley begins in the region of the volar plate of the metacarpophalangeal joint and extends to the level of the base of the proximal phalanx. The A2 pulley arises from the volar aspect of the proximal part of the proximal phalanx and extends to the junction of the middle and distal thirds of the proximal phalanx. The superficialis tendon divides beneath this pulley. The A3 pulley extends for a short distance over the region of the proximal interphalangeal joint. The A4 pulley is in the midportion of the middle phalanx and the A5 pulley is in the region of the distal interphalangeal joint.

Intrinsic Interosseous Ligaments

These ligaments are important in maintaining a normal functional and anatomical relationship to the proximal carpal row. They connect the bones of the proximal carpal row by thick dorsal and volar components with a thinner central, less important, membranous portion.

Scapholunate Ligament

The scapholunate ligament (SL) has three components consisting of dorsal, mid, and volar portions. The dorsal component of the SL is considered to be the most important in maintaining stability (Figure 6.6c).[1,4] The dorsal fibers are oriented transversally across the joint, where they form a thick bundle. The membranous fibers course obliquely and peripherally from the scaphoid to the lunate. These fibers attach to bone and articular cartilage. The volar fibers course obliquely between the volar portion of the lunate and scaphoid.

Lunotriquetral Ligament

The lunotriquetral ligament (LT) a thin, horseshoe-shaped structure (Figure 6.6b).[1] Like the SL ligament, this smaller ligament also has three components. The volar and dorsal portions attach directly to bone, while the midportion attaches to the hyaline articular cartilage of the joint.

Triangular Fibrocartilage Complex

The triangular fibrocartilage complex (TFCC) is composed of the dorsal and volar radioulnar ligaments, articular disc or triangular fibrocartilage (TFC), ulnolunate ligament, ulnotriquetral ligament, ulnar collateral ligament, and meniscus homologue.[1,8] It is classified as part of the extrinsic carpal ligament group.[8] The dorsal and volar radioulnar ligaments reinforce the peripheral portion of the articular disc, which is thinned centrally and thickened peripherally. The TFC has a variable appearance and attaches to the sigmoid notch of the radius and to the ulnar styloid process (Figure 6.6c). The ulnolunate ligament extends from the volar radioulnar ligament to the volar aspect of the lunate; the ulnotriquetral ligament originates ulnar to the ulnolunate ligament and attaches to the volar aspect of the triquetrum. The ulnar collateral ligament represents a thickening of the capsule that extends from the ulnar styloid process to the triquetrum and pisiform. The meniscus homologue does not represent a distinct structure but is composed of connective tissue that forms distal to the ulnar aspect of the TFC, between the dorsal radioulnar ligament and the radial aspect of the ECU tendon. It is separated from the TFC by an opening to the prestyloid recess.

Extrinsic Interosseous Ligaments

The carpal ligaments play an important part in the biomechanics of the wrist and may vary from subject to subject. The dorsal ligaments include the dorsal radiotriquetral ligament, dorsal ulnotriquetral ligament, dorsal scaphotriquetral ligament, and radial and ulnar collateral ligaments (Figure 6.5a). The volar or palmar ligaments include the radioscaphocapitate ligament, radiolunotriquetral ligament, radioscapholunate ligament, ulnolunate ligament, palmar ulnotriquetral ligament, and palmar scaphotriquetral ligament (Figure 6.5b).

Technique

The patient's examination is usually tailored to the site of the suspected abnormality. A systematic approach will be illustrated to include dorsal, volar, medial, and lateral examination of the wrist, followed by dedicated evaluation of the hand and fingers.[9,10]

Wrist

Dorsal Approach

The dorsal approach is used to examine the extensor tendons, the intrinsic scapholunate and lunotriquetral ligaments, and the dorsal extrinsic ligaments. The muscles of the hand and wrist are listed in Table 6.1. The patient is usually positioned comfortably in a chair facing the sonologist with the elbow flexed, arm in pronation, and wrist in a neutral position or slightly flexed, resting on a roll of towel or sponge. An overview of the wrist position for ultrasound evaluation is provided in Table 6.2.

Table 6.1. Muscles of the Wrist and Hand.

Muscle	Origin	Insertion	Main action
Abductor pollicis longus	Middle one-third of the posterior surface of the radius, interosseous membrane, midportion of the posterolateral ulna	Radial side of the base of the first metacarpal	Abducts and extends the thumb at the carpometacarpal joint
Abductor pollicis brevis	Flexor retinaculum, scaphoid, trapezium	Proximal phalanx thumb	Abducts the thumb
Adductor pollicis	Oblique head: capitate and base of the second and third metacarpals Transverse head: shaft of the third metacarpal	Base of the proximal phalanx thumb	Adducts the thumb
Extensor pollicis longus	Interosseous membrane and middle part of the posterolateral surface of the ulna	Base of the distal phalanx of the thumb	Extends the thumb at the interphalangeal joint
Extensor pollicis brevis	Interosseous membrane and the posterior surface of the distal radius	Base of the proximal phalanx of the thumb	Extends the thumb at the metacarpophalangeal joint
Extensor indicis	Interosseous membrane and the posterolateral surface of the distal ulna	Tendon joins the tendon of extensor digitorum to the second digit; both tendons insert into the extensor expansion	Extension of the index finger

Flexor digiti minimi brevis	Hook of hamate and flexor retinaculum	Proximal phalanx of the fifth digit	Flexes the carpometacarpal and metacarpophalangeal joints of the fifth digit
Flexor pollicis brevis	Flexor retinaculum, trapezium	Proximal phalanx of the first digit	Flexes the carpometacarpal and metacarpophalangeal joints of the thumb
Flexor pollicis longus	Anterior surface of the radius and interosseous membrane	Base of the distal phalanx of the thumb	Flexes the metacarpal and interphalangeal joints of the thumb
Dorsal interosseous muscles hand	Four muscles each arising from two adjacent metacarpal heads	Base of the proximal phalanx and the extensor expansion on the lateral side of the second digit, lateral and medial sides of the third digit, and medial side of the fourth digit	Flex the metacarpophalangeal joints, extend the proximal and distal interphalangeal joints of digits 2–4, abduct digits 2–4
Palmar interosseous muscles hand	Three muscles arising from the palmar surface of the shafts of metacarpals 2, 4, and 5	Base of the proximal phalanx and extensor expansion of the medial side of digit 2 and lateral side of digits 4 and 5	Flexes the metacarpophalangeal and extends the proximal and distal interphalangeal joints and adducts digits 2, 4, and 5 toward the midline of the third digit
Palmaris brevis	Fascia overlying the hypothenar eminence, transverse carpal ligament	Skin of the palm near the ulnar border of the hand	Draws the skin of the ulnar side of the hand toward the center of the palm
Lumbrical	Flexor digitorum profundus tendons of digits 2–5	Extensor expansion on the radial side of the proximal phalanx of digits 2–5	Flex the metacarpophalangeal joints, extend the proximal and distal interphalangeal joints of digits 2–5
Opponens digiti minimi	Hook of hamate and flexor retinaculum	Shaft of the fifth metacarpal	Opposes the fifth finger, i.e., draws the little finger forward

Table 6.2. Position for Ultrasound Evaluation of Muscles.

Muscle	Position examined
Abductor pollicis longus	Wrist in neutral position using radial approach
Extensor pollicis brevis	
Abductor pollicis brevis	
Adductor pollicis	Dorsal approach using oblique angle between bases of the first and second metacarpals with thumb extended
Extensor pollicis longus	Compartment 3: Dorsal approach on the ulnar side of Lister's tubercle
Extensor indicis	Compartment 4: Dorsal approach with common extensor tendons; move index finger to isolate the tendon
Flexor digiti minimi brevis	Volar approach with the hypothenar component of the hand
Flexor pollicis brevis	Volar approach with the thenar component of the hand
Flexor pollicis longus	Volar approach at the level of the carpal tunnel
Dorsal interosseous muscles of the hand	Dorsal approach at the level of the metacarpal heads
Palmar interosseous muscles of the hand	Volar approach at the level of the metacarpal shafts
Palmaris brevis	Volar approach at the medial aspect of the palm
Lumbrical	Volar approach at the level of the metacarpal shafts
Opponens digiti minimi	Volar approach at the hypothenar compartment of the hand

Extensor Tendons

The examination should begin at Lister's tubercle, the most useful bony landmark. Once located, the tendons on the radial aspect of the tubercle represent extensor carpi radialis brevis closer to the tubercle and extensor carpi radialis longus closest to the thumb, compartment 2 (Figure 6.7a and b). The position of the transducer continues in a radial direction and moves to the radial aspect of the distal wrist midway between the dorsal and volar aspect to identify the extensor pollicis brevis and the abductor pollicis longus, respectively (Figure 6.7c).

The transducer is then repositioned over Lister's tubercle. The extensor pollicis longus tendon is on the immediate ulnar aspect of the tubercle and comprises compartment 3 (Figure 6.7d). Confirmation that the correct tendon had being identified can be determined by dynamically abducting the thumb and seeing the tendon move in unison. Continuing in an ulnar direction, the common extensor complex, including the extensor indicis, is visualized (compartment 4) (Figure 6.8a).

The extensor indicis, compartment 5, lies just medial to compartment 4 (Figures 6.7a and 6.8b). This tendon can be confirmed by dynamically extending the fifth finger. Finally, the transducer is positioned along the ulnar aspect midway between the dorsal and volar aspects of the wrist to view the extensor carpi ulnaris, compartment 6. Dynamic scanning is necessary at this point to exclude subluxation of this tendon (Figures 6.7a and 6.9a). When

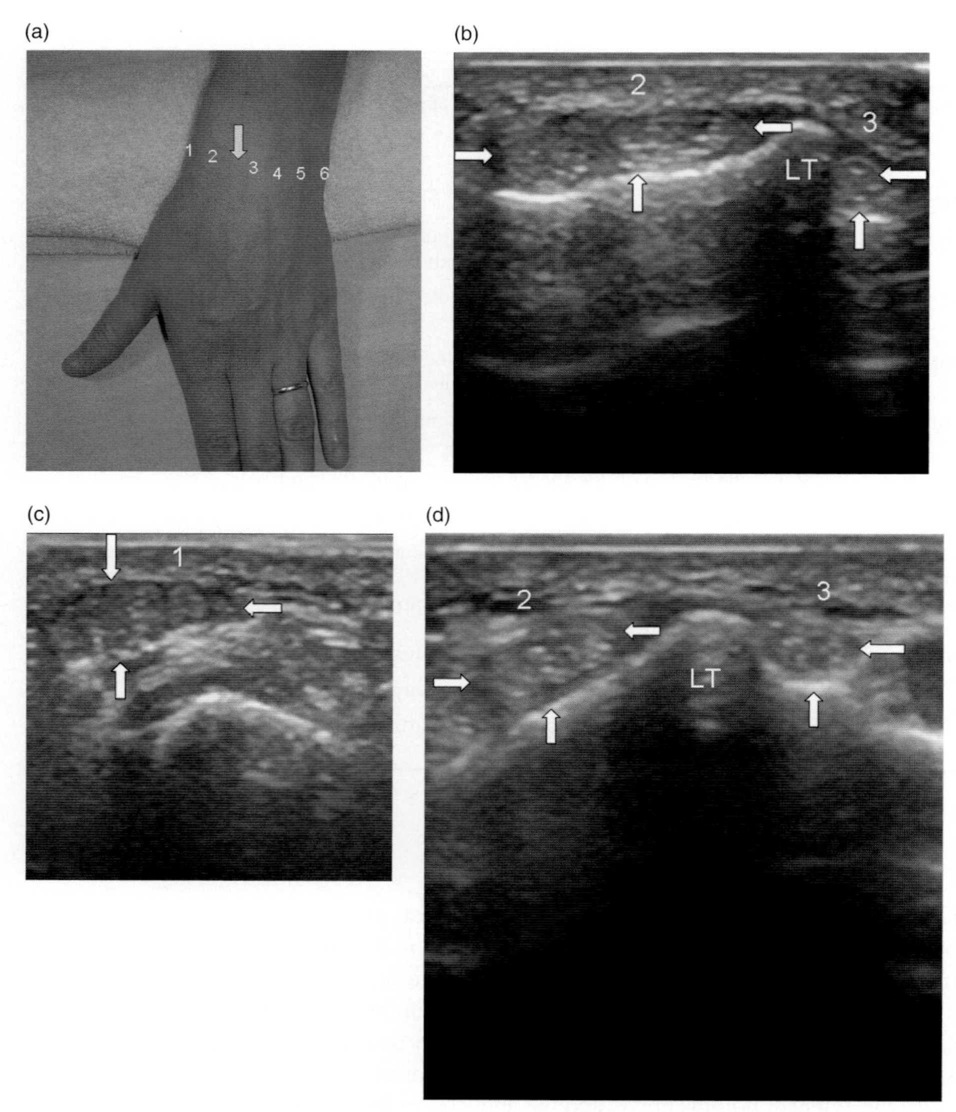

Figure 6.7. **(a)** Probe position for compartments 1 to 6. **(b)** Axial image of the wrist showing compartment 2 on the radial side of Lister's tubercle (LT) and compartment 3 on the ulna aspect (arrows). **(c)** Axial ultrasound image showing compartment 1. **(d)** Axial image showing compartment 3 on the ulna aspect of Lister's tubercle (LT) and compartment 2 on the ulna aspect.

evaluating each compartment, the probe should be rotated to view the tendons in both the short and long axis (Figure 6.9b).

Ligaments

Intrinsic Ligaments

The patient remains in the same position as described for the extensor tendons. The intrinsic SL and LT ligaments are easier to visualize on the dorsal aspect (Figure 6.10a). Unlike magnetic resonance imaging (MRI), the mid and volar aspect of the ligaments are incompletely seen on the ultra-

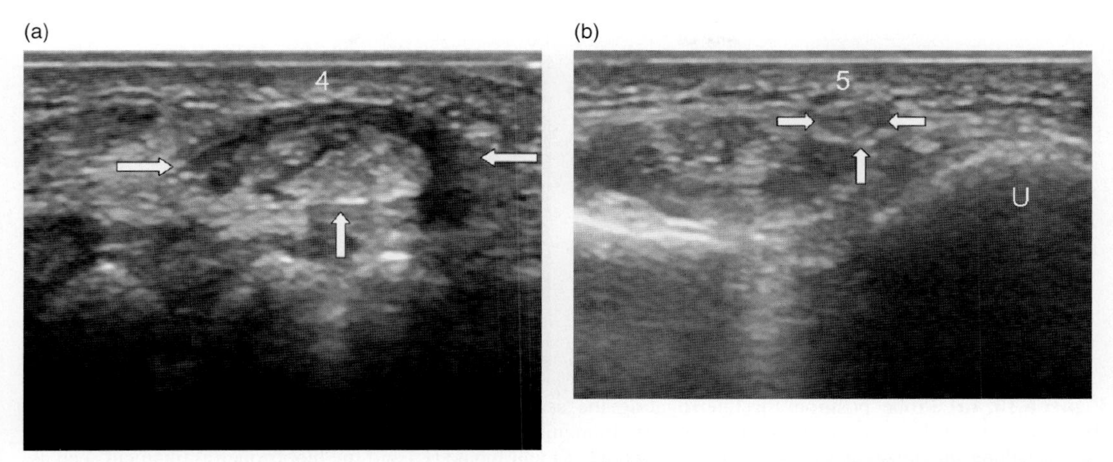

Figure 6.8. (**a**) Axial image showing compartment 4 (arrows). (**b**) Axial image showing compartment 5 (arrows). Distal ulna (U).

sound. The examination should begin by locating Lister's tubercle in the transverse plane[11] and then slowly moving distally until the SL ligament is visualized as an echogenic, well-defined triangle between the scaphoid and lunate (Figure 6.10b).[12] The ligament should be visualized in the neutral position or in slight extension. If extreme flexion is used, the ligament may appear hypoechoic, resulting in a false-positive disruption. Visualization of the ligament too far proximally can also give a false-positive result. Careful comparison with the opposite side is mandatory. At this point, the scaphoid should be assessed in both the short and long axis to exclude any occult fracture in symptomatic patients. The LT ligament is seen by moving the probe transversely toward the triquetrum until the echogenic ligament is identified between the lunate and triquetrum (Figure 6.10).

Extrinsic Dorsal Carpal Ligaments

These ligaments are visualized by using bony landmarks.[13] The patient is positioned as before but with the wrist in varying degrees of hyperflexion. After locating Lister's tubercle, the transducer is moved distally in the transverse plane

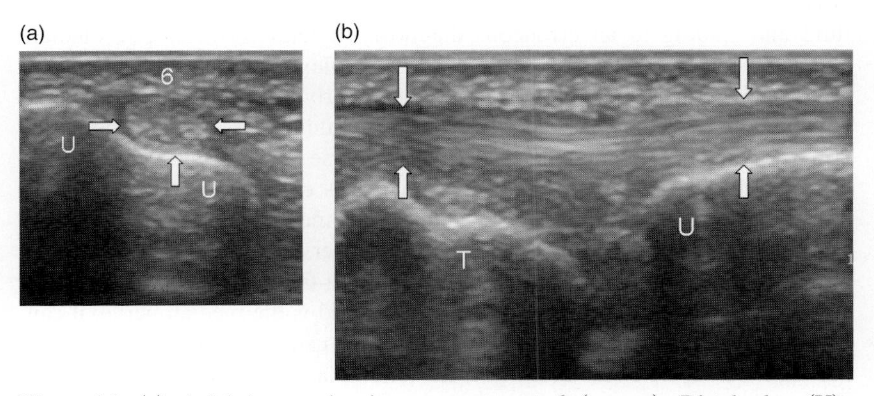

Figure 6.9. (**a**) Axial image showing compartment 6 (arrows). Distal ulna (U). (**b**) Sagittal image showing compartment 6 (arrows). Distal ulna (U). Triquetrum (T).

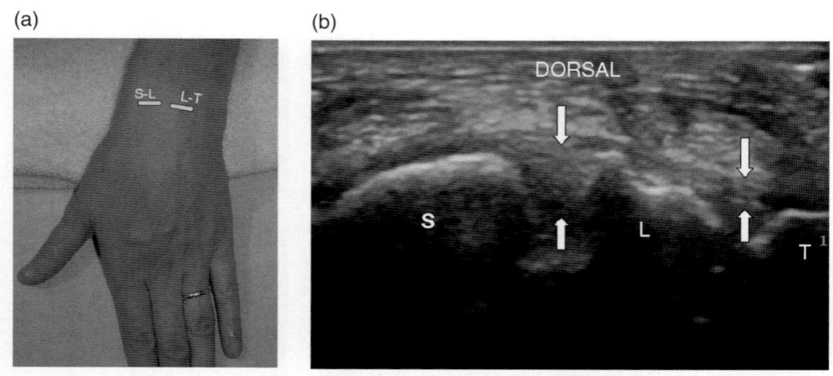

Figure 6.10. (**a**) Probe position for interrogating the scapholunate (SL) and lunotriquetral ligaments (LT). (**b**) Axial scan of the wrist showing the echogenic triangular appearance of the scapholunate ligament (SL) with the base along the dorsal aspect between the scaphoid (S) and lunate (L) and the lunotriquetral ligament seen as a linear band between the lunate (L) and triquetrum (T).

until the radial styloid is located. At this point, the transducer is angled obliquely along a plane parallel to the dorsal radiotriquetral ligament (Figure 6.11a and b). The probe is then shifted in an ulnar direction to locate the scaphoid and angled more parallel to assess the dorsal scaphotriquetral ligament (Figure 6.11a and c). The dorsal ulna triquetral ligament is shown by locating the probe in the long axis between the distal ulna and triquetrum (Figure 6.11d).

Volar Approach

The volar approach is used to evaluate the flexor tendons, median nerve and carpal tunnel, Guyon's canal and ulnar nerve,[9,10] and the volar SL[4,12] and volar extrinsic ligaments.[13] The patient is seated in a comfortable position facing the sonologist with the elbow flexed, forearm supinated, and wrist resting on a rolled up towel in mild hyperextension (Figure 6.12a.). The examination should be conducted in both the transverse and longitudinal planes.

Flexor Tendons and Carpal Tunnel

It is important once again to emphasize that the transducer should be perpendicular to the tendons, especially in the transverse plane, as the anisotropic effect will cause the tendons to appear hypoechoic, simulating synovial fluid and leading to an erroneous diagnosis of tenosynovitis. The median nerve is located superficial to the echogenic flexor tendons, and its size, shape, echogenicity, and relationship to the underlying tendons and overlying retinaculum should be noted.[6] The nerve should be assessed in both the transverse and longitudinal planes. In the transverse plane, the nerve resembles an "ovary" due to its multiple fascicles and it is closer to the radial half of the wrist (Figure 6.12b and c). Dynamic movement, including flexing and extending the fingers, shows that the median nerve is less mobile than the adjacent tendons and can be seen "bouncing" on the tendons below. If there is still doubt as to whether the structure identified is the median nerve, it can be traced proximally into the forearm where it can be seen emerging from between the superficialis and profundus tendon layers.

To further aid in the diagnosis of carpal tunnel syndrome, three quantitative measures are usually advocated. These include the circumference of the median nerve, maximum flattening ratio, and palmar displacement of the flexor

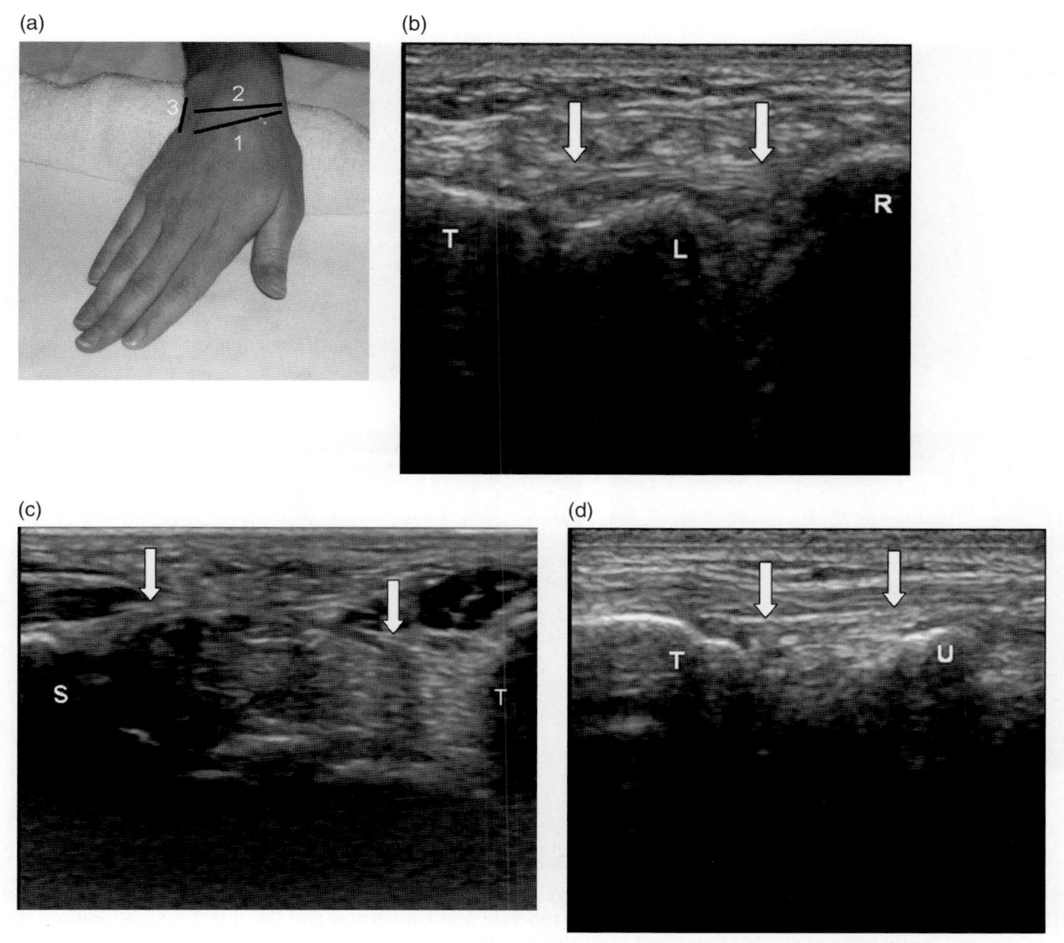

Figure 6.11. Dorsal extrinsic ligaments. **(a)** Probe position for evaluating the (1) radiotriquetral, (2) scaphotriquetral, and (3) dorsal ulnotriquetral ligaments with corresponding ultrasound images showing the dorsal extrinsic ligaments: **(b)** dorsal radiotriquetral, **(c)** dorsal scaphotriquetral, and **(d)** dorsal ulnotriquetral (arrows). Radius (R), scaphoid (S), lunate (L), triquetrum (T), and ulna (U).

retinaculum.[6] The circumference of the median nerve can be measured at the proximal and distal carpal tunnel in the transverse plane. The proximal carpal tunnel is defined in the transverse plane by the scaphoid tubercle and pisiform (Figure 6.12b) and the distal carpal tunnel is defined by the trapezium and the hook of hamate (Figure 6.12c). The mean cross-sectional area of the median nerve is usually obtained at the proximal carpal tunnel and should be no more than 10 mm.[6] The maximum flattening ratio of the nerve (the ratio of the maximum transverse diameter to its anteroposterior diameter) is best obtained in the transverse plane at the level of the hamate. This is at the level of the distal carpal tunnel and reflects the maximum flattening and constriction of the nerve between the flexor tendons and the transverse carpal ligament. A normal ratio should be less than 3.[6] A bifid median nerve, a normal variant usually accompanied by a persistent median artery, will give false-positive results.[4] The sonologist should be aware of this anomaly. The palmar displacement of the flexor retinaculum is measured by first drawing a line between the trapezium and hamate in

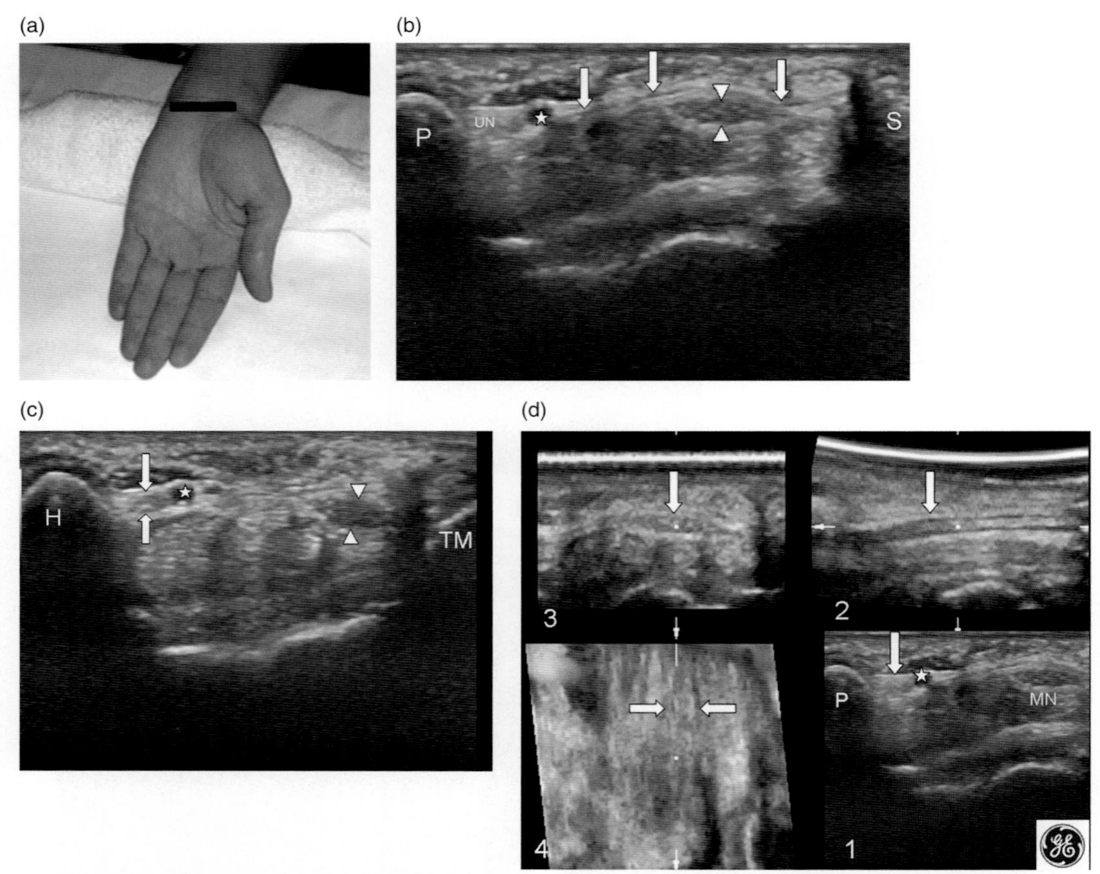

Figure 6.12. **(a)** Probe position for carpal tunnel. Bony landmarks should be used to locate the proximal tunnel defined in the transverse plane between the scaphoid tubercle and triquetrum and the distal tunnel between the trapezium and hook of hamate. **(b)** Axial image of the proximal carpal tunnel in the transverse plane between the scaphoid (S) and pisiform (P) showing the fascicular pattern of the median nerve resembling an "ovary" closer to the scaphoid (arrowheads) beneath the flexor retinaculum (arrows). Ulnar artery (asterisk). Ulnar nerve (UN). **(c)** Axial image of the distal carpal tunnel in the transverse plane between the trapezium (TM) and hamate (H) showing the median nerve (arrowheads) and ulnar nerve in Guyon's canal (arrows). Ulnar artery (asterisk). **(d)** Axial image acquired with 3-D ultrasound transducer demonstrating the ulnar nerve (arrow) in Guyon's canal adjacent to the pisiform (P) and medial to the ulnar artery (asterisk). Note the position of the median nerve (MN). Reformatted images in sagittal 2, axial 3, and coronal planes 4.

the transverse plane and then proceeding to measure the distance perpendicular to this line to the center of the flexor retinaculum. The normal palmar displacement should not exceed 4.0 mm.[6]

Insider Information 6.3

The most useful measurement of the median nerve remains the cross-sectional diameter. The cross-sectional measurement of the median nerve should not exceed 10 mm^2 at the proximal carpal tunnel. A bifid median nerve cannot be accurately assessed.

Guyon's Canal

The ulnar artery and nerve in Guyon's canal should be visualized in both the transverse and longitudinal planes (Figure 6.12c and d). The bony landmarks include the pisiform proximally and hook of hamate distally. It is easiest to first locate the ulnar artery and then proceed to locate the nerve.

Volar Intrinsic Ligaments

The palmar intrinsic scapholunate and lunotriquetral ligaments can be investigated by positioning the wrist palm up in hyperextension.[13] The scaphoid is then located in the long axis, at which point the transducer is swiveled 90° into the transverse plane, moving in an ulnar or medial direction to locate the scapholunate ligament. Continuing in a more ulnar direction, the lunotriquetral ligament is identified.

> **Insider Information 6.4**
> The SL ligament should be examined in a neutral position or slight extension, not in flexion, which can give false-positive results.

Volar Extrinsic Ligaments

The volar extrinsic ligaments are best defined by using bony landmarks.[13] The distal radius and scaphoid are first located in the long axis, and then the transducer is rotated in a slightly oblique direction to identify the capitate and radioscaphocapitate ligament (Figure 6.13a and c). The probe can then be rotated in a more horizontal direction to identify the radiolunotriquetral ligament, again using the appropriate bony landmarks (Figure 6.13a and d). To identify the radioscapholunate, ulnolunate, and ulnotriquetral ligaments, the patient's wrist is placed in hyperextension. The transducer is initially positioned at the ulnocarpal joint and moved slowly from medial (ulna) to lateral (radial) to visualize in succession the ulnotriquetral (Figure 6.13a and e), the ulnolunate, and the scaphotriquetral ligaments (Figure 6.13b and f). The triquetral and lunate bones are useful landmarks in identifying the ulnotriquetral and ulnolunate ligaments.

Volar-Ulnar

The structures best visualized along the ulnar aspect include the triangular fibrocartilage (TFC) and extensor carpi ulnaris, compartment 6, previously discussed under the dorsal extensor tendons.

Triangular Fibrocartilage Complex

The patient is positioned as before, sitting comfortably and facing the examiner with elbow flexed, forearm in pronation, and wrist in mild radial deviation. The extensor carpi ulnaris (ECU) tendon is used as an acoustic window.[14] The linear array multifrequency hockey stick 9- to 12-MHz probe is preferred, but if more penetration is required to identify the radial tip of the articular disc, the larger linear array 7- to 13-MHz probe may be necessary. The gain should be increased until the attachment of the tip to the radius is clearly visible.

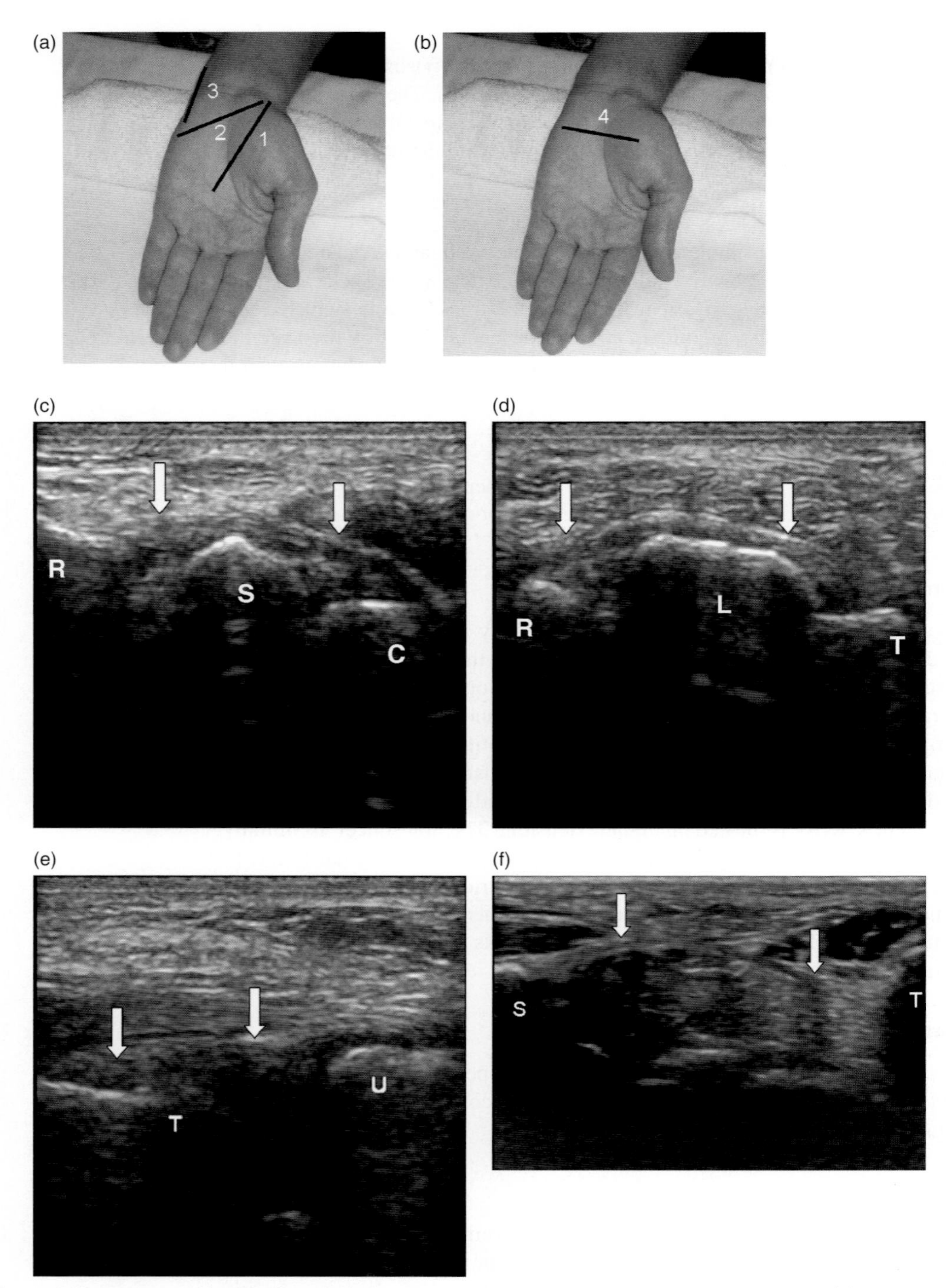

Figure 6.13. Probe positioning (**a** and **b**) for the evaluation of the volar extrinsic ligaments: (1) radioscaphocapitate, (2) radiolunotriquetral, (3) ulnotriquetral, and (4) volar scaphotriquetral ligaments. (**c, d, e,** and **f**) Corresponding ultrasound images showing the volar (1) radioscaphocapitate, (2) radiolunotriquetral, (3) ulnotriquetral, and (4) scaphotriquetral ligaments (arrows). Radius (R), scaphoid (S), lunate (L), triquetrum (T), capitate (**c**), and ulna (U).

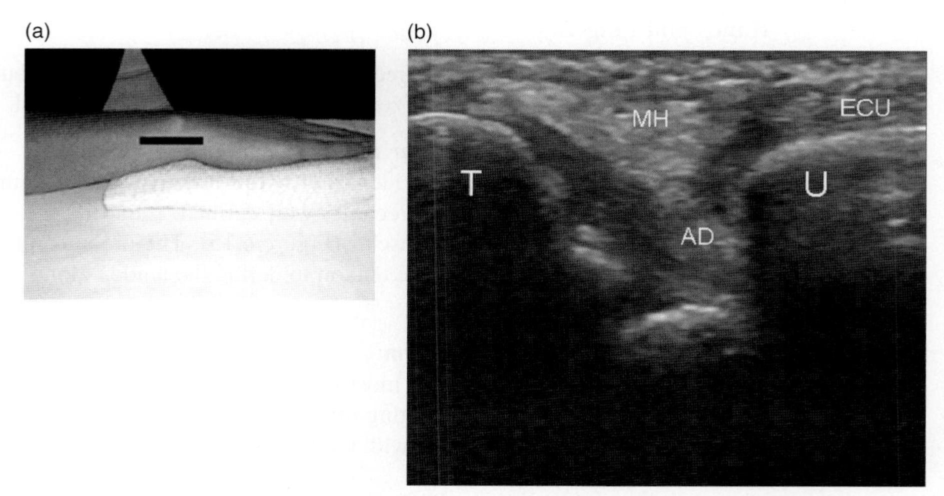

Figure 6.14. (**a**) Probe position for examining the triangular fibrocartilage (TFC). (**b**) Long axis of the TFC showing the meniscus homologue (MH) and articular disc (AD). The MH is often mistaken for the articular disc due to incorrect imaging. The extensor carpi ulnaris (ECU) tendon is used as a window.

Scanning is performed initially in the long axis after locating the bony landmarks. Locating the bony landmarks includes finding the distal ulna proximally and triquetrum distally, then angling the probe toward the radial aspect, and finally sweeping toward the ulnar aspect of the articular cartilage (Figure 6.14a). A hyperechoic triangle, the TFC, should be seen with the base closest to the ECU and apex attaching to the radius (Figure 6.14b). Careful comparison with the opposite side is necessary for diagnosis of subtle tears. It is important not to mistake the more proximal homologue, which also has a triangular echogenic appearance similar to the articular disc (Figure 6.14b). A hypoechoic line can often be seen between the homologue and the true articular disc. This is a pitfall that can result in the erroneous diagnosis of a false tear. In the transverse plane, it is important to examine the ECU for pathology that can account for the patient's pain.

Insider Information 6.5
The ECU tendon should be used as a window to assess the TFC. The tip of the TFC, which resembles an echogenic triangle, should be traced to the tip of the radius. Do not mistake the meniscus homologue for the TFC. The ECU should be examined dynamically to exclude subluxation. Pathology to the ECU can simulate a tear to the TFC.

Volar-Radial

The structures evaluated include the abductor pollicis longus and brevis, compartment 1, as previously described, and the scaphoid in the long axis for occult fractures. After first identifying Lister's tubercle in the transverse plane, the probe is swept distally until the scaphoid is identified. The probe is then swiveled in a longitudinal oblique plane until the whole length of the scaphoid is identified.

Hands and Fingers

Small linear transducers with a frequency of 10 MHz or higher should be used as these will allow the focal zones to be brought up to skin level.

Hypothenar Eminence and Flexor Pollicis Longus

The flexor pollicis longus is best identified within the hypothenar eminence in the transverse plane as a hyperechoic, well-defined, rounded structure in the adjacent, more hypoechoic muscles (Figure 6.15). The probe can then be swiveled along the long axis of the tendon to define the tendon along its long axis from origin to insertion.

Flexor Tendons and Pulley System

Rupture of flexor tendons occurs most commonly in the fingers; ultrasound has a role in the diagnosis and staging of tears. Pulley injuries are often found in rock climbers or in association with tendon rupture, also well demonstrated using ultrasound.

In the examination for tendon injury, the tendons are followed from the myotendinous junction to the point of tendinous insertion in both the long axis and transverse planes. It is prudent to first identify the bony anatomical landmarks, which include the metacarpal heads, metacarpophalangeal joint, proximal interphalangeal (PIP) joint, and distal interphalangeal (DIP) joint, from proximal to distal in the long axis (Figure 6.16a and b) and then proceed to view the tendons in both planes. The decussation of the flexor digitorum superficialis (FDS) and profundus (FDP) is usually identified at the proximal aspect of the proximal phalanx (Figure 6.16c), where the FDS splits around the FDP and then reforms more distally before insertion at the base of the middle phalanx (Figure 6.16d). The abnormal side should always be compared to the normal side in a suspect tear. The A3 and A5 pulleys are not usually identified during routine investigation.[4,7] The A2 pulley can usually be seen in the sagittal and axial planes as a hyperechoic

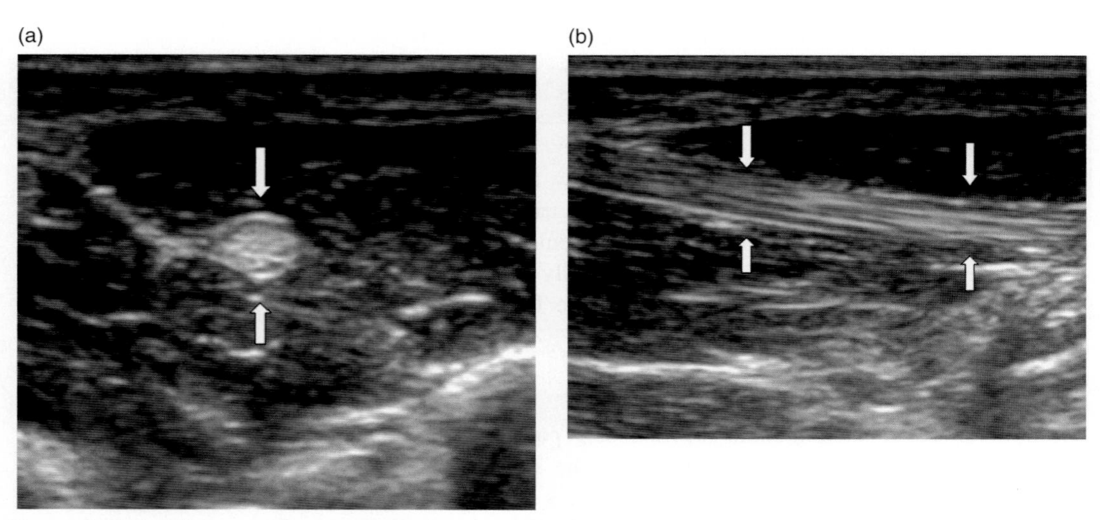

Figure 6.15. (a, b) Transverse image of the flexor pollicis longus within the hypothenar eminence seen as a well-defined hyperechoic rounded structure on a transverse scan and a classic fibrillar structure (arrows) on a longitudinal scan against the more hypoechoic muscle.

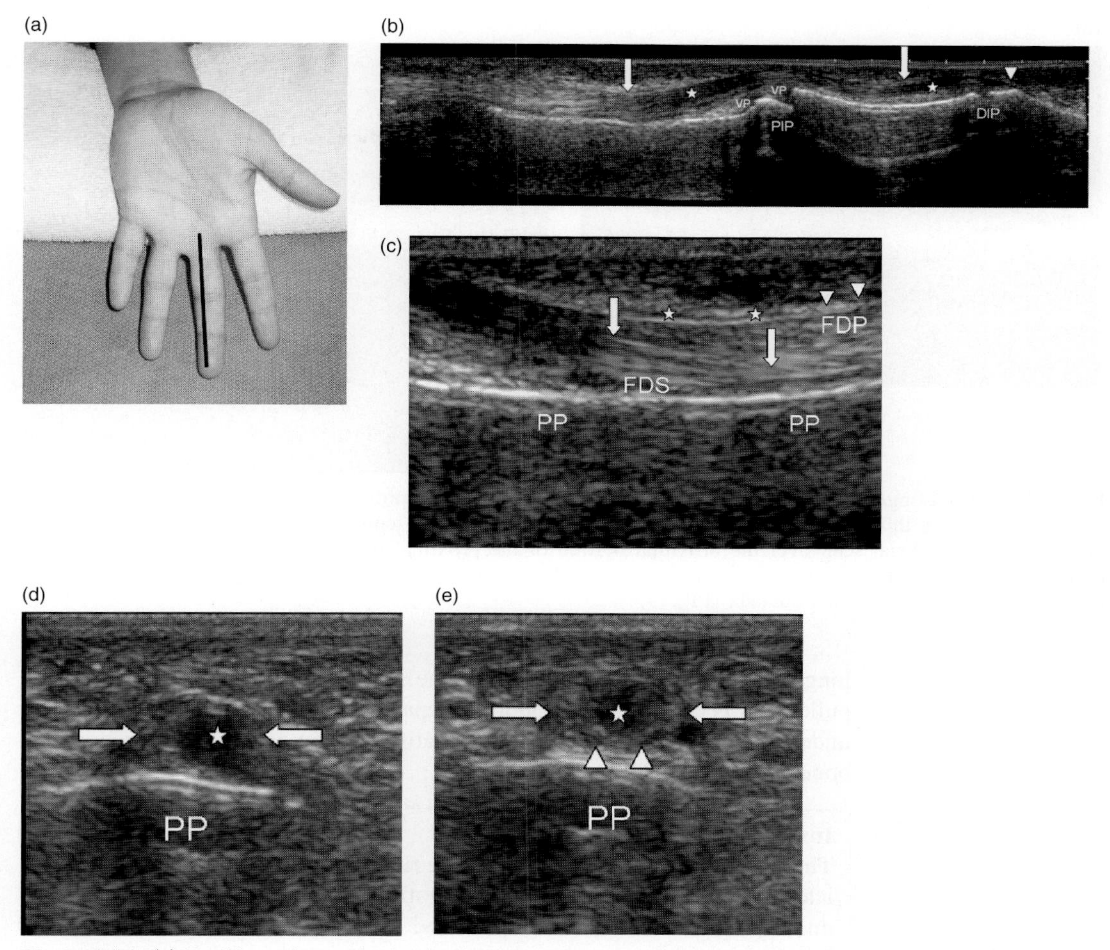

Figure 6.16. **(a)** Position of a probe in the long axis for the evaluation of the flexor tendons. **(b)** Extended field of view (EFOV) in the long axis showing the flexor digitorum profundus (FDP) (arrows) extending across the proximal interphalangeal joint (PIP) and distal interphalangeal joint (DIP) before attaching to the base of the distal phalanx. Note areas of anisotropy (asterisks). Volar plate (VP). **(c)** Long axis of the proximal phalanx showing decussation of the flexor digitorum superficialis (FDS) with fibers extending dorsally toward the attachment (arrows) and the flexor digitorum profundus (FDP) becoming more superficial (arrowheads). Proximal phalanx (PP). Note the hypoechoic second anular pulley (asterisks). Axial images over the midpoint of the proximal phalanx showing **(d)** the split of the hyperechoic FDS (arrows) around the hypoechoic FDP (asterisk) and **(e)** the reformation of the FDS deep to the profundus more distally (arrowheads) before insertion at the base of the middle phalanx. Proximal phalanx (PP).

area of focal synovial thickening at the proximal third of the proximal phalanx (Figure 6.17).[4,7] The A4 pulley may also be detected in the sagittal and axial planes as a focal area of synovial thickening at the midpoint of the middle phalanx.[4,7]

In trigger fingers, the transducer should be placed in the longitudinal plane, usually at the level of the distal metacarpals, using controlled extension against resistance. The tendon and/or tendon synovium can be seen caught under the A1 flexor pulley during dynamic real time motion. In suspect A2 pulley tears, controlled flexion against resistance is necessary with the transducer placed

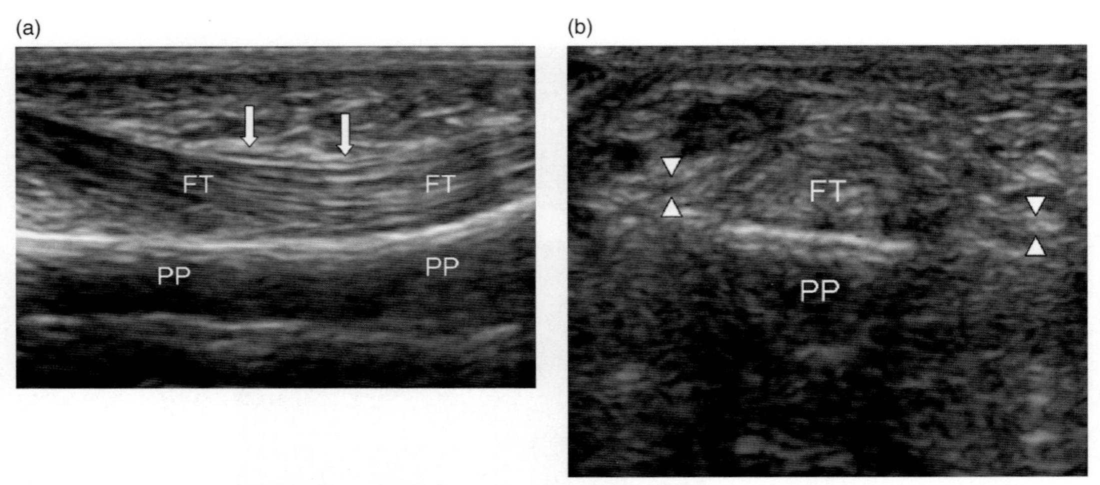

Figure 6.17. (**a**) Longitudinal scan over the proximal portion of the proximal phalanx showing the second annular pulley as a thin hypoechoic line (arrows) anterior to the flexor tendon. Flexor tendons (FT). Proximal phalanx (PP). (**b**) Axial scan over the proximal portion of the proximal phalanx showing the second annular pulley as a thin hypoechoic line that extends to the sides of the base of the proximal phalanx (arrowheads). Flexor tendons (FT). Proximal phalanx (PP).

longitudinally and transversely over the PIP joint and proximal phalanx. A pulley tear is confirmed by abnormal separation of the flexor tendon from the underlying echogenic bony cortex, creating a large gap between tendon and bone and a bowstring appearance.[15]

> **Insider Information 6.6**
> The flexor and extensor tendons of the fingers should be examined dynamically. A pulley injury will see the flexor tendon displaced from the underlying phalanx, resembling a bow.

Extensor Tendons

The extensor tendons are examined in the same fashion as the flexor tendons, identifying the previously described bony landmarks. More gel should be applied, and the gains should be adjusted as structures are more superficial.

In the case of dorsal hood injuries (an injury of the ligamentous support structure of the extensor tendon over the knuckles), the transducer is positioned in the transverse plane over the metacarpophalangeal joints and, in some patients, the proximal web spaces to identify the extremely thin radial and ulnar sagittal slips of the dorsal hood. Dynamic assessment is then made in the transverse plane during flexion and extension. In the case of a dorsal hood injury, subluxation of the extensor tendon is more pronounced during finger flexion and especially well demonstrated using a clenched fist.

Collateral Ligaments

In the assessment of the collateral ligaments, the transducer is positioned along the long axis of the medial and lateral joint capsules.

Ulnar Collateral Ligament of the Thumb

The ulnar collateral ligament (UCL) can be assessed in the long axis by placing the transducer along the superior aspect of the thumb across the first metacarpophalangeal joint (Figure 6.18a) and then in the transverse plane by crossing the first web space.[8] The medial aspect of the first metacarpal is identified at the origin of the ligament. The ligament is then traced in the long axis crossing the ulnar aspect of the first metacarpophalangeal joint (Figure 6.18b). Careful comparison with the normal side should always be undertaken. To identify a displaced ligament, the transducer should be placed over the first web space between the first and second metacarpal heads with the thumb in maximal abduction (Figure 6.18a). Two muscle layers will then be visible. The more superficial muscle is the dorsal interosseous muscle and the deeper muscle is the adductor, which ends laterally in the adductor aponeurosis (Figure 6.18c).

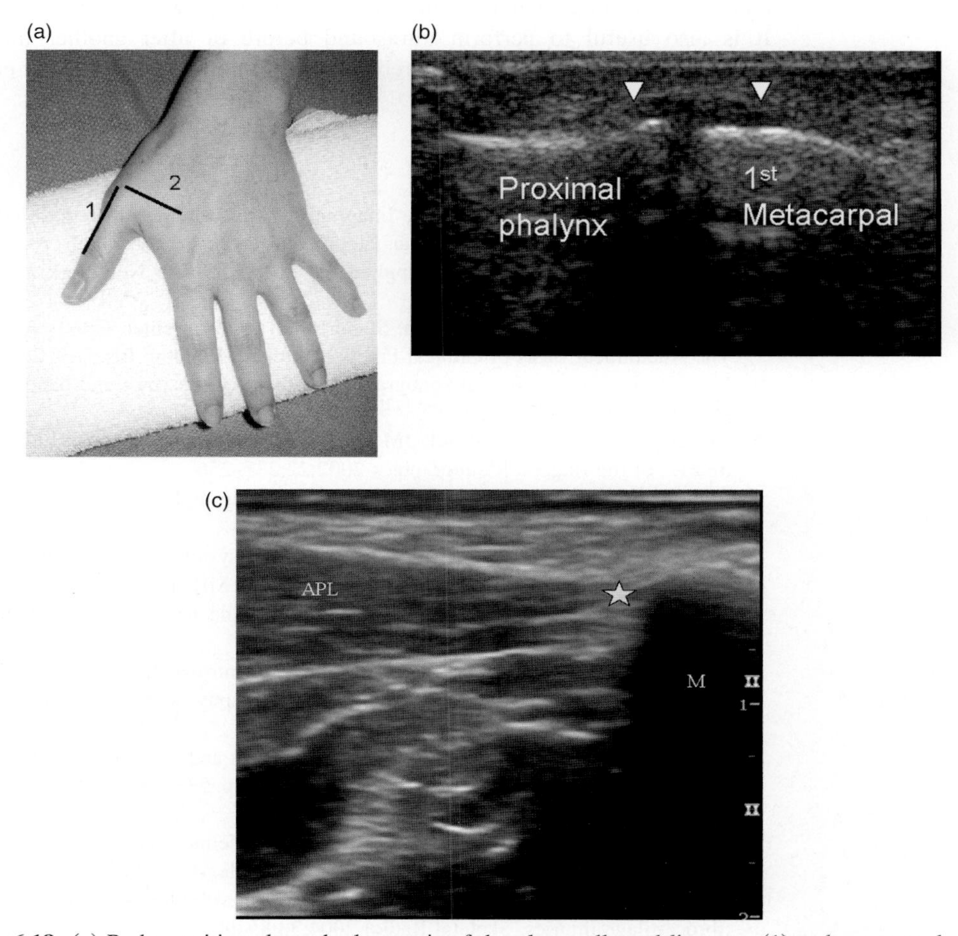

Figure 6.18. **(a)** Probe position along the long axis of the ulnar collateral ligament (1) and transversely across the first web space between metacarpal heads (2) to evaluate the integrity of the ligament and for exclusion of a Stener's lesion. **(b)** Longitudinal image showing a normal ulnar collateral ligament (arrowheads) traversing the first metacarpophalangeal joint of the thumb. **(c)** Normal first web space showing the adductor pollicis longus (APL) and normal adductor aponeurosis attachment (asterisk) at the base of the first metacarpal (M). In the event of a Stener's lesion the retracted ligament presents as a hypoechoic lesion between the base of the first metacarpal and APL (location of the asterisk) anterior to the aponeurosis.

The normal UCL and undisplaced torn UCL remain deep to the aponeurosis. With a Stener's lesion, the displaced and ruptured UCL stump is seen above or superficial to the aponeurosis.[16] Transverse oblique images demonstrate the displaced ligament as a small, rounded structure or lesion adjacent to the medial aspect of the extensor pollicis longus tendon above or superficial to the aponeurosis.

Imaging Protocols

Imaging protocols are tailored to the clinical question. We will routinely include any new area involving symptoms that have since had a previous clinical review. A standard study of the wrist is outlined in the Appendix. Until you are comfortable with musculoskeletal ultrasound of the wrist and hand we recommend that a full examination be performed in each case. It is also useful to perform ultrasound before or after another imaging modality, for example, MRI, whereby normal anatomy and pathology can be compared.

References

1. Stoller DW. Magnetic Resonance Imaging in Orthopedics and Sports Medicine, 2nd ed., pp. 851–904. Philadelphia: Lippincott–Raven, 1997.
2. Last RJ. Anatomy Regional and Applied, 6th ed., pp. 78–106. New York: Churchill Livingstone, 1978.
3. Johnson D, Ellis H, eds. Wrist. In: Standring S, editor-in-chief. Gray's Anatomy. The Anatomical Basis of Clinical Practice, 39th ed. London: Elsevier, 2005.
4. Lee JC, Healey JC. Normal sonographic anatomy of the wrist and hand. Radiographics 2005;25:1577–1590.
5. Clavero JA, Alomar X, Monill JM et al. MR imaging of ligament and tendon injuries of the fingers. Radiographics 2002;22:237–256.
6. Chen P, Maklad N, Redwine M, Zelitt D. Dynamic high-resolution sonography of the carpal tunnel. AJR 1997;168:533–537.
7. Hauger O, Chung CB, Lektrakul N et al. Pulley system in the fingers; normal anatomy and simulated lesions in cadavers at MR imaging, CT, and US with and without contrast material distention of the tendon sheath. Radiology 2000;217:201–212.
8. Brown RB, Fliszar E, Cotton A et al. Extrinsic and intrinsic ligaments of the wrist: Normal and pathologic anatomy at MR arthrography with three compartment enhancement. Radiographics 1998;18:667–674.
9. van Holsbeeck MT. Sonography of the elbow, wrist and hand. In: van Holsbeeck M, Intracaso JH, eds. Musculoskeletal Ultrasound, pp. 531–571. St. Louis: Mosby, 2001.
10. Lee D. Wrist. In: Chhem RK, Cardinal E, eds. Guidelines and Gamuts in Musculoskeletal Ultrasound, pp. 107–124. New York: Wiley-Liss, 1999.
11. Finlay K, Lee R, Friedman L. Ultrasound of intrinsic wrist ligaments and triangular fibrocartilage injuries. Skeletal Radiol 2004;33:85–90.
12. Jacobson JA, Oh E, Prospeck T et al . Sonography of the scapholunate ligament in four cadaveric wrists: Correlation with MR arthrography and anatomy. AJR 2002;179:523–527.
13. Boutry N, Lapegue F, Masi L et al. Ultrasonographic evaluation of normal extrinsic and intrinsic carpal ligaments; preliminary experience. Skeletal Radiol 2005;34:513–521.

14. Keogh CF, Wong AD, Wells NJ et al. High-resolution sonography of the triangular fibrocartilage: Initial experience and correlation with MRI and arthroscopic findings. AJR 2004;182:333–336.
15. Martinoli C, Bianchi S, Nebiolo M et al. Sonographic evaluation of digital annular pulley tears. Skeletal Radiol 2000;29:387–391.
16. O'Callaghan BI, Kohut G, Hoogewoud H. Gamekeeper thumb; identification of the Stener leison with US. Radiology 1994;182:477–480.

Section 3

The Lower Limb

7

The Adult Hip

John O'Neill and Gandikota Girish

Assessments of joint effusion and synovial proliferation have been the predominant indications for ultrasound of the adult hip joint. The surrounding structures were often difficult to visualize because of their deep location and complex anatomy[1] Advances in musculoskeletal ultrasound, however, including transducer technology and operator experience from the more commonly imaged joints, have significantly increased the ability of ultrasound to assess the hip joint and surrounding soft tissue structures. Ultrasound and magnetic resonance imaging (MRI) are complimentary imaging modalities, each offering unique advantages. Ultrasound offers a dynamic real-time study in multiple planes with immediate comparison to the contralateral side. This has proven particularly useful in the evaluation of dynamic pathologies such as the snapping hip syndrome. Direct patient contact allows maneuvers that elicit symptoms to be evaluated while performing the ultrasound study.

Clinical Indications

Ultrasound is most commonly used in the evaluation of a painful hip, which has a wide array of etiologies. Tendon pathology, including tear, tendonopathy, and avulsions and muscle injuries such as tears and intramuscular hematomas can be assessed. Femoral triangle pathology includes incidental femoral and inguinal hernias, pseudoaneurysm, lymphadenopathy, and saphena varix. Periarticular masses include cystic lesions such as abscess, hematoma, ganglion, and bursae. Solid masses can be assessed for cystic or calcific/ossific components, internal and perilesional vascularity, and location in both static and dynamic evaluation and can guide biopsy or aspiration where appropriate. Assessment of the postoperative hip includes joint effusion and periarticular collections.

Ultrasound is gaining an increasing role in the evaluation of rheumatological diseases and the presence and extent of synovial proliferation. Assessment of joint effusion can be difficult to separate from synovial proliferation, and Doppler evaluation may be useful. Comparison with the contralateral hip joint is important. Ultrasound-guided aspiration can be performed to confirm the effusion and for fluid analysis. Other synovial pathologies, including synovial chondromatosis and pigmented villonodular synovitis, can be visualized, but their full intraarticular extent, particularly in the posterior aspect of the joint, requires alternative imaging modalities such as MRI. Peripheral femoral head articular defects and crystal deposition, as in chondrocalcinosis, may be seen. Visualized cortical bone, for example, the femoral neck cortex anteriorly and laterally, can be evaluated for erosions or fractures.

The anterior superior labrum, the commonest site for labral pathology, can be visualized with ultrasound, as can intraarticular loose bodies that usually collect inferiorly. There is an extensive array of bursae surrounding the hip joint. Bursae located around the greater trochanter are commonly evaluated, as is the iliopsoas bursa. The snapping hip syndrome may be symptomatic or asymptomatic, internal or external. Internal and anterior snapping hip is usually caused by the iliopsoas tendon, and lateral and external snapping hip by the iliotibial band or gluteus maximus. Intraarticular pathology, such as a labral tear or loose body, can cause a clicking of the hip and should also be considered where appropriate.

The evaluation of the above clinical indications will depend on the patient's habitus and the experience of the sonologist. A good working knowledge of anatomy and technique is required. As always, the ease of comparison with the contralateral side is one of the main advantages of ultrasound and should be generously employed.

Technical Equipment

An array of transducers can be utilized to evaluate the adult hip. Body habitus plays a significant role in probe selection. A 9- to 15-MHz linear array transducer may be used on many patients, but a linear 7-MHz transducer may have to be used in a patient with ample subcutaneous tissue. On some occasions, we have also resorted to curved array probes, 3.5–5 MHz, traditionally used for abdominal imaging. Do not hesitate to use a combination of probes if required to perform the study.

Anatomy

Surface Anatomy

The inguinal ligament can be felt deep to the oblique skin crease, which it forms at the junction of the anterior abdominal wall and the thigh. It attaches laterally to the anterior superior iliac spine, which lies at the anterior margin of the iliac crest, and pubic tubercle medially, felt as a bony protuberance on the upper border of the pubis (Figure 7.1a).[2,3] Medial to the pubic tubercle lies the palpable pubic crest and the adjacent symphysis pubis. The pulsations of the femoral artery can be felt at the midpoint between the anterior superior iliac spine and the pubic symphysis. Medial to the femoral artery lies the femoral vein, and lateral to the artery is the femoral nerve.

The femoral triangle is an inverted triangle with its base along the oblique skin crease, the lateral margin formed by the sartorius as it extends obliquely across the thigh, and the medial margin by the adductor longus. It is best

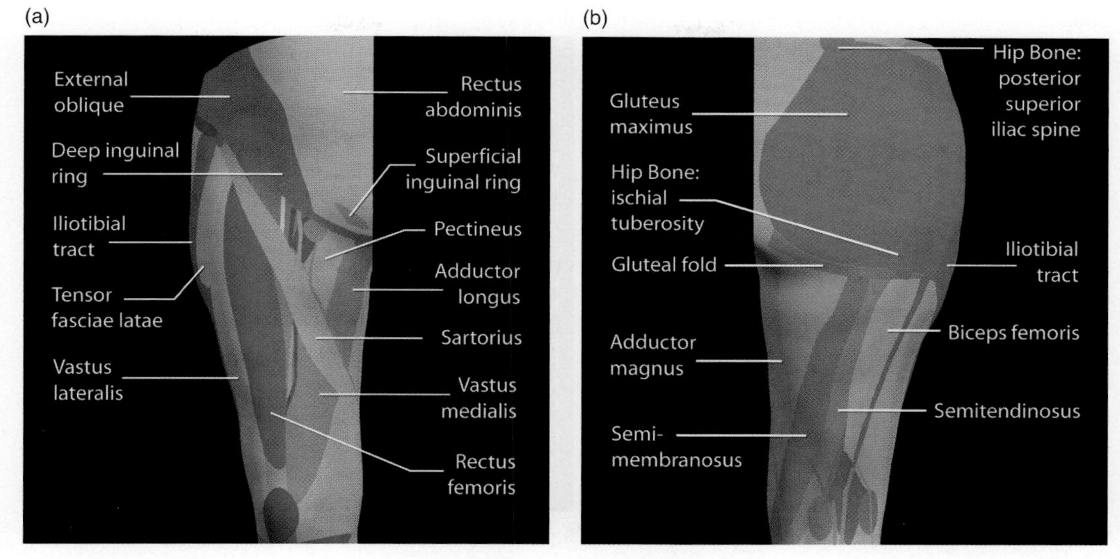

Figure 7.1. Surface anatomy of the hip: **(a)** anterior and **(b)** posterior views.

identified as a shallow depression in the frog-lateral position with the leg externally rotated and abducted just below the oblique skin crease.[3,4] It contains the femoral vasculature, femoral nerve, and lymphatics. The iliac crest can be easily felt as a smooth, bony outline extending posterolaterally from the anterior superior iliac spine. It terminates posteriorly in the form of a bony prominence, the posterior superior iliac spine. The ischial tuberosity is felt posteriorly in the lower inner aspect of the buttock (Figure 7.1b). It is easier to palpate when the hips are flexed as it then emerges from beneath the gluteus maximus. The greater trochanter of the femur is palpable as a prominent eminence along the posterolateral aspect of the proximal thigh.

Bones and Hip Joint

The hip joint is a synovial ball-and-socket joint with the spherical head of the femur (ball) articulating with the acetabulum (socket) of the pelvis.[2] The proximal femur is composed of a head, neck, and the greater and lesser trochanters. The femoral head, unlike the humeral head, is mostly covered by hyaline cartilage, except focally along the medial aspect of the femoral head (Figure 7.2a). This bare area is called fovea capitis femoris, which is the site of proximal attachment of the ligamentum teres.[2] It appears as a flattened band enclosed within a synovial membrane. Distally it extends as two bands, one on either side of the acetabular notch. This is not visualized by ultrasound. The head is directed medially, anteriorly, and superiorly. The femoral neck has a flattened pyramidal shape that narrows centrally. The entire anterior surface and part of the posterior surface of the neck are intraarticular in nature. This narrow neck is, in part, responsible for the wide range of motion at this joint. The neck of the femur is inclined at an angle of approximately 125° with the shaft. The superior border is short and thick and ends laterally at the greater trochanter; the inferior border is long and narrow and ends at the

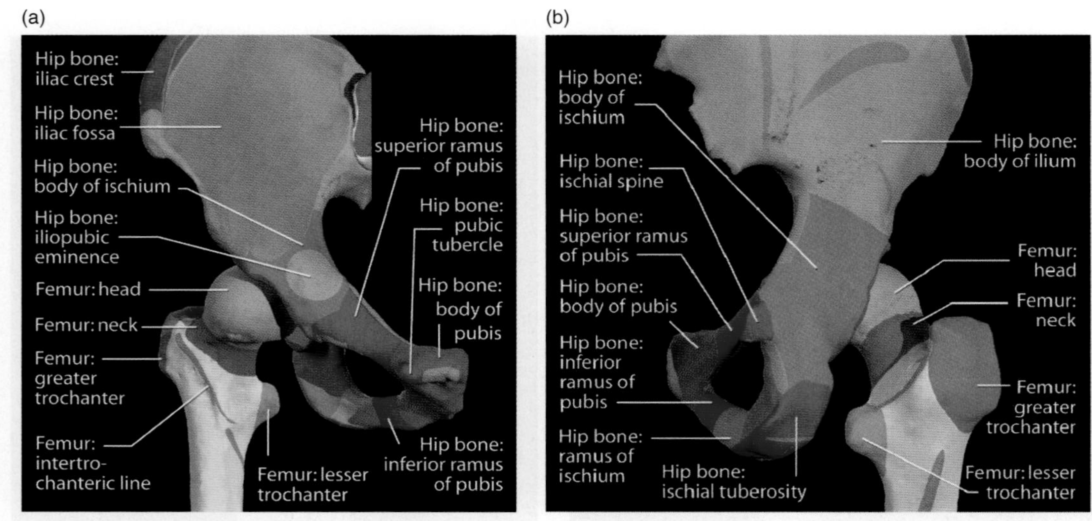

Figure 7.2. The important bony landmarks around the hip joint: **(a)** anterior and **(b)** posterior views.

lesser trochanter. The greater trochanter, the larger of the two eminences, is a prominent quadrangular protuberance seen along the superolateral aspect of the proximal femur at the junction of the neck and shaft. It has an internal and external surface and multiple borders for the attachment of a large number of tendons (Figure 7.2).

The lesser trochanter, site of attachment of the distal iliopsoas tendon, is a bony projection at the junction of the neck and shaft of the femur, and is variable in size. It is located along the posteromedial aspect of the proximal thigh and lies inferior to the greater trochanter. The intertrochanteric line extends from the greater trochanter to the lesser trochanter anteriorly and is the site of attachment of the anterior capsule. Posteriorly, the intertrochanteric crest connects the two trochanters.[2]

The acetabulum is a cup-shaped cavity that is angled laterally, inferiorly, and anteriorly. It is formed by the contribution of all three bones of the pelvis. The medial portion is formed by the pubis, the superior portion by the ilium, and the lateral and inferior portion by the ischium. It is covered with hyaline cartilage and is not amenable to ultrasound evaluation. It has a thick, strong, and uneven rim where the labrum attaches.[2] The deep acetabular notch is a circular, nonarticular depression at the bottom of the acetabular cavity that is continuous with the acetabular fossa. The acetabular notch is transformed into a foramen by the transverse acetabular ligament. Neurovascular structures enter the joint through this foramen. The ligamentum teres attaches to the margins of the acetabular notch.[2] Its cavity is deepened by a peripheral rim of fibrocartilage, termed the labrum. This explains the increased stability of the hip joint when compared to the shoulder joint, which of course comes at the expense of mobility. The stability is further enhanced by three strong ligaments, a tough enclosing fibrous capsule, and strong surrounding musculature. The acetabular labrum is deficient inferiorly where it is replaced by the transverse acetabular ligament. Only the anterior superior portion of the labrum is well-visualized sonographically.

Insider Information 7.1
The capsule of the hip joints extends anteriorly to the intertrochanteric line and posteriorly to the midportion of the femoral neck. This is helpful to remember for joint aspiration or injection.

Capsule and Synovial Membrane

The capsule extends anteriorly from the acetabulum to the intertrochanteric line and posteriorly from the acetabulum to the midportion of the femoral neck, approximately 1.25 cm proximal to intertrochanteric crest. This is an important point to remember when injecting into or aspirating the hip joint. The synovial membrane lines the capsule and is reflected along the neck of the femur. The capsule is strengthened by three strong ligaments: the iliofemoral, the ischiofemoral, and the pubofemoral.[5]

Muscles and Tendons

There is significant overlap between the description of muscles of the hip and thigh regions. This chapter describes the muscles and tendons that are predominantly localized to the hip or are common etiologies of hip pain; the remaining muscles and tendons are evaluated in Chapter 8. The origin, insertion sites, and action of these tendons and muscles are detailed in Table 7.1 and Figure 7.3. The hip muscles can be divided into several different groups: anterior, medial, posterior, and gluteal/lateral (Table 7.2)

The sartorius and rectus femoris are anterior (Figures 7.3a, and 7.4a).[4] The sartorius is a ribbon-shaped muscle that originates just below the anterior superior iliac spine and inserts at the medial surface of the proximal tibia as part of the pes anserinus. Its origin is anteromedial to the rectus femoris, which arises from two heads. The straight head originates from the anterior

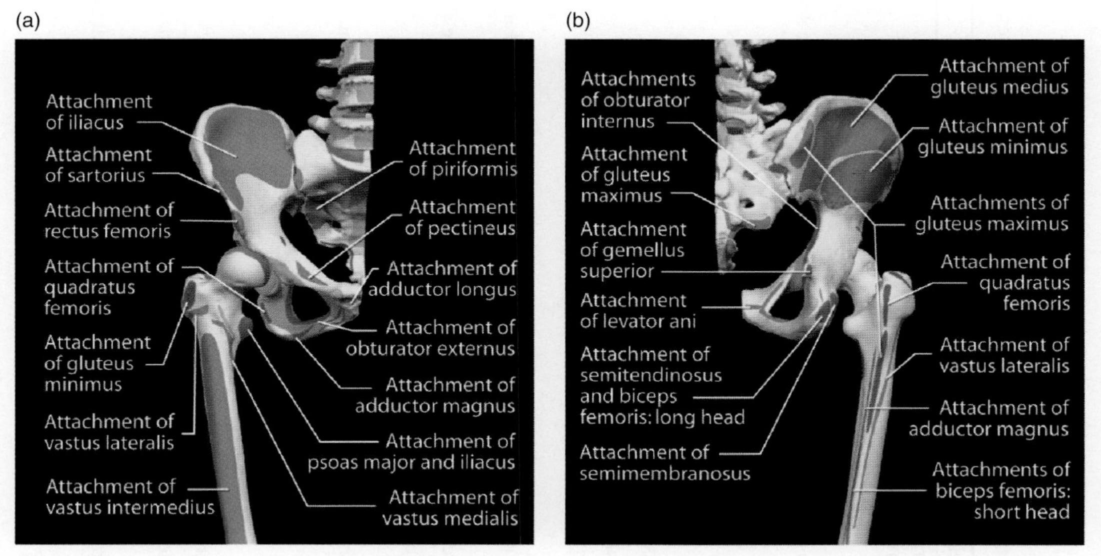

Figure 7.3. The muscle origin (red) and insertion (blue) points of the muscles around the hip joint: **(a)** anterior and **(b)** posterior views.

Table 7.1. Origin, Insertion, and Action of Hip Muscles.

Muscle	Origin	Insertion	Action
Anterior group			
Sartorius	Anterior superior iliac spine	Proximal medial shaft of tibia (pes anserinus)	Hip—flexion, abduction and lateral rotation of thigh Knee—flexion of leg
Rectus femoris	Straight head—anterior inferior iliac spine Reflected head—ilium above acetabular rim	Patella—via quadriceps tendon and patellar ligament to tibial tuberosity	Knee—extension Hip—flexion of thigh
Psoas	T12–L5 vertebrae and transverse processes	Lesser trochanter	Hip—flexion and medial rotation
Iliacus	Iliac fossa	Lesser trochanter	
Medial group			
Gracilis	Body and inferior Ramus pubis	Proximal medial shaft of tibia (pes anserinus)	Hip—adduction of thigh Knee—flexion of legand medial rotation
Pectineus	Pubis—pectineal line and superior part of ramus	Pectineal line inferior to lesser trochanter	Hip—flexion, Adduction, and medial rotation of thigh
Adductor longus	Body of pubis—inferior to pubic crest	Linea aspera—middle third	Hip—adduction of thigh
Adductor brevis	Pubis—body and inferior ramus	Linea aspera—upper third and pectineal line	Hip—adduction of thigh
Adductor magnus	Adductor portion— ischiopubic ramus	Adductor portion—linea aspera, gluteal tuberosity	Adductor portion—adduction and medial rotation of thigh
	Hamstring portion—ischial Tuberosity—inferior and lateral quadrant	Hamstring portion—adductor tubercle	Hamstring portion—extension of thigh
Posterior group			
Semitendinosus	Ischial tuberosity—upper inner quadrant	Proximal medial shaft of tibia (pes anserinus)	Extension of thigh, flexion and medial rotation of knee
Semimembranosus	Ischial tuberosity—upper outer quadrant	Medial condyle of tibia, fascia over popliteus and oblique popliteal ligament	Extension of thigh, flexion and medial rotation of knee

Biceps femoris	Long head—ischial tuberosity (upper and inner quadrant) Short head—lateral aspect of supracondylar ridge of femur, linea aspera middle third	Styloid process of head of fibula, lateral tibial condyle and lateral collateral ligament	Extension of thigh, flexion and lateral rotation of leg
Gluteal			
Gluteus maximus	Ilium—posterior to gluteal line, iliac crest, sacrum—lateral mass, sacrotuberous ligament and coccyx	Iliotibial tract and gluteal tuberosity of femur	Hip—extension and external rotation Knee actions are via iliotibial tract
Gluteus medius	Ilium between posterior and anterior gluteal lines	Greater trochanter—posterolateral surface	Hip—abduction and medial rotation
Gluteus minimus	Ilium between anterior and inferior gluteal lines	Greater trochanter—anterior surface	Hip—abduction and medial rotation
Tensor fascia latae	Anterior iliac crest, anterior superior iliac spine	Iliotibial band	Hip—abduction, medial rotation, and flexion of thigh Knee—assists gluteus maximus in maintaining knee extension
Iliotibial band	Fascia lata, tensor fascia latae	Gerdy's tubercle tibia	Hip—flexion, Abduction, and medial rotation Knee—lateral stabilization
Obturator externus	Obturator membrane—outer surface and adjacent pubis and ischium	Greater trochanter—trochanteric fossa along the medial surface	Hip—lateral rotation
Obturator internus	Inner surface obturator membrane, ischiopubic rami	Greater trochanter—medial surface	Hip—lateral rotation, abduction of thigh and stabilization
Piriformis	Sacrum-2,3,4 costotransverse bars and greater sciatic notch	Greater trochanter—superior border	Hip—lateral rotation of thigh and stabilization
Gemellus superior	Ischial spine	Greater trochanter—medial surface	Hip—lateral rotation and stabilization
Gemellus inferior	Ischial tuberosity—upper border	Greater trochanter— medial surface	Hip—lateral rotation and stabilization
Quadratus femoris	Ischial tuberosity—lateral surface	Quadrate tubercle of femur	Hip—lateral rotation and stabilization

inferior iliac spine, and the reflected head originates from the ilium, above the acetabular rim, and immediately joins the fibers of the straight head.

The iliopsoas and pectineus compose the medial group (Figure 7.4a). The psoas major originates proximally from transverse processes of L1–L5, vertebral bodies of T12–L5, and intervening intervertebral discs. Distally it forms a conjoint tendon with the iliacus. The iliacus originates from the iliac fossa within the pelvis and inserts along with the psoas tendon onto the lesser trochanter of the femur.

The pectineus is a flat quadrangular muscle that forms the floor of the femoral triangle. The femoral vasculature lies superficial and lateral to the pectineus and is a helpful landmark to remember when localizing the muscle. The pectineus originates from the pectineal line of the pubis and between the pubic tubercle and iliopectineal eminence, and inserts on a line passing between the linea aspera and lesser trochanter of the femur.[4] The adductors and gracilis are reviewed in Chapter 8 (Figure 7.4b).

The gluteal/lateral group is comprised of the triad of gluteal muscles, the maximus, medius, and minimus; the tensor fascia latae; iliotibial tract; piriformis; gemellus superior; gemellus inferior; obturator externus; obturator internus; and quadratus femoris (Figure 7.4c–e). The most superficial muscle in the gluteal region is the gluteus maximus. It is the main muscle forming the contour of the buttock. It is a very thick, bulky muscle arising from the posterior gluteal line on the ilium, posterior third of the iliac crest, aponeurosis of the erector spinae, sacrotuberous ligament, and lower portions of the sacrum and coccyx. The whole muscle fibers of the upper portion and the superficial fibers of the lower portion of the muscle form a tendon that passes laterally to blend with the iliotibial tract. The deep fibers of the lower portion insert on the gluteal trochanter.

The gluteus medius is a thick muscle that is superficial along its anterior two-thirds. Its posterior third lies deep to the gluteus maximus. The gluteus medius originates between the iliac crest and posterior and anterior gluteal lines. It extends distally, forming a tendon that inserts on the lateral surface of the greater trochanter of the femur. The smallest among the gluteus muscles, the gluteus minimus, is deepest of all. It originates between the anterior and

Table 7.2. Muscles of the Hip and Thigh.

Anterior group	Medial group	Posterior group	Gluteal/lateral group
Sartorius[a]	Iliopsoas[a]	Biceps femoris	Gluteus maximus[a]
Rectus femoris[a]	Pectineus[a]	Semitendinosus	Gluteus medius[a]
Vastus lateralis	Gracilis	Semimembranosus	Gluteus minimus[a]
Vastus intermedius	Adductor longus		Piriformis[a]
Vastus medialis	Adductor brevis		Tensor fascia lata
	Adductor magnus		Iliotibial tract
			Gemellus superior[a]
			Gemellus inferior[a]
			Obturator externus[a]
			Obturator internus[a]
			Quadratus femoris[a]

[a]Denotes those muscles detailed in this chapter. The remaining muscles are reviewed in Chapter 8.

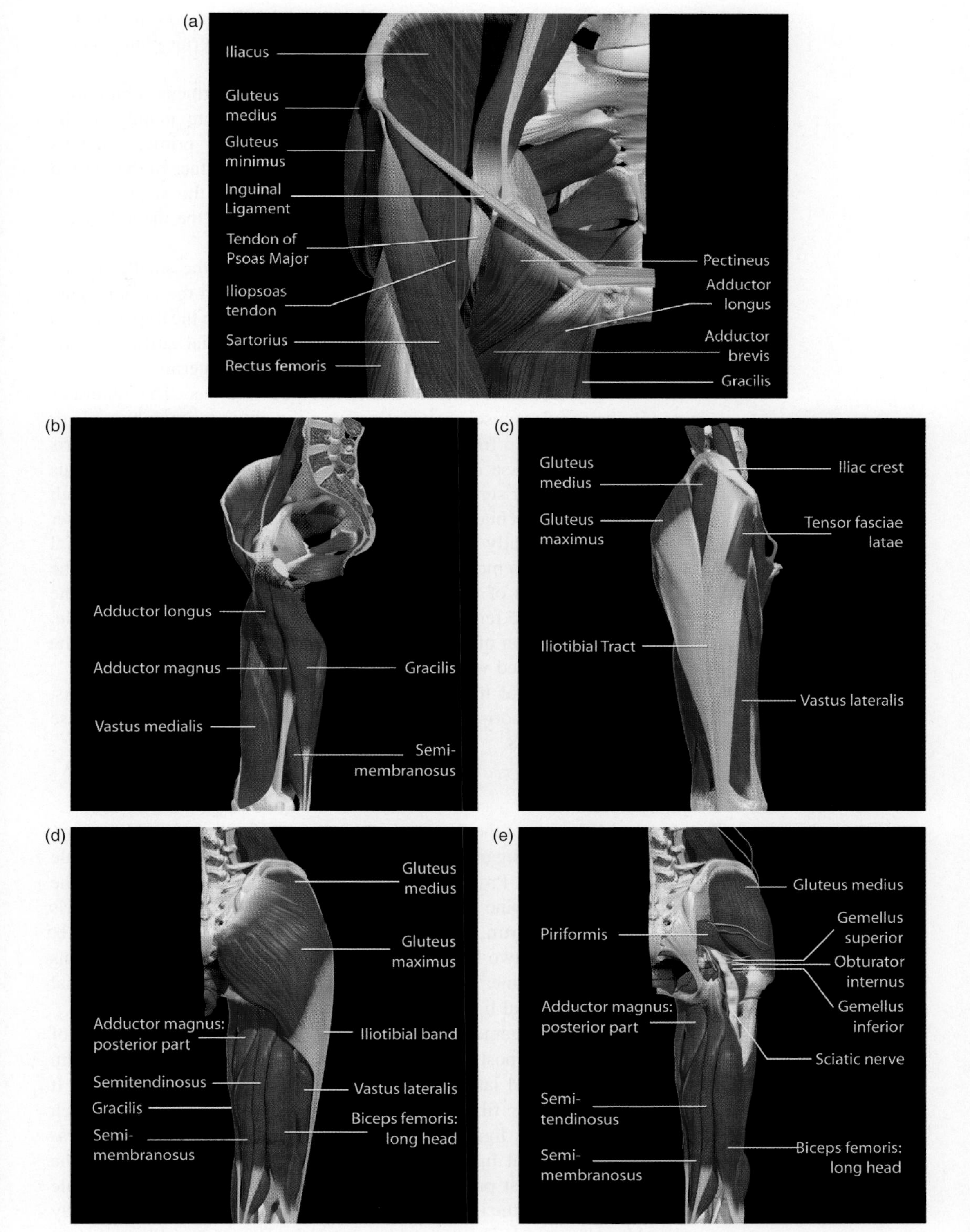

Figure 7.4. The muscles around the hip joint: **(a)** anterior c, **(b)** medial, **(c)** lateral, **(d)** posterior view, and **(e)** posterior view with gluteus maximus removed.

inferior gluteal lines on the ilium. Distally, its tendon inserts on the anterior surface of the greater trochanter.[4] Deep branches of the superior gluteal nerve and vessels lie between the gluteus medius and minimus.

All of the short muscles around the hip joint—the pectineus, obturators, piriformis, gemelli, and the quadratus femoris—contribute mainly to the stability and integrity of the hip rather than acting as primary movers (Figure 7.4e). The piriformis originates from the anterior surface of the sacrum and passes through the greater sciatic notch superior to the sciatic nerve. Distally the tendon attaches to the greater trochanter along the medial aspect of its upper surface.

There are two gemelli muscles: the gemellus superior, the smaller of the two, and the gemellus inferior. The former originates from the ischial spine over its dorsal surface. The gemellus inferior originates from the upper portion of the ischial tuberosity. Both attach distally to the medial surface of the greater trochanter along with the tendon of the obturator internus.

There are two obturator muscles, externus and internus. The obturator externus is a triangular muscle originating from the obturator membrane over its outer surface and also from the adjacent pubic and ischial rami. It inserts into the trochanteric fossa of the greater trochanter. The obturator internus originates from the inner surface of the obturator membrane. It passes through a groove between the ischial spine and tuberosity, extends through the lesser sciatic foramen, and finally inserts onto the greater trochanter over its medial surface. The quadratus femoris is a quadrilateral muscle originating from the upper and outer aspects of the ischial tuberosity. It extends posterior to the hip joint and neck of the femur and finally inserts into the quadrate tubercle. It helps in lateral rotation of the thigh at the hip joint.[4] Figure 7.5 details the axial anatomy as obtained with MRI.

The posterior group of muscles, better known as the hamstring muscles, includes the biceps femoris, semitendinosus, and semimembranosus. These are detailed in Chapter 8.

Ligaments

The strongest ligament of the three main ligaments is the iliofemoral ligament, which is a Y-shaped ligament adherent to the anterior articular capsule (Table 7.3, Figure 7.6). Proximally it is attached to the undersurface of the anterior inferior iliac spine just below the attachment of the rectus femoris and adjacent acetabular rim, in close approximation to the underlying labrum. Inferiorly it extends as two bands that attach to the upper and lower portions of the intertrochanteric line.[5] Along the anterior aspect of the hip, the proximal portion of the iliofemoral ligament can be localized sonographically.

The ischiofemoral ligament is a triangular, strong band, the majority of which blends with the posterior joint capsule. It extends from the ischium medially and is attached laterally to the midportion of the femoral neck. It blends with the circular fibers of the capsule, the zona orbicularis, which encircle the neck.[5] This ligament cannot be satisfactorily assessed by ultrasound. The pubofemoral ligament is attached to the superior ramus of the pubis and obturator crest proximally and is adherent to the inferior capsule and the vertical band of the iliofemoral ligament.[5] This ligament is also poorly visualized by ultrasound. The transverse acetabular ligament and ligamentum teres are detailed in the prior section on the hip joint.

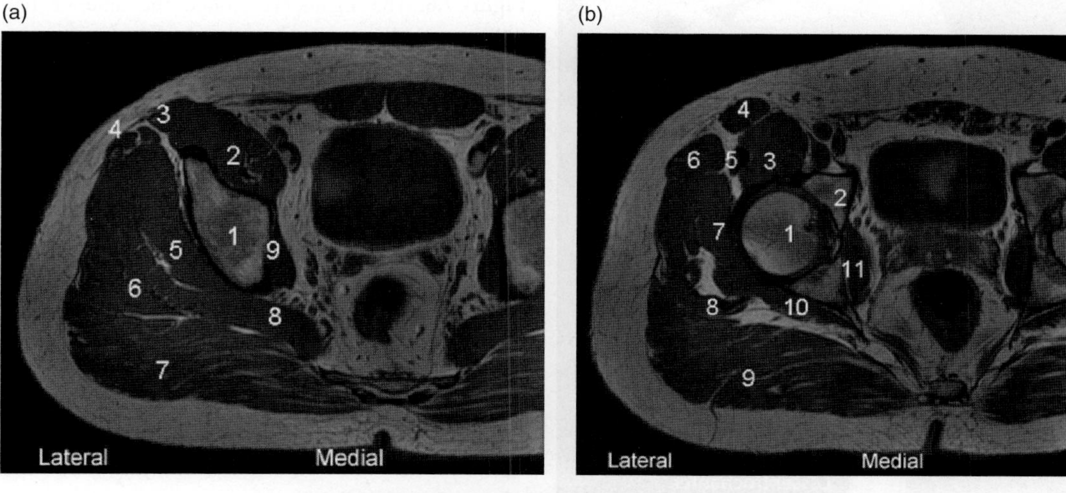

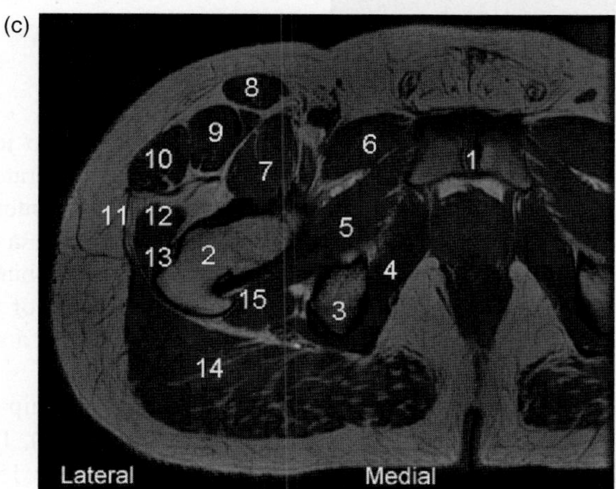

Figure 7.5. Axial T1-weighted MRI anatomy. **(a)** Superior to hip joint: 1–acetabulum, 2–iliopsoas muscle and tendon, 3–sartorius, 4–tensor fascia lata, 5–gluteus minimus, 6–gluteus medius, 7–gluteus maximus, 8–piriformis, 9–obturator internus. **(b)** At the level of the hip joint: 1–femoral head, 2–anterior acetabular column, 3–iliopsoas, 4–sartorius, 5–rectus femoris, 6–tensor fascia lata, 7–gluteus minimus, 8–gluteus medius, 9–gluteus maximus, 10–piriformis, 11–obturator internus. **(c)** Below the level of the hip joint: 1–pubic symphysis, 2–femoral neck, 3–ischium, 4–obturator internus, 5–obturator externus, 6–adductor longus, 7–iliopsoas, 8–sartorius, 9–rectus femoris, 10–tensor fascia lata, 11–iliotibial band, 12–gluteus medius, 13–gluteus minimus, 14–gluteus maximus, 15–quadratus femoris.

Table 7.3. Hip Joint Ligaments.

Iliofemoral ligament[a]
Ischiofemoral ligament
Pubofemoral ligament
Ligamentum teres
Transverse acetabular ligament

[a]Can normally be visualized under ultrasound.

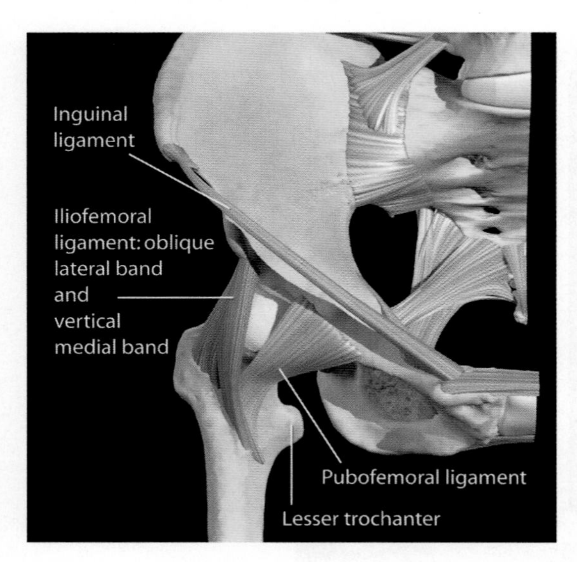

Figure 7.6. The ligaments around the anterior hip joint.

Bursae

There are a vast number of bursae around the hip joint. The better known bursae will be described here. Three bursae separate the gluteus maximus tendon from the surrounding structures: the trochanteric bursa of the gluteus maximus from the greater trochanter, the ischial bursa of the gluteus maximus from the ischial tuberosity, and the gluteofemoral bursa from its tendon and that of the vastus lateralis. The trochanteric bursa of the gluteus medius lies between its tendon and the greater trochanter, with a similar interposition for the trochanteric bursa of the gluteus minimus.

The iliopsoas bursa is situated between the hip joint capsule and the posterior portion of the iliopsoas tendon (Table 7.4). This is a large bursa that communicates with the hip joint in approximately 15% of individuals. It is very important to recognize that it is a virtual space that is not readily seen unless it is distended by fluid or thickening of the bursal wall.

Nerves

The sciatic nerve is the largest nerve in the body and supplies the muscles of the leg and foot as well as adductor and extensor compartments of the thigh. It exits the pelvis, below the piriformis, via the greater sciatic notch and lies in turn on the superior gemellus, obturator internus, inferior gemellus, and

Table 7.4. Major Greater Trochanteric and Hip Joint Bursae.

Trochanteric bursa, ischial bursa,
and gluteofemoral bursae of the gluteus maximus
Trochanteric bursa of the gluteus medius
Trochanteric bursa of the gluteus minimus
Iliopsoas bursa[a]

[a]Can communicate with the hip joint.

quadratus femoris muscles (Figure 7.4e). It lies lateral to the ischial tuberosity, which can be a useful bony landmark in locating this nerve. From here the nerve proceeds distally into the thigh.

The femoral nerve supplies the extensor compartment. It enters the thigh deep to the inguinal ligament and lateral to the femoral artery. It divides almost immediately into superficial and deep divisions (see Chapter 12, Figure 12.13a).

Technique

Ultrasound of the hip is divided into anterior, medial, lateral, and posterior approaches. The examination targets the region of symptoms. We do not routinely, therefore, perform a full evaluation of all quadrants. One of the great advantages of ultrasound is direct patient contact; this should always be utilized. A brief pertinent clinical history should be obtained. Patients can often localize the site of symptoms and indicate if there have been any changes since they were last seen by the referring clinician. They can often describe and reproduce movements responsible for symptoms, such as the snapping hip syndrome. Ask a patient who finds a certain movement particularly painful to demonstrate the movement on the contralateral side first; this helps to limit the number of times the movement is required on the symptomatic side, particularly if the movement is painful. It is also possible to palpate over the area of snapping prior to imaging to help localize the area of pathology. The asymptomatic side should also be used for anatomic correlation. Knowledge of the surface anatomy and the use of bony landmarks are very useful in providing a structured reproducible approach.

Proper patient positioning is crucial for a good examination as well as patient comfort (Table 7.5). It is essential that the patient be informed of what the examination entails prior to the study and to be aware of the patient's personal comfort level. Correct transducer position in relation to the underlying structure to be examined is the key to achieving good diagnostic images. Subtle changes in angulation of the transducer can influence the information obtained. Structures should always be evaluated in their orthogonal planes.

Insider Information 7.2
It is essential to inform the patient of what the examination entails prior to the study and to be aware of the patient's personal comfort level.

Table 7.5. Muscle Groups and Position for Ultrasound Examination.

Muscle group	Position for ultrasound study	Muscle group	Position for ultrasound study
Anterior group	Supine, with toes approximating each other	*Posterior group*	Prone, leg extended
Medial group	Supine, leg externally rotated and abducted	*Gluteal/lateral group*	Lateral decubitus, extended leg

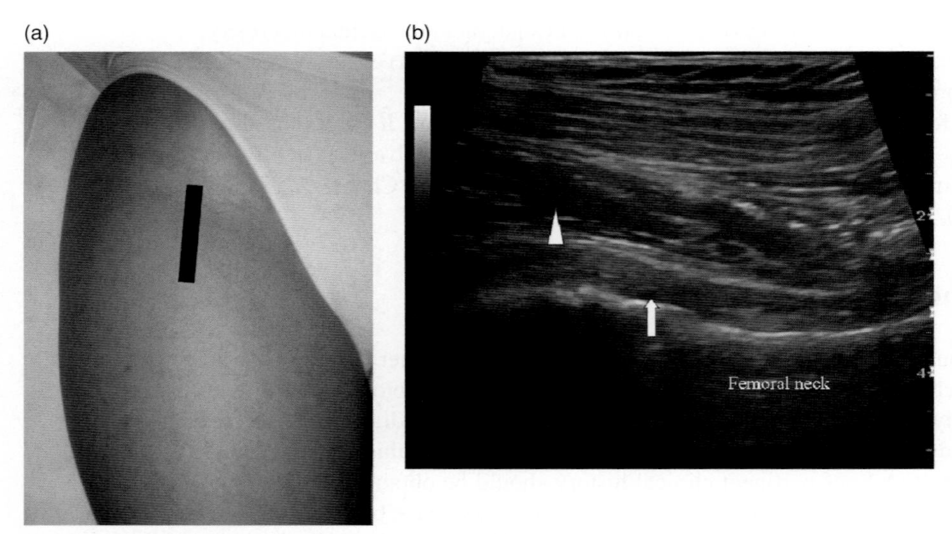

Figure 7.7. Femoral neck: **(a)** transducer position and **(b)** corresponding ultrasound image demonstrating the hyperechoic line of the anterior surface of the femoral neck, the overlying capsulosynovial tissue and joint space (arrow), and directly superficial to the joint capsule, the iliopsoas (arrowhead).

Anterior

The patient lies supine with the hips and knees extended. Place the transducer in a sagittal oblique plane parallel to the long axis of the femoral neck (Figure 7.7). The latter lies lateral to the palpable pulsations of the femoral artery. The hyperechoic continuous line of the bony cortex of the neck of the femur should be clearly visible, with the overlying thin hyperechoic band of the joint capsule (Figure 7.7). Moving the transducer superiorly, the anterior cortical margin of the acetabulum is seen. The hyperechoic rounded surface of the femoral head has a thin hypoechoic rim of hyaline articular cartilage (Figure 7.8).

The anterior superior labrum can be visualized sonographically as a triangular, echo-bright structure extending inferiorly from the acetabulum and draping over the femoral head (Figure 7.9). It lies in close proximity to the

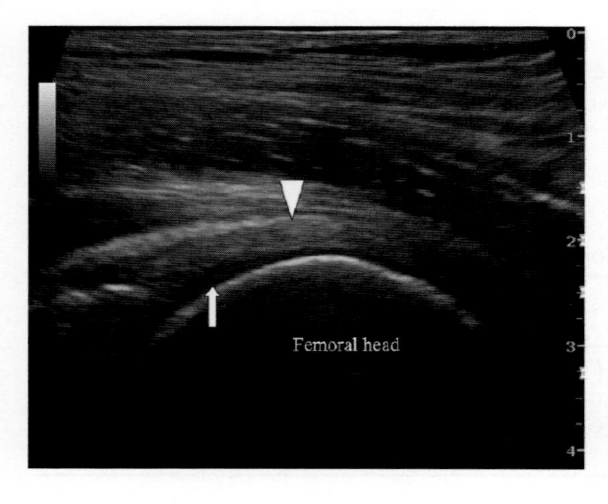

Figure 7.8. Ultrasound image of the longitudinal axis of the femoral head and articular cartilage (arrow) with the overlying iliofemoral ligament (arrowhead).

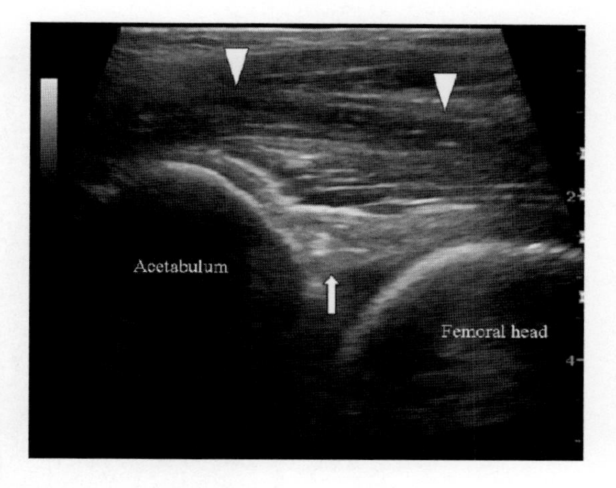

Figure 7.9. Ultrasound image of the longitudinal axis of the femoral head demonstrating the labrum (arrow) with the overlying rectus femoris (arrowheads).

overlying iliofemoral ligament (Figure 7.8). On ultrasound only the anterior superior labrum is satisfactorily visualized. Fortunately, most symptomatic tears involve this portion of the labrum.

Joint effusion and synovial pathology are best visualized at the junction of the femoral neck and head. The capsule that normally embraces the neck is pushed further away when there is a joint effusion. The capsulosynovial thickness normally measures 5 mm or less (Figure 7.7). An increase in distance between the cortex femoral neck and the capsule of the joint, with loss of concavity of the anterior capsule, is seen with effusion or synovitis without effusion. This should be correlated with the contralateral side.

The rectus femoris has two proximal attachment sites as described in the anatomy section. The transducer is placed longitudinally along the femoral head and neck and then moved laterally and superiorly until a bony protuberance is seen: the anterior inferior iliac spine (Figure 7.10a). Hypoechogenicity just inferior to the anterior inferior iliac spine and deep to the straight head of rectus femoris fibers represents anisotropy of the fibers of the reflected head (Figure 7.10b). The sartorius originates at the anterior superior iliac spine (Figure 7.11). It is superficial and anterior to the hip joint and runs obliquely from the lateral to the medial aspect of the thigh, forming the lateral border of the femoral triangle. Knowledge of origin and insertion points is essential for the correct identification of muscles and tendons and subsequent transducer alignment.

The iliopsoas tendon is a combination of two muscles; the majority of the muscular portion is derived from the iliacus, and the tendinous portion is from the psoas. It exits the pelvic brim inferior to the inguinal ligament and courses anteromedial to the hip joint to attach to the lesser trochanter. The muscle is best seen in the longitudinal plane when the pennate structure is appreciated. The tendon overlies the labrum medially (Figure 7.12). The tendon portion is a hyperechoic band running in the posterior aspect of the iliopsoas muscle with a considerable amount of muscle directly anteriorly. In cross section, the oval tendon can be identified by rocking the probe to take advantage of anisotropy (Figure 7.13). Attachment to the lesser trochanter can be difficult to identify in this position. Reposition the patient into the frog-lateral position, hip externally rotated and the knee flexed to 45°. Place the probe transversely over the proximal shaft of the femur and slowly move

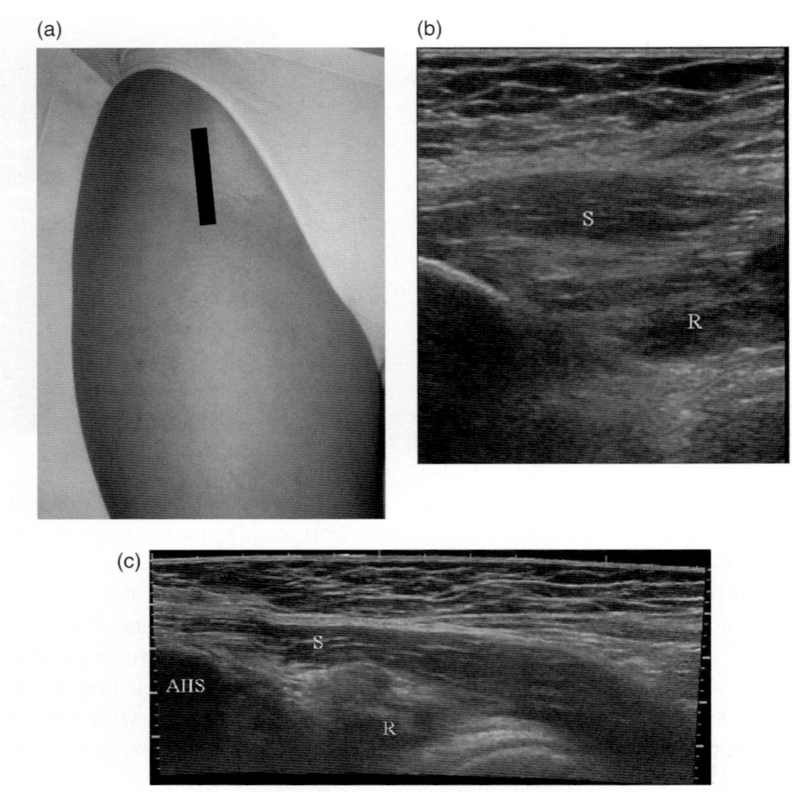

Figure 7.10. Rectus femoris: **(a)** transducer position and **(b)** corresponding ultrasound image in the longitudinal axis demonstrating the origin straight (S) and reflected (R) heads of the rectus femoris from the anterior inferior iliac spine (AIIS) and between the AIIS and acetabulum, respectively; **(c)** extended field of view demonstrating anisotropy of the reflected head.

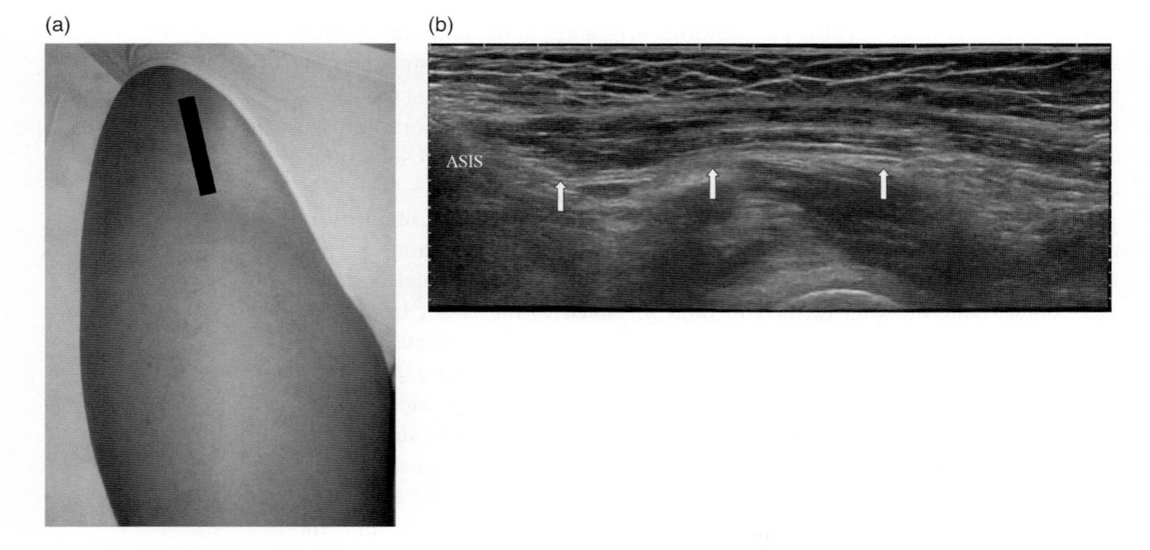

Figure 7.11. Sartorius: **(a)** transducer position and **(b)** corresponding ultrasound image in the longitudinal axis of the sartorius (arrows) arising from the anterior superior iliac spine (ASIS).

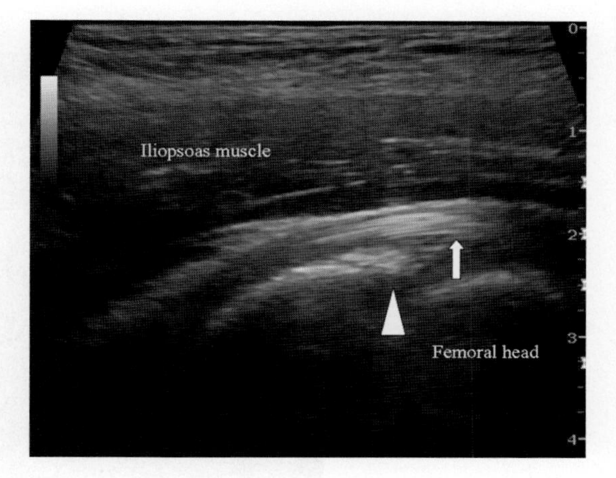

Figure 7.12. Ultrasound image of the longitudinal axis of the iliopsoas. The hyperechoic tendon (arrow) lies deep to the hypoechoic muscle. The labrum can be identified deep to the tendon (arrowhead).

the probe superiorly. A bony protuberance is noted along the inner medial aspect of the proximal femur, the lesser trochanter. The attachment of the iliopsoas tendon is best visualized by turning the transducer clockwise along the direction of the iliopsoas tendon (Figure 7.14).

The iliopsoas bursa, when distended, can be seen between the iliopsoas tendon and the joint capsule along the medial aspect of the hip joint. It is imaged in transverse and longitudinal planes in a fashion similar to that used for the iliopsoas tendon. As mentioned before, it is a virtual space and hence not easily seen unless it is distended by fluid or thickening of the bursal wall. Ultrasound guidance has been actively used for iliopsoas bursa injections.[6,7]

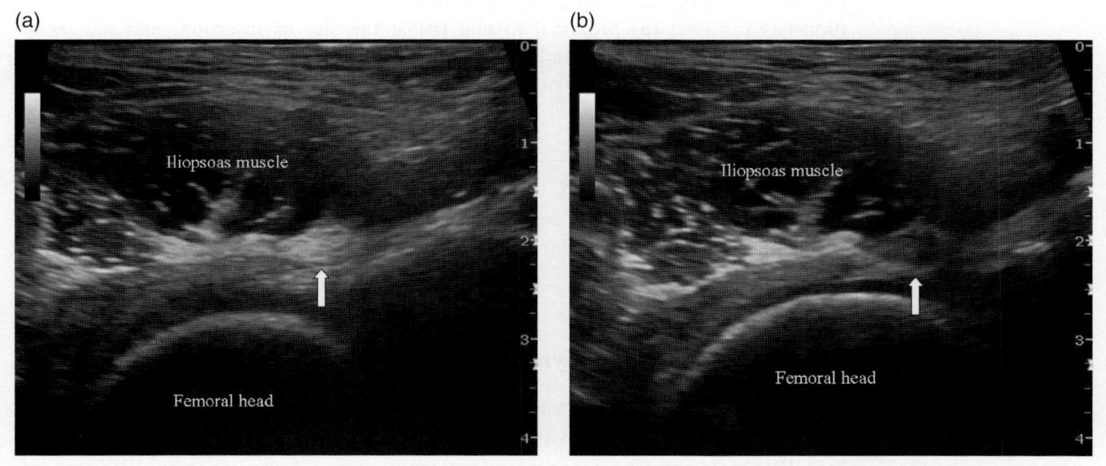

Figure 7.13. Anisotropy of the iliopsoas tendon. **(a)** Normal transverse ultrasound image of the iliopsoas tendon (arrows) with the ultrasound beam perpendicular to the tendon. **(b)** The same position as **(a)** with the transducer angled 5–10°; thus the ultrasound beam is no longer perpendicular and the hyperechoic tendon becomes hypoechoic.

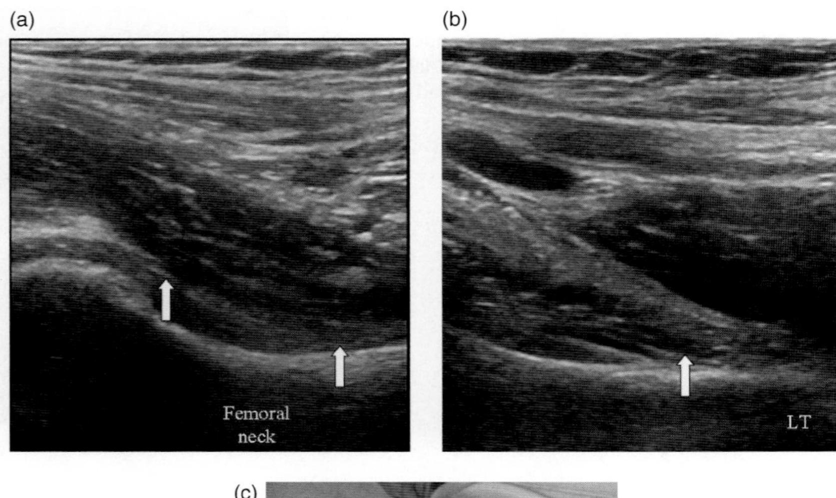

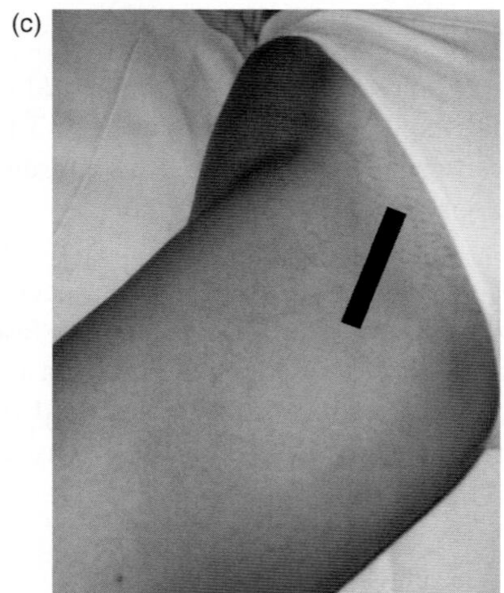

Figure 7.14. Iliopsoas tendon: ultrasound image in the longitudinal plane of the iliopsoas (arrows) (**a**) proximal to and (**b**) at the site of insertion onto the lesser trochanter (LT). (**c**) Corresponding transducer position for image (**b**).

Insider Information 7.3
The iliopsoas tendon is a combination of two muscles; the majority of the muscular portion is derived from the iliacus and the tendinous portion from the psoas.

Internal Snapping Hip Syndrome

There are many causes of snapping or clicking at the hip joint, and defined as an audible sound of varable intensity produced during motion of the hip. Etiology may be internal or external. One of the important causes of internal snapping is snapping of the iliopsoas tendon as it passes over the superior pubic bone. Various maneuvers have been described to elicit the snapping. It is best, however, to ask the patient to perform the maneuver

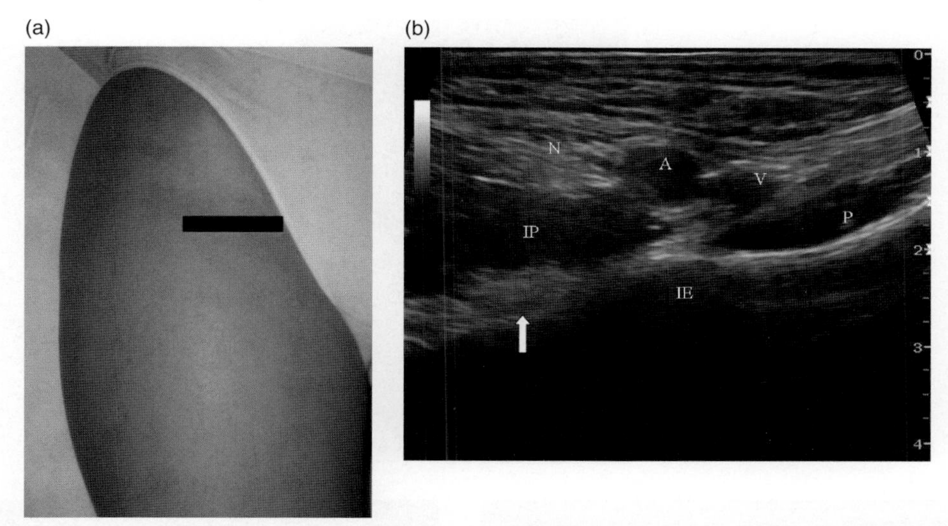

Figure 7.15. Femoral neurovascular bundle: **(a)** transverse ultrasound image and **(b)** transducer position. A, common femoral artery; V, common femoral vein; N, femoral nerve; IP, Iliopsoas; P, pectineus; IE, iliopectineal eminence; arrow, psoas tendon.

that reproduces the snapping. It generally involves extending a semiflexed and abducted hip. Dynamic imaging, often using extension and external rotation, can also be used to evaluate for internal snapping of the hip.[8] The transducer is placed transversely over the psoas tendon, taking great care to keep the iliopectineal eminence and the psoas tendon visualized at all times (Figure 7.15). Recent evidence contradicts initial reports of the tendon snapping over the iliopectineal eminence, and it is now thought that the tendon moves laterally and anteriorly over part of the iliacus muscle on hip flexion, abduction and external rotation.[9] On return to normal position there may be a sudden snap as the iliacus muscle releases the tendon.[9] When present, the iliopsoas tendon and muscle move abruptly with a palpable snap; it is advisable not to blink.

Femoral Triangle

Sometimes pathology involving the neurovascular structures of the femoral triangle can mimic hip pathology. The femoral vein, artery, and nerve can be identified in that order medial to lateral (Figure 7.15). On sonography, the femoral nerve is most easily seen in cross section and appears as several small, hypoechoic spaces, each surrounded by a hyperechoic thin rim. These are the individual nerve bundles encased in connective tissue. Lymph nodes can be identified adjacent to the neurovascular structures. Inflamed lymph nodes can be a source of groin pain.

Medial Structures

The patient is repositioned into the frog-lateral position, hip externally rotated and the knee flexed to 45°. The insertion of the iliopsoas tendon is best evaluated in this position. The pectineus, which lies medial to the palpable

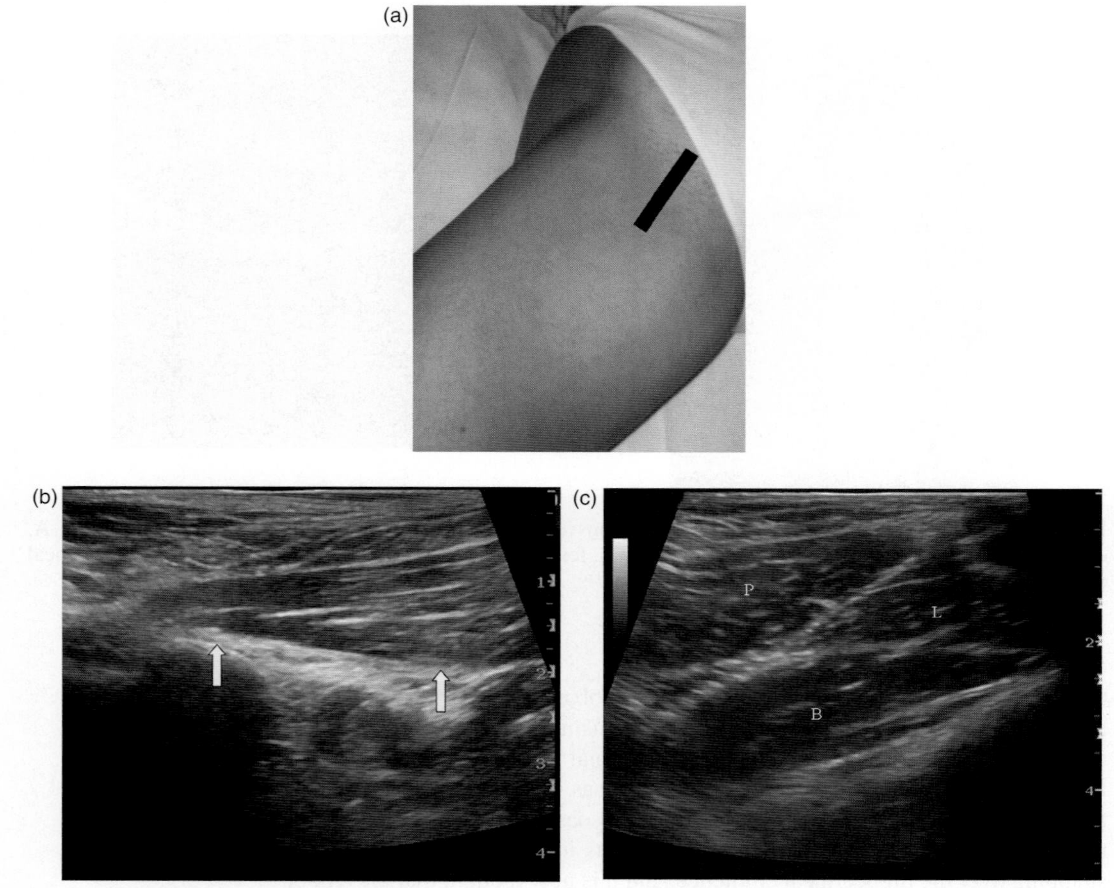

Figure 7.16. Pectineus muscle and tendon: **(a)** transducer position in the longitudinal plane, **(b)** corresponding ultrasound image of the pectineus (arrows) arising from the superior pubic ramus, and **(c)** transverse plane of the pectineus muscle belly. P, pectineus; L, adductor longus; B, adductor brevis.

pulsations of the common femoral artery, can be seen arising from the superior pubic ramus and is oriented inferiorly, laterally, and posteriorly to insert inferior to the lesser trochanter. The pectineus forms the floor of the femoral triangle (Figures 7.15 and 7.16). The evaluation of the gracilis and adductor tendons is described in detail in Chapter 8.

Lateral Structures

The patient is placed in the lateral decubitus position, symptomatic side up. Placing a pillow between the knees can increase patient comfort. The greater trochanter is the bony landmark of the lateral hip examination. The bony prominence of the greater trochanter is palpated. Place the transducer into a longitudinal plane with respect to the trochanter, which appears hyperechoic and rectangular with a somewhat irregular surface (Figure 7.17). There are a number of bursae that surround the greater trochanter and include the gluteus minimus, the gluteus medius anteriorly, and the gluteus maximus

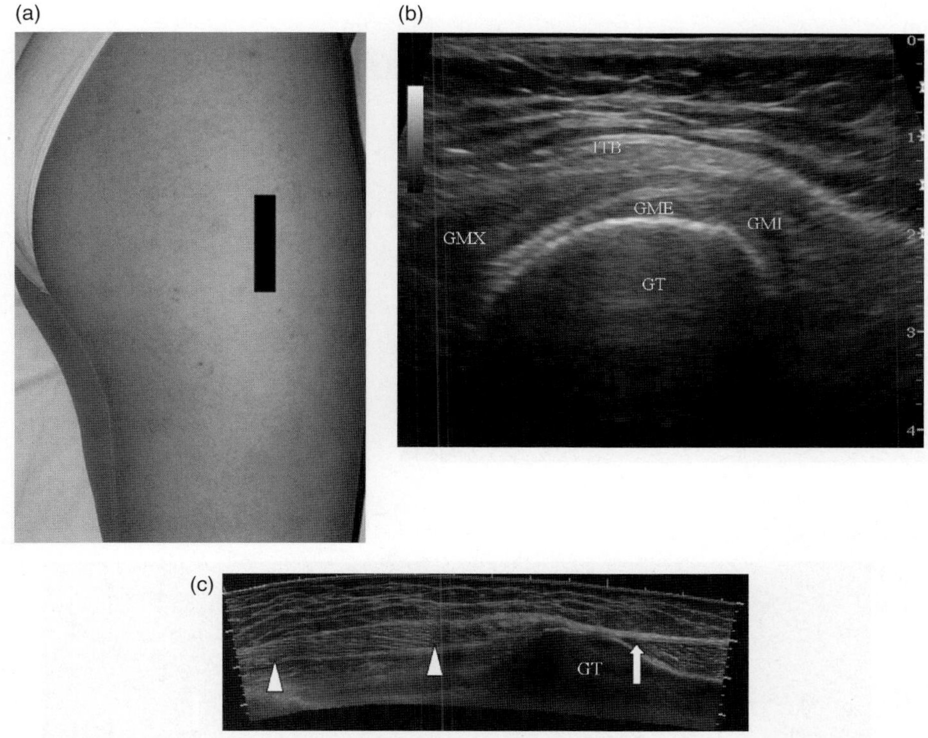

Figure 7.17. Greater trochanter: **(a)** transducer position in the coronal plane to the body and resulting **(b)** ultrasound image. **(c)** Longitudinal ultrasound image of the proximal iliotibial band (arrow) and tensor fascia lata (arrowhead). GT, greater trochanter; ITB, iliotibial band; GMX, gluteus maximus; GME, gluteus medius; GMI, gluteus minimus.

bursae posteriorly. Each is a potential space for fluid collection or thickening. The distal portion of the gluteus medius is seen at the level at which the iliotibial bands pass over the greater trochanter (Figure 7.17). Dynamic imaging with external rotation followed by extension may reveal a snapping gluteus maximus or iliotibial band over the greater trochanter.[9,10]

The gluteus maximus, medius, and minimus can be followed proximally from the greater trochanter to their individual origins (Figure 7.18). Their posteromedial components can also be assessed in the prone position. Detailed assessment may be limited due to patient habitus. The iliotibial band is seen as a hyperechoic band anterior to the greater trochanter. Once identified in the longitudinal plane it can be traced superiorly and slightly anteriorly (Figure 7.17c). The hypoechoic muscle of the tensor fasciae latae is enclosed in the hyperechoic fascia and can be traced proximally to its origin on the iliac crest.

Posterior Structures

The patient is placed prone with the legs and knees extended. The glutei can be assessed running obliquely and laterally to the greater trochanter for the gluteus minimus and medius, and the linea aspera in the case of

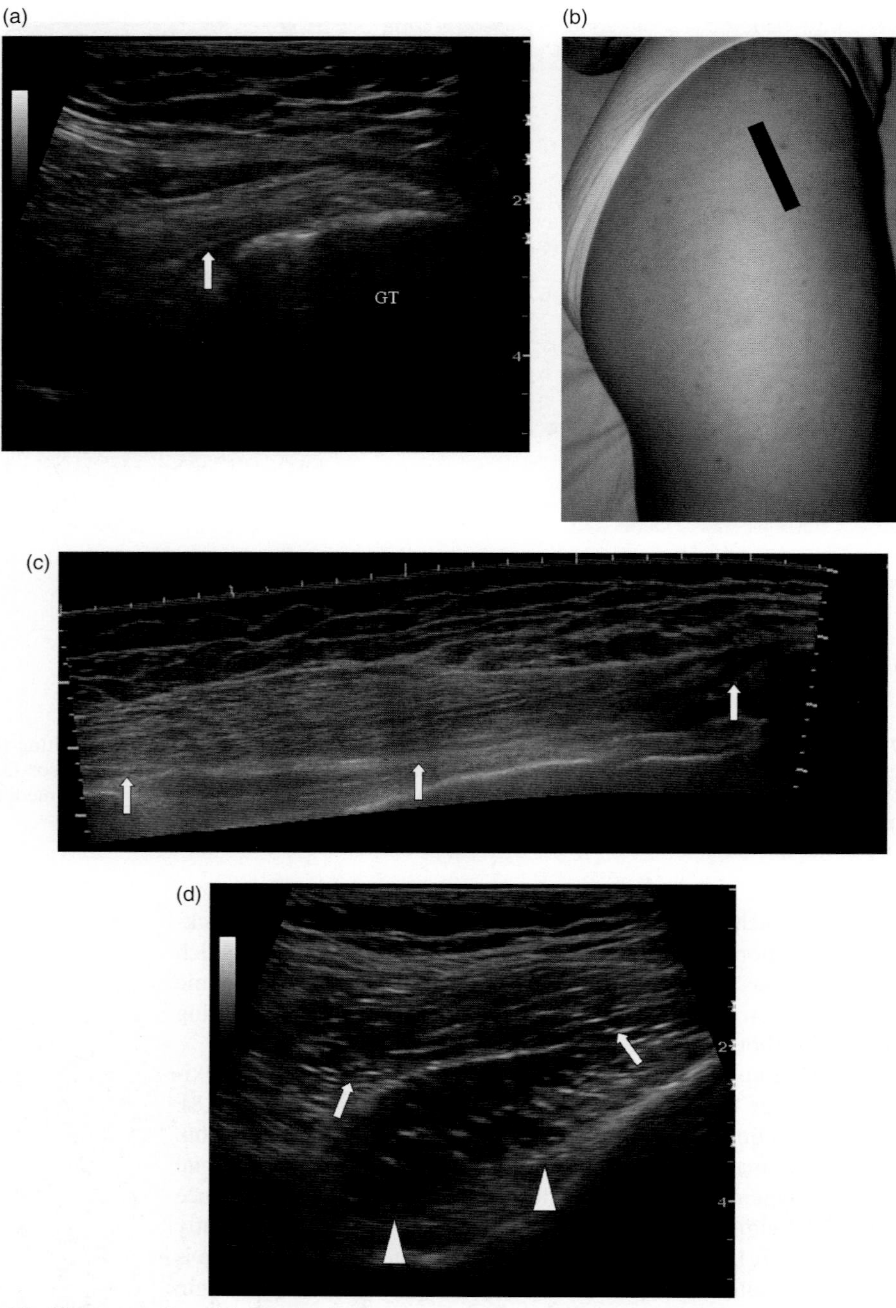

Figure 7.18. Gluteus medius. (**a**) Longitudinal ultrasound image of the gluteus medius (arrows) attachment to the greater trochanter (GT) and (**b**) corresponding transducer position. (**c**) Extended field of view ultrasound image of the gluteus medius muscle and tendon. (**d**) Transverse ultrasound image of the muscle belly of the gluteus medius superficial to that of the gluteus minimus.

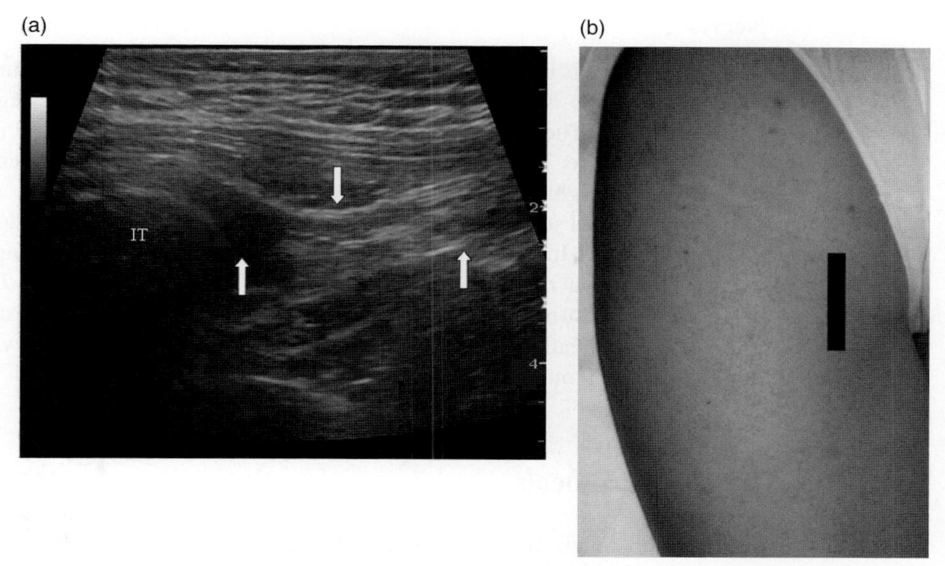

Figure 7.19. Ischial tuberosity (IT). (**a**) Longitudinal ultrasound image of the common tendon (arrows) of the biceps femoris and semitendinosus and corresponding (**b**) transducer position.

the gluteus maximus. The hamstrings, the long head of the biceps femoris, the semimembranosus, and semitendinosus arise from the ischial tuberosity (Figure 7.19). This is palpable as a bony prominence in the inferomedial aspect of the buttock as described in the surface anatomy section. The long head of the biceps femoris and the semitendinosus arise from a common tendon on the inferomedial aspect of the ischial tuberosity and the semimembranosus superolaterally. The tendons can be followed distally into the thigh as detailed in Chapter 8.

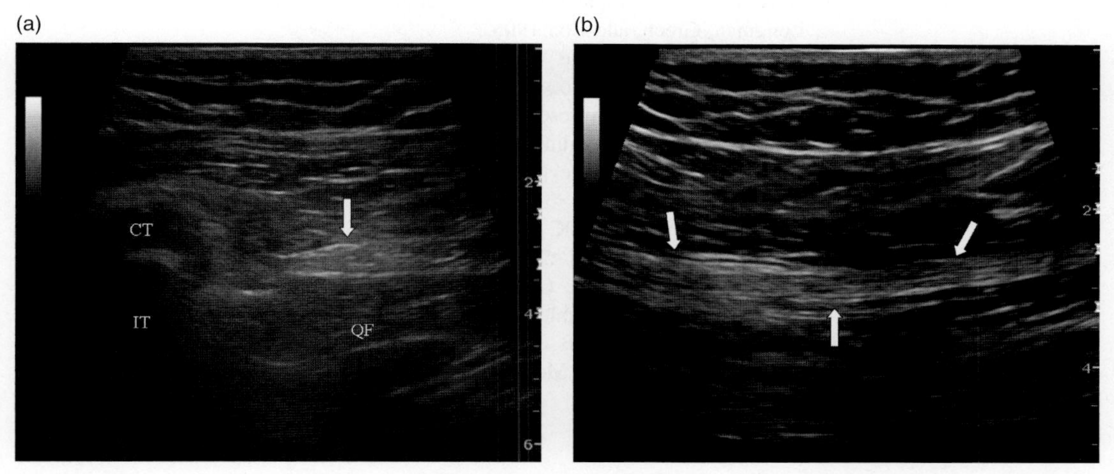

Figure 7.20. Sciatic nerve. (**a**) Transverse ultrasound image of the sciatic nerve (arrows) medial to the ischial tuberosity (IT) and origin of the common tendon (CT). QF, quadratus femoris. (**b**) Longitudinal ultrasound image of the sciatic nerve within the proximal thigh.

Nerves

The sciatic nerve is identified in the deep posterior hip, lateral to the hamstring attachment on the ischial trochanter. The patient is prone with the legs and knees extended. The sciatic nerve can be identified just lateral to the ischial trochanter (Figure 7.20a). The nerve runs between the superior gemellus muscle and the gluteus maximus. In cross section it appears as a multi-vesicular, rounded structure, with hypoechoic spaces surrounded by echogenic connective tissue. In the longitudinal plane, the nerve is tubular with multiple hyperechoic linear reflectors that run parallel to one another (Figure 7.20b). The hypoechoic structures between these lines are the actual nerve fascicles. The nerve is typically 5–9 mm in diameter. The femoral nerve was reviewed in the previous femoral triangle section.

Imaging Protocols

Examination of the hip is tailored to the area of concern and the adjacent compartments. It is important to evaluate structures adjacent to the site of the suspected abnormality as they may mimic hip-related pathology, for example, groin hernias, pathology of the lower rectus sheath. A large number of structures are not limited to the hip region and have proximal and distal extensions that may also be referred to the hip. The standard ultrasound imaging protocol is summarized in the Appendix.

References

1. Cho KH, Park BH, Yeon KM. Ultrasound of the adult hip. Semin Ultrasound CT MRI 2000;21(3):214–230.
2. Gray H. The Complete Gray's Anatomy, 16th ed, pp. 300–321. London: Longman, Green, and Co., 1905.
3. Snell R. The lower limb. In: Clinical Anatomy, 7th ed., pp. 704–706. Philadelphia: Lippincott Williams & Wilkins, 2004.
4. Gray H. The Complete Gray's Anatomy, 16th ed., pp. 540–558. London: Longman, Green, and Co., 1905.
5. Gray H. The Complete Gray's Anatomy, 16th ed., pp. 397–402. London: Longman, Green, and Co., 1905.
6. Adler RS, Buly R, Ambrose R et al. Diagnostic and therapeutic use of sonography-guided iliopsoas peritendinous injections. AJR 2005;185:940–943.
7. Blankenbaker DG, Tuite MJ. The painful hip: New concepts. Skeletal Radiol 2006;35:352–370.
8. Cardinal E, Buckwalter K, Capello W et al. US of the snapping iliopsoas tendon. Radiology 1996;198:521–522.
9. Deslandes M, Guillin R, Cardinal E et al. The snapping iliopsoas tendon: New mechanisms using dynamic ultrasound. AJR 2008;190:576.
10. Choi Y, Lee S, Song B et al. Dynamic sonography of external snapping hip syndrome. J Ultrasound Med 2002;21:753–758.

8

The Adult Thigh

John O'Neill and Gandikota Girish

The thigh region is more commonly evaluated as an extension of a study involving the adjacent joints, the hip and knee. Occasionally an examination will be dedicated to the thigh, which extends between the hip and knee joints, usually in the evaluation of a soft tissue mass, muscle, or tendon injury. One particular advantage of ultrasound in this region, given the large area involved, is the ability to localize the site of symptoms and then trace the pathology proximally or distally in real time. In addition, as this is a relatively uncommon region to study, direct comparison with the contralateral side can be very helpful in delineating normal anatomy from pathology. Ultrasound evaluation can be limited by patient habitus and depth of pathology.

Clinical Indications

Tendons can be affected by a wide array of pathology including tendonopathy, partial and complete tears, and avulsions. The parent muscle may be affected by hematomas; partial or complete posttraumatic tears; muscle hernias, which may be only intermittent; or intramuscular masses. Intramuscular masses should be assessed for cystic versus solid components, intralesional and perilesional flow on Doppler, and dynamic changes with contracture muscle, including changes in hemodynamics and the relationship to the surrounding neurovascular bundles. In addition, ultrasound can guide biopsy to the most appropriate solid component, thereby avoiding significant vessels. In general, all biopsies should be performed in consultation with a surgeon and should avoid routes through adjacent compartments.

An inflamed bursa, particularly around the greater trochanter, can be a common site of symptoms. This is often associated with tendonosis or a partial tear of the adjacent glutei tendons. In addition, this is also the location for one of the causes of snapping hip where the iliotibial band and/or gluteus maximus snaps across the greater tuberosity. Fluid collections, including hematomas and abscesses, can involve any compartment. Musculoskeletal infections that can be assessed with ultrasound include pyomyositis, soft tissue abscess, infective tenosynovitis and bursitis, osteomyelitis, and septic arthritis and necrotizing fasciitis.[1]

The femur lies deep, and a detailed review depends on patient habitus. We occasionally use ultrasound in the assessment of orthopedic hardware with suspected superimposed infection and evaluate for surrounding fluid collections. If present, they can be aspirated under ultrasound guidance. Other interventional procedures include soft tissue mass or bone biopsy. The latter usually requires cortical involvement to localize the appropriate site. All biopsies of masses should be in consultation with a surgeon.

The sciatic nerve is the dominant nerve within the thigh and is amenable for assessment of local pathology including neuropathy, entrapment, and primary lesions such as neuromas.

Technical Review

The choice of ultrasound transducer will depend on the region being evaluated and the habitus of the patient. In general, the transducer is chosen that will offer the highest resolution at the depth of the structure being evaluated. This may be a linear multifrequency 9- to15-MHz transducer for superficial structures such as the quadriceps tendon; deep structures may require a curvilinear 5-MHz transducer. A combination of probes can be used if required to perform the study. Structures are evaluated in orthogonal planes.

Anatomy

There is significant overlap of anatomy between the thigh and that of the hip and knee regions as detailed in Chapters 7 and 9, respectively. For the most part we will try and prevent repetition, but a certain amount is required to convey a full anatomical description.

Surface Anatomy

The surface landmarks of the proximal thigh and hip, as well as the knee, have been detailed in Chapters 7 and 9, respectively. The greater trochanter of the femur is palpable as a prominent eminence along the posterolateral aspect of the proximal thigh. The anterior group of muscles, the quadriceps femoris, forms the prominent muscle bulk over the anterior surface of the thigh. The rectus femoris forms the anterior border of the proximal and mid thigh and extends distally as the palpable quadriceps tendon. The vastus medialis and lateralis form the smooth soft tissue contour to the medial and lateral aspects of the anterior thigh, respectively (Figure 8.1a).

The femoral triangle has been described in Chapter 7. Distal to the apex of this triangle is the adductor canal. This is also known as the subsartorial canal; the sartorius forms its roof. It is bounded laterally by the vastus medialis and posteriorly by the adductor longus and magnus. The adductor muscles can be seen as a soft tissue contour on the medial side of the proximal thigh. The iliotibial tract forms a groove on the anterolateral aspect of the thigh, extending from the iliac crest to the proximal end of the tibia, when the thigh is extended. Posteriorly, the upper thigh is covered by the gluteus maximus, with the contours of the adductor magnus and the iliotibial tract forming the medial and lateral boundaries, respectively. The gluteal fold lies transversely at the lower level of the buttock. The ischial tuberosity can be palpated at

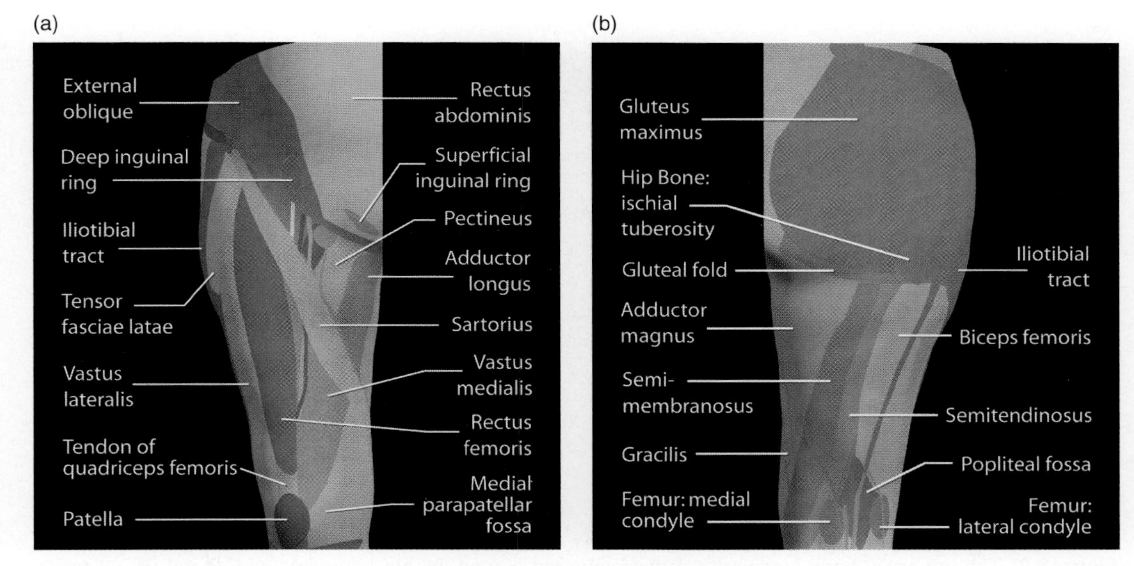

Figure 8.1. Surface anatomy of the thigh: **(a)** anterior and **(b)** posterior views.

the inner and lower portion of the buttock just proximal to the gluteal fold. Distally within the popliteal fossa, the lateral border is formed by the biceps femoris, palpated as a taut tendon in the semiflexed knee, and the medial border by the semitendinous and semimembranosus tendons (Figure 8.1b).

Bones

Femur

The anatomy of the proximal and distal femur is detailed in Chapter 7 (the hip) and Chapter 9 (the knee). We will concentrate here on the shaft of the femur. The femur is the single bone of the thigh and the largest bone in the body. The proximal femur is composed of a head, neck, and the greater and lesser tuberosities at the junction of the neck and shaft (Figure 8.2a). The shaft of the femur is almost cylindrical, narrowing toward its center and becoming flattened distally.[2] It has three borders—the linea aspera and two lateral borders—and three surfaces—anterior, internal, and external. The shaft is generally smooth except for the posterior border, the linea aspera (Figure 8.2b). This is a prominent, longitudinal ridge within the mid-shaft with an internal and external lip. Superiorly, the linea aspera diverges into three ridges that extend to the greater and lesser tuberosities, and to the spiral line of the femur.[2] Distally the linea aspera also diverges out, in this case forming two ridges: the medial and lateral supracondylar ridges. The two lateral borders extend from the greater and lesser trochanters to the anterior aspects of the medial and lateral condyles.

Distally the femur forms into two large condyles, medial and lateral, with a smooth intervening depression anteriorly and the trochlea and the large intercondylar notch posteriorly. The femur articulates with the patella anteriorly and the tibia inferiorly as outlined in Chapter 9.

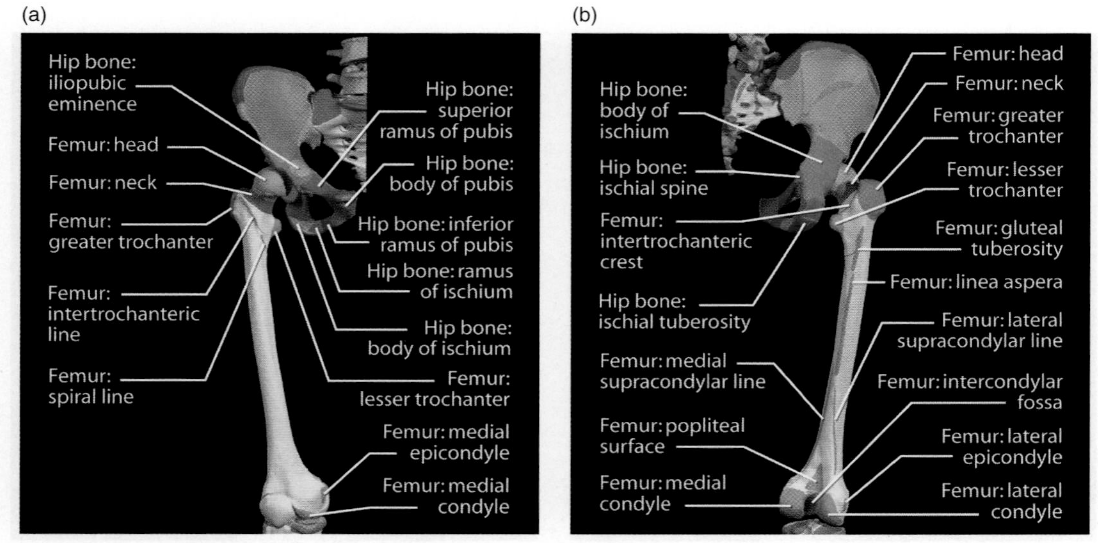

Figure 8.2. The important bony landmarks of the femur and around the hip joint: (**a**) anterior and (**b**) posterior views.

> **Insider Information 8.1**
> The femur has three borders—the linea aspera and two lateral borders—and three surfaces—anterior, internal, and external.

Fascia and Compartments

The deep fascia of the thigh, the fascia lata, is extensive and encloses the muscles of the thigh. It is of variable thickness, being thicker superolaterally and around the knee. It attaches superiorly and inferiorly to a large array of bony prominences. It encloses two muscles: the tensor fascia lata and the gluteus maximus.[3] From its deep surface, two intermuscular septa emerge, the thin medial and the stronger lateral septa, which insert onto the linea aspera and its superior and inferior extensions. The medial septum separates the anterior and medial compartments; the lateral septum separates the anterior and posterior compartments. A smaller septum, the posteromedial intermuscular septum, separates the medial and posterior compartments. These septae also serve as sites of partial origin to adjacent musculature.[3]

> **Insider Information 8.2**
> Two main intermuscular septa extend inward from the deep fascia of the thigh—the medial and the lateral septa—and separate the anterior and medial compartments and the anterior and posterior compartments, respectively. A smaller septum, the posteromedial intermuscular septum, separates the medial and posterior compartments.

Muscles and Tendons

Muscles of the thigh are subdivided into groups: the anterior group, medial group, posterior group, and gluteal group (Table 8.1). The gluteal group exists

Table 8.1. Muscles of the Hip and Thigh.

Anterior group	Medial group	Posterior group	Gluteal/lateral group
Sartorius[a]	Iliopsoas	Biceps femoris[a]	Gluteus maximus
Rectus femoris[a]	Pectineus	Semitendinosus[a]	Gluteus medius
Vastus lateralis[a]	Gracilis[a]	Semimembranosus[a]	Gluteus minimus
Vastus intermedius[a]	Adductor longus[a]		Piriformis
Vastus medialis[a]	Adductor brevis[a]		Tensor fascia lata[a]
	Adductor magnus[a]		Iliotibial band[a]
			Gemellus superior
			Gemellus inferior
			Obturator externus
			Obturator internus
			Quadratus femoris

[a] Denotes those muscles detailed in this chapter.

essentially at the level of the hip joint and is reviewed in Chapter 7. The origin, insertion, and action of the different muscles and tendons are summarized in Table 8.2 and Figure 8.3.

Anterior Group

The anterior group of muscles includes the sartorius and the quadriceps femoris.[3] The quadriceps femoris consists of four muscles: the rectus femoris, vastus lateralis, vastus intermedius, and vastus medialis (Figures 8.4a and 8.5). These muscles form the soft tissue contour of the anterior surface of the thigh. The sartorius is a strap-shaped, band-like muscle that arises from the anterior superior iliac spine and passes obliquely across the thigh from lateral to medial to insert over the upper inner surface of the proximal tibia as a broad aponeurosis. This insertion is anterior to the insertion sites of the remainder of the pes anserinus, the gracilis and semitendinous tendons, with which it partly blends. The rectus femoris is the most superficial muscle of the quadriceps femoris, arising from two heads: the straight head and the reflected head. This muscle lies in the midline superficial to the vastus intermedius.

The vastus intermedius, as its name implies, lies between the vastus lateralis and vastus medialis and lies deep to the rectus femoris. Its musculotendinous origin is distal to the rectus femoris and forms the deeper portion of the quadriceps tendon in the midline. These two components are separable by ultrasound almost to the point of insertion onto the patella. The vastus lateralis originates from a broad aponeurosis and is the largest among the quadriceps femoris. The muscle mass ultimately forms a flat tendon that inserts on the lateral border of the patella and contributes to the formation of the quadriceps tendon. Some of its fibers also blend with the knee joint capsule and iliotibial tract. The vastus medialis distally forms an aponeurosis inserting on to the medial aspect of the patella with fibers contributing to the quadriceps tendon.[3] The quadriceps tendon, formed by the union of the aponeuroses of four muscles of the quadriceps group, contains the largest sesamoid bone of the

Table 8.2. Muscles of the Hip and Thigh: Origin, Insertion, and Main Actions.

Muscle	Origin	Insertion	Action
Anterior group			
Sartorius	Anterior superior iliac spine	Proximal medial shaft of tibia (pes anserinus)	Hip—flexion, abduction, and lateral rotation of thigh Knee—flexion of leg
Rectus femoris	Straight head—anterior inferior iliac spine Reflected head—ilium above acetabular rim	Patella—via quadriceps tendon and patellar ligament to tibial tuberosity	Knee—extension Hip—flexion of thigh
Vastus lateralis	Proximal portion of intertrochanteric line, greater trochanter, lateral aspects of linea aspera, supracondylar ridge, and intermuscular septum	Patella—via quadriceps tendon and patellar ligament to tibial tuberosity	Knee—leg extension
Vastus intermedius	Shaft of femur—anterior and lateral portion above condyles	Patella—via quadriceps tendon and patellar ligament to tibial tuberosity	Knee—leg extension
Vastus medialis	Distal portion of intertrochanteric line, spiral line, medial aspect of linea aspera and intermuscular septum	Patella—via quadriceps tendon and patellar ligament to tibial tuberosity	Knee—leg extension and stabilization of patella
Medial group			
Gracilis	Body and inferior Ramus pubis	Proximal medial shaft of tibia (pes anserinus)	Hip—adduction of thigh Knee—flexion of leg and medial rotation
Pectineus	Pubis—pectineal line and superior part of ramus	Pectineal line inferior to lesser trochanter	Hip—flexion, Adduction, and medial rotation of thigh
Adductor longus	Body of pubis—inferior to pubic crest	Linea aspera—middle third	Hip—adduction of thigh
Adductor brevis	Pubis—body and inferior ramus	Linea aspera—upper third and pectineal line	Hip—adduction of thigh
Adductor magnus	Adductor portion—ischiopubic ramus Hamstring portion—ischial Tuberosity—inferior and lateral quadrant	Adductor portion—linea aspera, gluteal tuberosity Hamstring portion—adductor tubercle	Adductor portion—adduction and medial rotation of thigh Hamstring portion—extension of thigh
Posterior group			
Semitendinosus	Ischial tuberosity—upper inner quadrant	Proximal medial shaft of tibia (pes anserinus)	Extension of thigh, flexion and medial rotation of knee

Semimembranosus	Ischial tuberosity—upper outer quadrant	Medial condyle of tibia, fascia over popliteus and oblique popliteal ligament	Extension of thigh, flexion and medial rotation of knee
Biceps femoris	Long head—ischial tuberosity (upper and inner quadrant) Short head—lateral aspect of supracondylar ridge of femur, linea aspera middle third	Styloid process of head of fibula, lateral tibial condyle and lateral collateral ligament	Extension of thigh, flexion and lateral rotation of leg
Gluteal			
Gluteus maximus	Ilium—posterior to gluteal line, iliac crest, sacrum—lateral mass, sacrotuberous ligament and coccyx	Iliotibial tract and gluteal tuberosity of femur	Hip—extension and external rotation Knee actions are via iliotibial tract
Gluteus medius	Ilium between posterior and anterior gluteal lines	Greater trochanter—posterolateral surface	Hip—abduction and medial rotation
Gluteus minimus	Ilium between anterior and inferior gluteal lines	Greater trochanter—anterior surface	Hip—abduction and medial rotation
Tensor fascia latae	Anterior iliac crest, anterior superior iliac spine	Iliotibial band	Hip—abduction, medial rotation, and flexion of thigh Knee—assists gluteus maximus in maintaining knee extension
Iliotibial band	Fascia lata, tensor fascia latae	Gerdy's tubercle tibia	Hip—flexion, Abduction, and medial rotation Knee—lateral stabilization
Obturator externus	Obturator membrane—outer surface and adjacent pubis and ischium	Greater trochanter—trochanteric fossa along the medial surface	Hip—lateral rotation
Obturator internus	Inner surface obturator membrane, ischiopubi crami	Greater trochanter—medial surface	Hip—lateral rotation, abduction of thigh and stabilization
Piriformis	Sacrum-2,3,4 costotransverse bars and greater sciatic notch	Greater trochanter—superior border	Hip—lateral rotation of thigh and stabilization
Gemellus superior	Ischial spine	Greater trochanter—medial surface	Hip—lateral rotation and stabilization
Gemellus inferior	Ischial tuberosity—upper border	Greater trochanter— medial surface	Hip—lateral rotation and stabilization
Quadratus femoris	Ischial tuberosity—lateral surface	Quadrate tubercle of femur	Hip—lateral rotation and stabilization

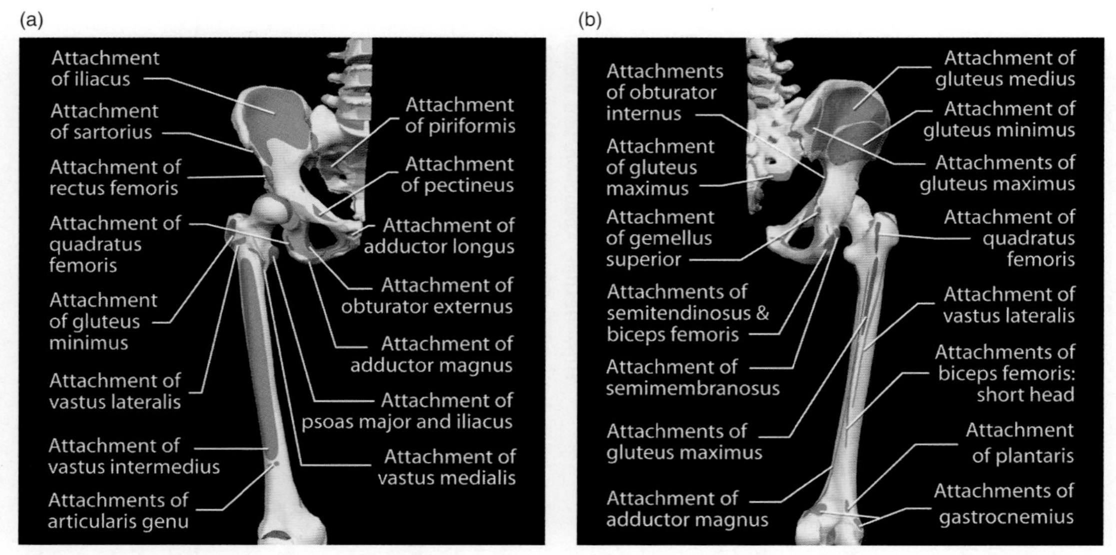

Figure 8.3. The muscle origin (red) and insertion (blue) points of the muscles of the thigh: (**a**) anterior and (**b**) posterior views.

body—the patella, or knee cap—before inserting into the tibial tuberosity via the patellar tendor.

Medial Group

The medial group, the adductors of the thigh, is composed of the gracilis, pectineus, and adductor longus, brevis, and magnus muscles (Figures 8.3a, 8.4b and 8.5). The gracilis has a flat, thin bandlike origin from the inferior pubic ramus and medial aspect of the body of the pubis, and passes straight

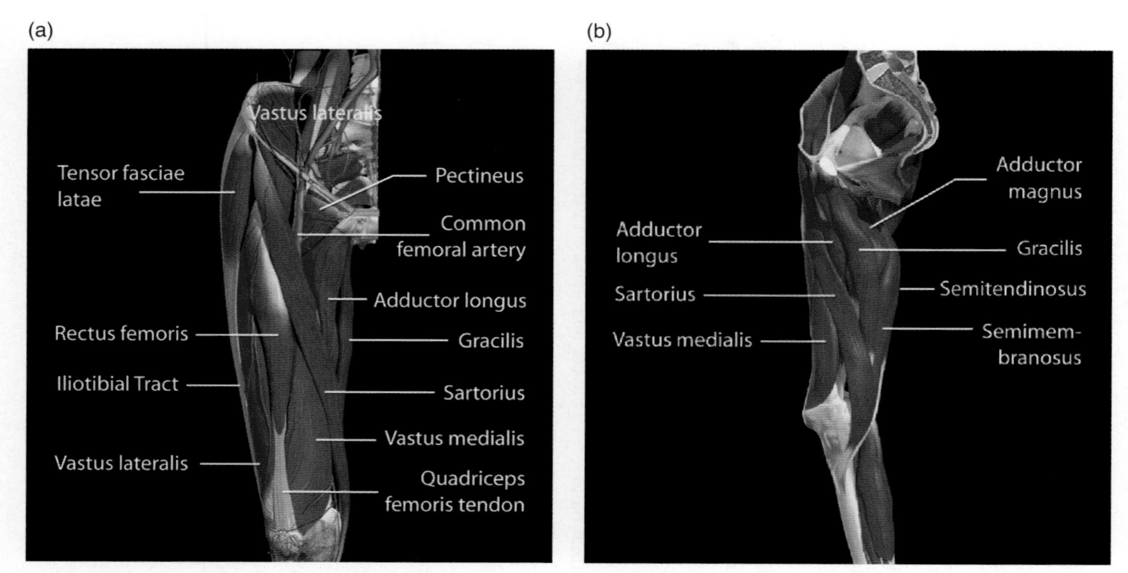

Figure 8.4. The muscles of the thigh: (**a**) anterior, (**b**) medial.

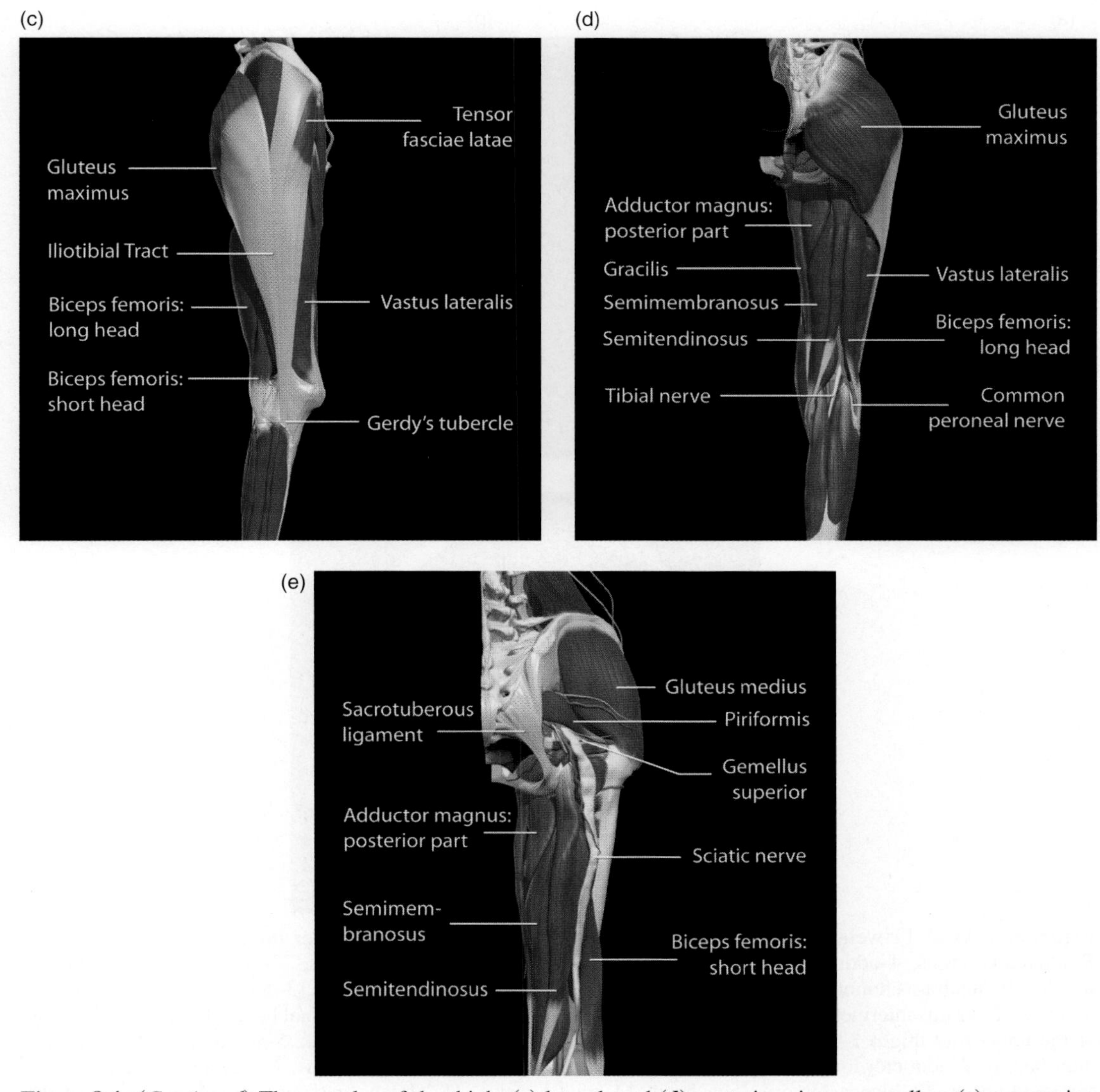

Figure 8.4. (*Continued*) The muscles of the thigh: **(c)** lateral, and **(d)** posterior views, as well as **(e)** a posterior view with the gluteus maximus removed.

down the medial aspect of the thigh. It takes a curve at the medial condyle of the tibia to insert into the medial aspect of the proximal shaft of the tibia, forming part of the pes anserinus. The insertion of the gracilis is overlapped by the sartorius, while it is overlapped by the semitendinous tendon, thus forming an appearance of a bird's foot, termed the pes anserinus. The pectineus is a quadrangular muscle forming the floor of the femoral triangle. This is reviewed in Chapter 7.

Among the three adductors, the adductor longus is the most anterior and superficial; it arises from the body of the pubis just medial to the pubic tubercle as a thin tendon and forms a broad, fleshy belly.[3] It inserts along the linea aspera between and blending with the vastus medialis and adductor

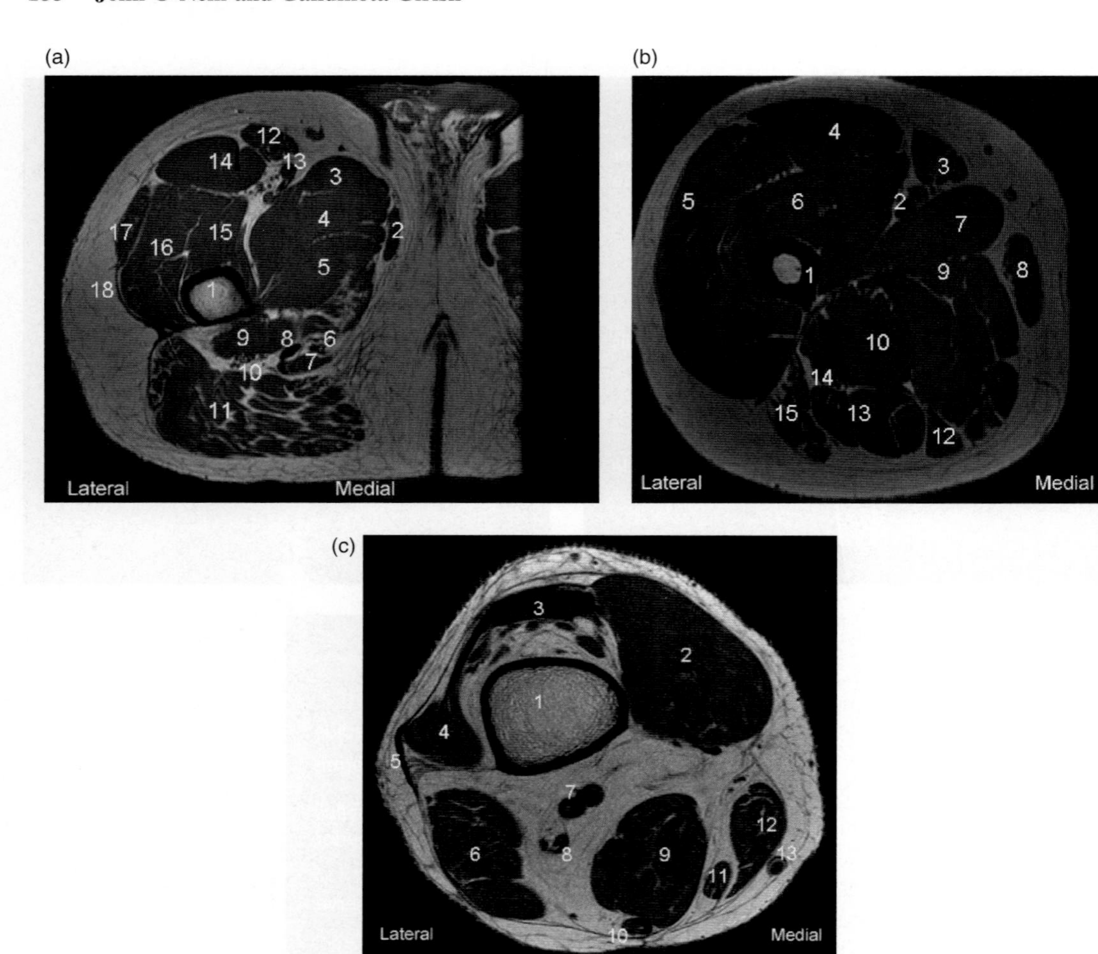

Figure 8.5. Axial T1-weighted MRI anatomy. (**a**) Axial at the level of the upper thigh: 1–femur, 2–gracilis, 3–adductor longus, 4–adductor brevis, 5–adductor magnus, 6–semimembranosus, 7–semitendinosus, 8–biceps femoris, 9–quadratus femoris, 10–sciatic nerve, 11–gluteus maximus, 12–sartorius, 13–femoral vessels, 14–rectus femoris, 15–vastus intermedius, 16–vastus lateralis, 17–tensor fascia lata, 18–iliotibial band. (**b**) Axial at the level of the upper/mid thigh: 1–femur, 2–femoral vessels, 3–sartorius, 4–rectus femoris, 5–vastus lateralis, 6–vastus intermedius, 7–adductor longus, 8–gracilis, 9–adductor brevis, 10–adductor magnus, 11–semimembranosus, 12–semitendinosus, 13–biceps femoris long head, 14–sciatic nerve, 15–gluteus maximus. (**c**) Axial image of the distal thigh: 1–femur, 2–vastus medialis, 3–quadriceps tendon, 4–vastus lateralis, 5–iliotibial tract, 6–biceps femoris, 7–popliteal vessels, 8–sciatic nerve, 9–semimembranosus, 10–semitendinosus, 11–gracilis, 12–sartorius, 13–greater saphenous vein.

magnus. Deep to it lies the adductor brevis, which runs down posterior to the longus and inserts on the upper third of the femur. The adductor magnus, as its name implies, is a large muscle, triangular in appearance. Its fibers from the ischial ramus insert into the linea aspera and on the medial supracondylar line proximally. The medial portion arising from the ischial tuberosity is also known as the hamstring portion of the adductor magnus, which inserts on the adductor tubercle along the medial condyle of the femur. There are four osseoaponeurotic openings forming tendinous arches for the passage of vessels. The largest provides passage for the femoral vessels, between the adductor canal and the popliteal space.[3]

Posterior Group

The posterior group of muscles is better known as the hamstring muscles of the thigh and constitutes the biceps femoris, semitendinosus, and semimembranosus muscles (Figures 8.4d and e, and 8.5).

The biceps femoris has two heads of origin. The long head forms a common tendon with the semitendinosus and arises from the upper medial surface of the ischial tuberosity. The long head continues as a muscle belly, which lies superficial to the sciatic nerve, with the majority of its fibers extending laterally to attach to the head of the fibula. The few remaining fibers attach to the lateral tibial condyle and the lateral collateral ligament. Just prior to the attachment, the biceps forms a conjoint tendon with the distal component of the lateral collateral ligament. The short head originates from the middle third portion of linea aspera and extends distally to join the aponeurosis of the muscle belly of the long head.

The semitendinosus forms a common tendon with the biceps femoris at its origin. It forms a fusiform muscle belly that gives rise to the distal tendon at the level of the mid thigh. This long tendon runs superficial to the semimembranosus muscle, passes around the medial condyle of the tibia and over the tibial collateral ligament, and finally inserts on the medial surface of the upper portion of the shaft of the tibia, forming a part of the pes anserinus attachment.

The semimembranosus arises as a long flat membranous tendon, hence the name, from the upper and lateral surface of the ischial tuberosity.[3] Immediately after its origin, the tendon runs medially, passing inferior to the common tendon of the semitendinosus and biceps femoris where some of the fibers intermingle with the common tendon. The proximal myotendinous junction is at the level of the mid thigh. Distally the main component of the tendon inserts at the tubercle on the posterior medial tibial condyle, and the remaining fibers attach to the oblique popliteal ligament, the medial margin of the tibia behind the tibial collateral ligament, and the fascia over the popliteus.

Gluteal/Lateral Group

The tensor fasciae latae originates from the outer surface of the anterior iliac crest, the anterior superior iliac spine, and the deep surface of fascia lata, and inserts—at the level of the middle and upper third of the thigh—between the two layers of the fascia lata. The fascia is then continued distally as the iliotibial band, a thin superficial structure that inserts on Gerdy's tubercle along the lateral condyle of the tibia (Figure 8.4a and c).[3] The gluteal/lateral group also comprises gluteal muscles: the maximus, medius, and minimus, piriformis, gemellus superior, gemellus inferior, obturator externus, obturator internus, and quadratus femoris (Table 8.2). This group has been reviewed in detail in Chapter 7.

Bursae

The bursae of the thigh are limited to the greater trochanteric and knee regions and are reviewed in Chapters 7 and 9.

Nerves

The femoral nerve has just entered the anterior thigh, under the inguinal ligament and lateral to the femoral artery, when it divides into superficial and deep branches. The deep branches supply the components of the quadriceps. The saphenous nerve is its main cutaneous branch.[4] The adductor compartment is supplied by the obturator nerve, which divides in the obturator notch into anterior and posterior branches. These branches are small and not clearly discernible on ultrasound.

The sciatic nerve passes lateral to the ischial tuberosity and proceeds distally into the posterior or hamstring compartment of the thigh, which it supplies (Figure 8.4d and e).

The proximal and distal portions are described in Chapters 7, 9, and 12. The distal bifurcation into the common peroneal and tibial nerve is usually within the posterior aspect of the lower one-third of the leg, but may occur as far proximal as the pelvis. The posterior cutaneous nerve exits the pelvis medial to the sciatic nerve, which it crosses, and extends distally superficial to the hamstring muscles. Again this nerve is difficult to fully visualize on ultrasound.

Technique

Ultrasound of the thigh is divided into anterior, medial, posterior, gluteal, and lateral approaches (Table 8.3). The examination involves the region of symptoms. Often the examination is an extension from the hip or knee study. As stated throughout this book, a brief pertinent clinical history should be obtained before the study. Patients can often localize the site of symptoms and indicate if there have been any changes since they were last seen by the referring clinician. They can often describe and reproduce movements responsible for symptoms.

First, ensure patient comfort and correct positioning. Knowledge of the surface anatomy and the use of bony landmarks can provide a structured reproducible approach. Structures should always be evaluated in their orthogonal planes. Obtaining images with an extended field of view will allow a full appreciation of the anatomy and pathology and may be particularly useful when reviewing the case at a later time with the referring clinician. The

Table 8.3. Muscle Groups and Position for Ultrasound Examination[a].

Muscle group	Position of ultrasound study	Muscle group	Position of ultrasound study
Anterior group	Supine, with toes approximating each other	*Posterior group*	Prone, leg extended
Medial group	Supine, leg externally rotated and abducted	*Gluteal/lateral group*	Lateral decubitus, straight leg

[a]Tendons extending to the knee may require repositioning for the evaluation of their distal components, as detailed in Table 9.3.

examination of structures as they extend about the knee or thigh is further detailed in the appropriate chapters.

Insider Information 8.3
A structured reproducible approach to an ultrasound study is aided by knowledge of the surface anatomy and the use of bony landmarks.

Anterior

The patient lies supine with the hip extended and mild flexion of the knee. The patella is palpable over the anterior aspect of the knee joint and is a good bony landmark for ultrasound evaluation of the anterior aspect of the thigh. The quadriceps tendon inserts onto the superior border of the patella (Figure 8.6). Place the transducer in the longitudinal plane of the quadriceps tendon, which is seen as a thick hyperechoic band. This is then traced proximally into the lower thigh where first the musculotendinous junction of the vastus intermedius is seen, deep to the rectus femoris tendon and superficial to the hyperechoic femoral cortex (Figure 8.7). The vastus intermedius muscle appears as a thick, hypoechoic structure on the anterior and lateral aspect of the femur. Often the two separate tendons of the rectus femoris and vastus intermedius can be followed distally, with a hyperechoic plane representing the tendinous fibers from the vastus medialis and lateralis, separating the tendons, close to the point of joint insertion, which gives the tendon a trilaminar appearance.[5] The rectus femoris musculotendinous junction lies slightly more proximally.

The vastus medialis and lateralis lie medially and laterally, respectively. Place the transducer in a sagittal oblique orientation on the medial aspect of the proximal patella. The hyperechoic aponeurosis of the vastus medialis is

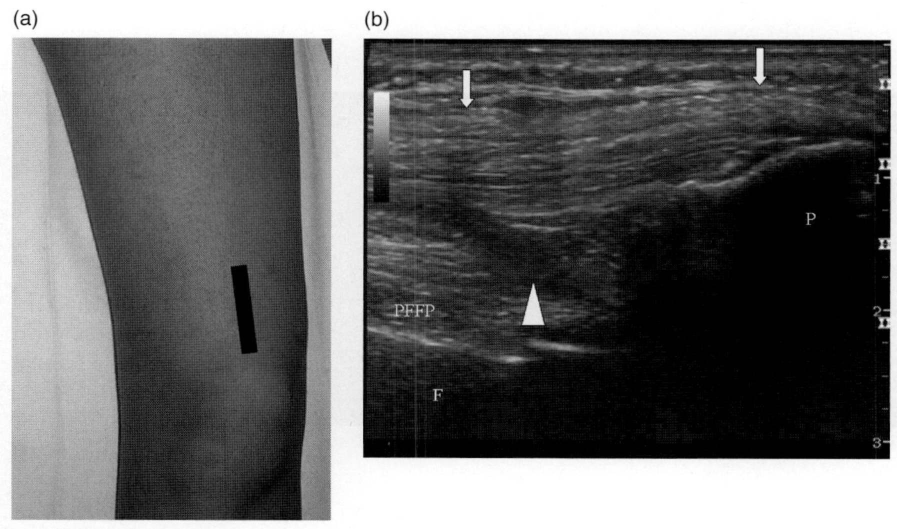

Figure 8.6. Quadriceps tendon: **(a)** transducer placement and **(b)** corresponding ultrasound image in the longitudinal axis of the quadriceps tendon (arrows), suprapatellar recess (arrowhead). P, patella; F, femur; PFFP, prefemoral fat pad.

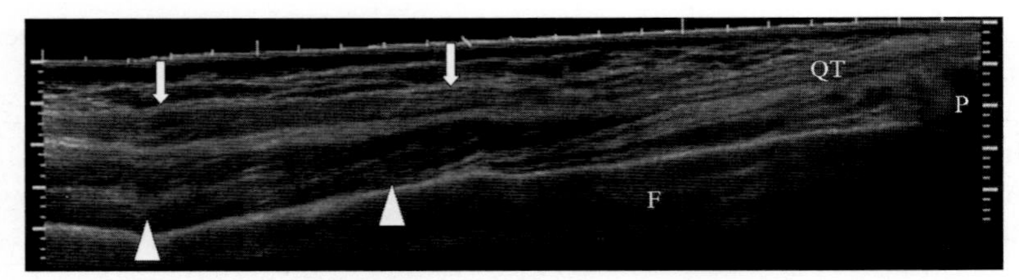

Figure 8.7. Rectus femoris tendon (arrows) and vastus intermedius muscle (arrowheads): longitudinal, extended field of view ultrasound image of the distal anterior thigh. Note that the rectus femoris is the first to form its tendon. P, patella; F, femur; QT, quadriceps tendon.

identified inserting into the medial aspect of the patella with some of its fibers also contributing to the quadriceps tendon (Figure 8.8). The same technique is repeated for the vastus lateralis. Once the tendons are correctly identified, they can be traced proximally to the appropriate muscle bellies in orthogonal planes.

> **Insider Information 8.4**
> The quadriceps tendon has a trilaminar appearance formed, superficial to deep, by the rectus femoris tendon, the vastus medialis and lateralis uniting in the midline and posteriorly, and the vastus intermedius tendon.

Medial

The pubis is an important landmark when assessing the medial hip joint. The pubic bone provides the origin for the adductors of the hip and is often the site of sports-related groin injury involving the proximal adductor attachment. More distally, the adductor insertion avulsion syndrome can be

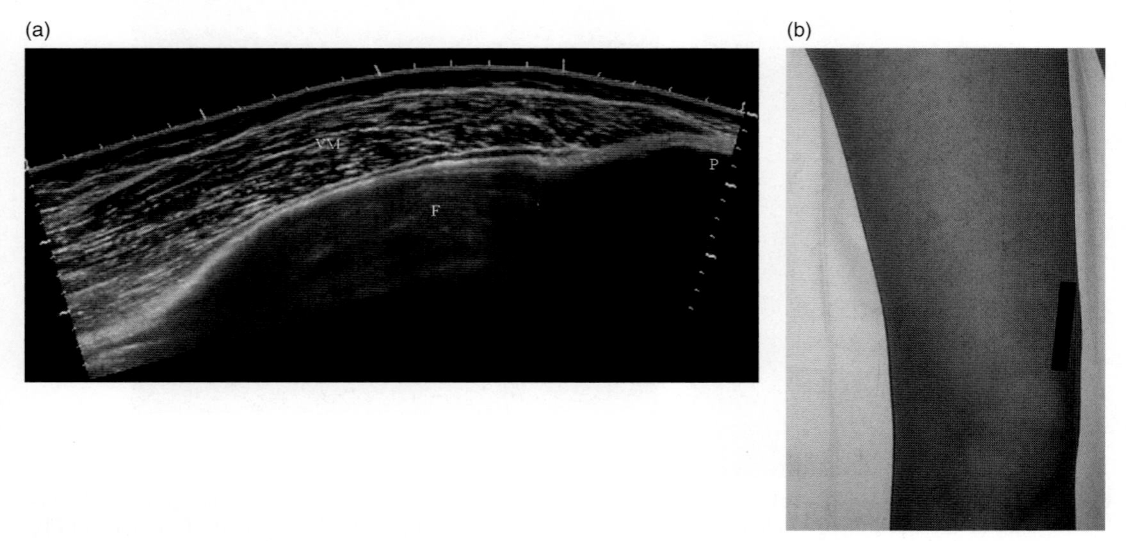

Figure 8.8. Vastus medialis (VM): **(a)** extended field of view ultrasound image in the longitudinal axis of the vastus medialis and **(b)** its corresponding transducer position. P, patella; F, femur.

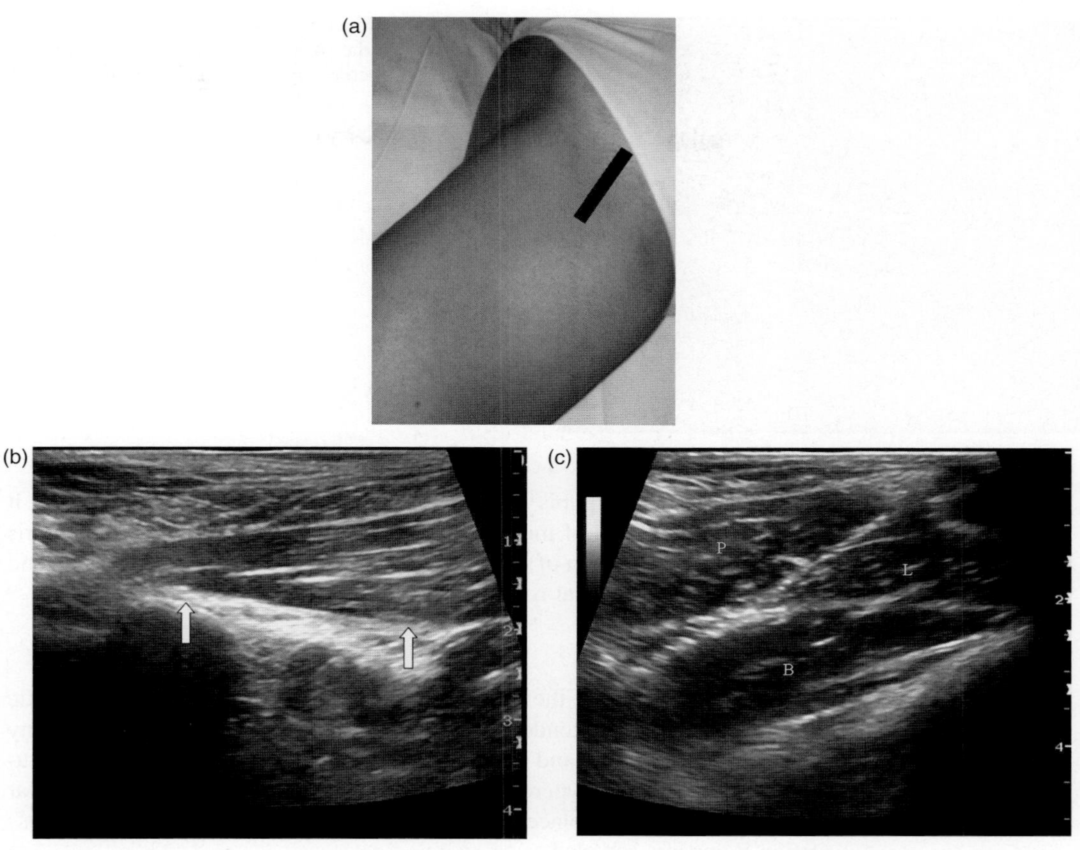

Figure 8.9. Pectineus muscle and tendon: **(a)** transducer position in the longitudinal plane, **(b)** the corresponding ultrasound image of the pectineus (arrows), and **(c)** the transverse plane of the pectineus muscle belly. P, pectineus; L, adductor longus; B, adductor brevis.

evaluated with ultrasound to assess traction periostitis, bone remodeling, and possible stress fracture.[6]

The medial thigh is best evaluated with the patient supine, the leg externally rotated and abducted. Medial musculatures of the thigh include the gracilis, pectineus, and adductor muscles (Table 8.2). Knowledge of origin and site of insertion are essential in obtaining a correct transducer position in the longitudinal axis of the muscle.

The transducer is placed in a transverse plane with the lateral margin on the palpable femoral artery. Directly medial to the artery lies the femoral vein, beside which the superficial hypoechoic muscle belly of the pectineus can be seen (Figure 8.9). The pectineus can be seen arising from the superior pubic ramus and is oriented inferiorly, laterally, and posteriorly to insert inferior to the lesser trochanter. Turn the transducer 90° to obtain the longitudinal view of this muscle. Directly deep to this muscle lie the adductor longus, brevis, and magnus, in that order (Figure 8.10). These muscles and tendons are best evaluated in their longitudinal plane initially and followed to their respective sites of insertion. Medial and superficial to the adductors, the hypoechoic gracilis is identified extending from the hyperechoic cortex of the body and

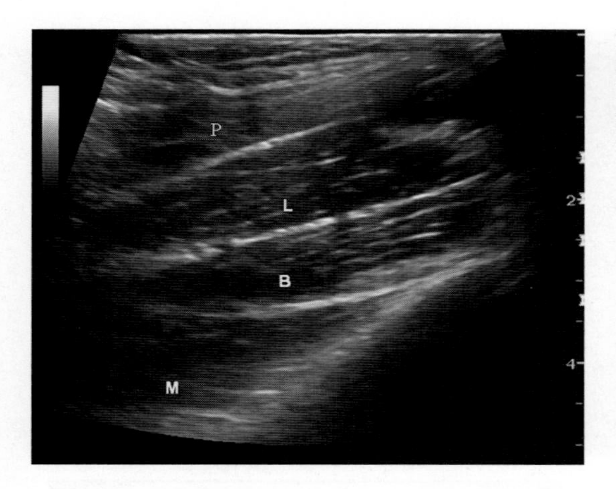

Figure 8.10. Adductor muscles: a longitudinal ultrasound image in the plane of the muscles. L, adductor longus; B, adductor brevis; M, adductor magnus; P, pectineus.

inferior ramus of the pubis to the medial proximal tibia. Sonographically it appears as a thin band of muscle less than half the size of the rectus femoris (Figure 8.11). Evaluation of its distal portion will require the patient to extend the leg with mild external rotation as detailed in Chapter 9.

Lateral and Gluteal

The patient is placed in the lateral decubitus position with the symptomatic side up and the leg extended. The greater trochanter is an excellent bony landmark in this region and is easily palpable. On ultrasound, in the longitudinal plane, it appears hyperechoic and rectangular with a somewhat irregular surface. The probe is placed in a coronal orientation to the hip. In cross section it appears rounded.

The iliotibial band is most easily located at the lateral aspect of the proximal tibia inserting on to Gerdy's tubercle (Figure 8.12).[7] It can then be followed proximally to the greater trochanter. The tensor fasciae latae is seen extending distally from the iliac crest toward the greater trochanter where it attaches to the hyperechoic iliotibial band (Figure 8.13). At the same level posteriorly,

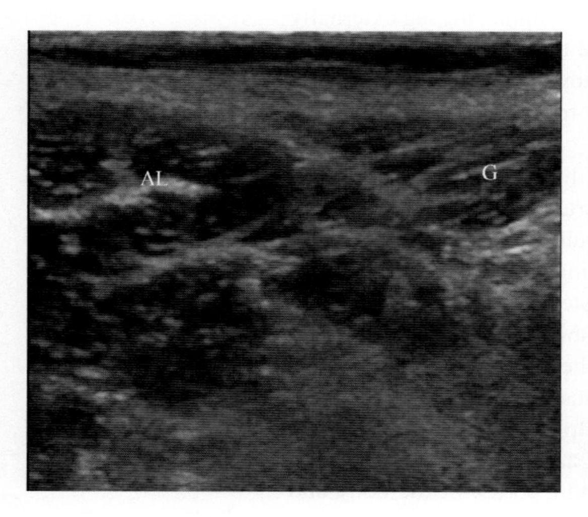

Figure 8.11. Gracilis: a transverse ultrasound image of the proximal gracilis muscle (G) close to its origin with the adjacent adductor longus (AL) muscles.

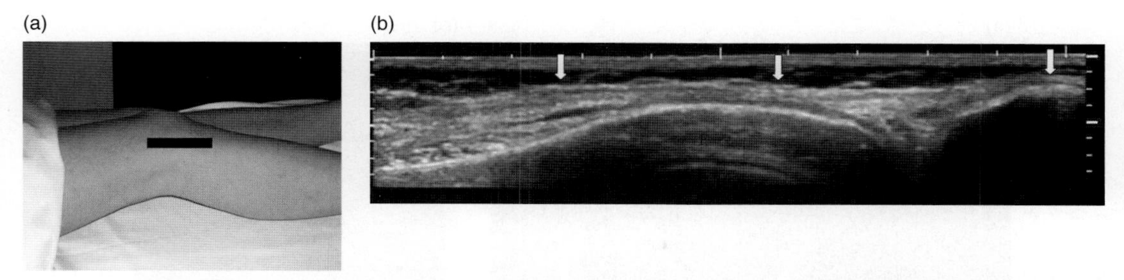

Figure 8.12. Iliotibial band (ITB): the distal ITB (arrows) at its insertion onto Gerdy's tubercle tibia. **(a)** Transducer position and its corresponding **(b)** extended field of view ultrasound image.

the superior fibers of the gluteus maximus join the iliotibial band superficial to the posterior aspect of the greater trochanter. Dynamic imaging with the probe placed transversely along the posterolateral aspect of the greater trochanter and with external rotation or extension of a semiflexed hip may reveal a snapping gluteus maximus or iliotibial band over the greater trochanter.[8] It is best to ask the patient to reproduce the same movement that causes clicking while performing dynamic scanning. The glutei are evaluated as described in Chapter 7.

Posterior

The patient is placed in a prone position. The main bony landmark of the posterior hip is the ischial tuberosity, which is seen as a prominent hyperechoic structure deep to the overlying musculature in the sagittal plane. The long head of the biceps femoris, the semimembranosus, and semitendinosus make up the hamstrings and originate from different portions of the ischial tuberosity. Hamstring muscle complex injury can be readily assessed by ultrasound and is comparable to magnetic resonance imaging (MRI).[9] The conjoint attachment of the biceps femoris and the semitendinosus can be identified when the probe is placed in the longitudinal plane along the inferomedial aspect of the ischial tuberosity (Figure 8.14). The distal attachment of the biceps femoris is also in the form of a conjoint tendon, this time with the lateral collateral ligament prior to its attachment over the styloid process of the fibular head. The semimembranosus arises from the superolateral aspect of the ischial tuberosity, hence the probe should be placed along the lateral aspect of the ischial tuberosity, and then it immediately dives deep to the conjoint tendon of the rectus femoris and semitendinosus where it can be difficult to identify. The muscle belly of the semimembranosus is located deep to the tendon of the semitendinosus in the mid and distal thigh (Figure 8.15).

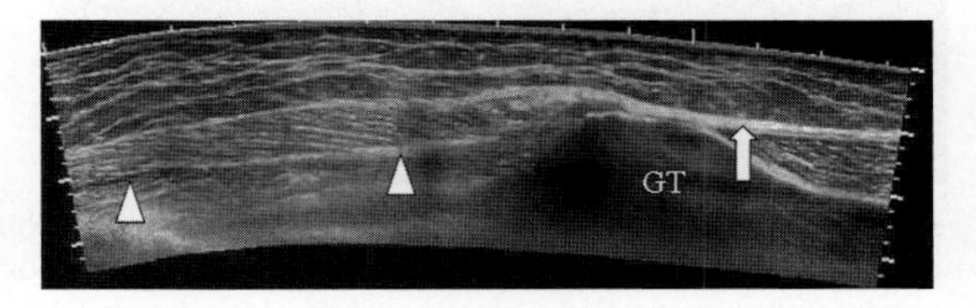

Figure 8.13. Longitudinal ultrasound image of the proximal iliotibial band (arrow) and the tensor fascia lata (arrowhead). GT, greater trochanter.

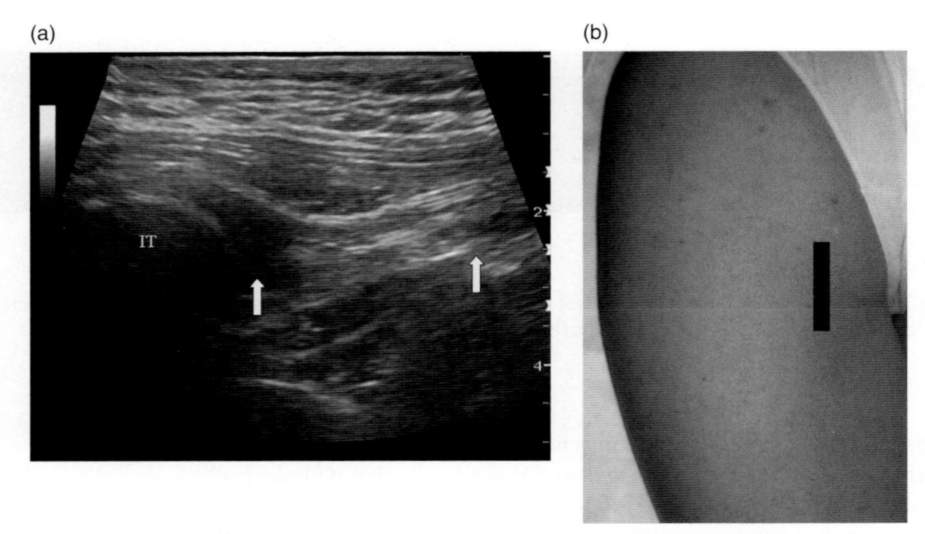

Figure 8.14. Ischial tuberosity (IT): **(a)** a longitudinal ultrasound image of the common tendon (arrows) of the biceps femoris and semitendinosus and **(b)** its transducer position.

Bursae

The bursae of the proximal thigh are reviewed in Chapter 7.

Nerves

The sciatic nerve is identified in the deep posterior hip lateral to the hamstring attachment on the ischial tuberosity. It can be identified just lateral to the ischial tuberosity. In cross section it appears as a multivesicular, rounded structure with hypoechoic spaces surrounded by echogenic connective tissue (Figures 8.15 and 8.16). In the longitudinal plane, the nerve is tubular with multiple hyperechoic linear reflectors that run parallel to one another. Once

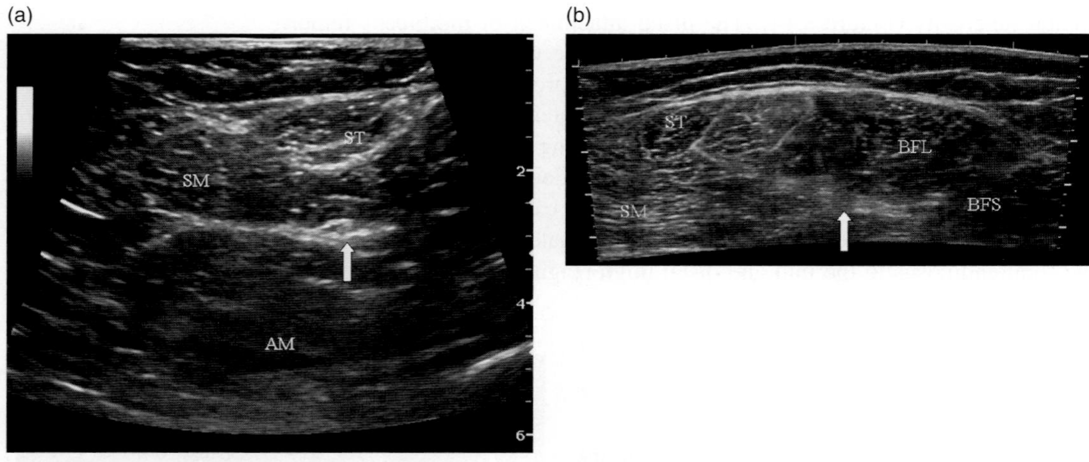

Figure 8.15. Posterior mid thigh: **(a)** a transverse ultrasound image of the posteromedial aspect of the mid thigh and **(b)** a transverse extended field of view of the mid post thigh. Arrow, sciatic nerve; ST, semitendinosus; SM, semimembranosus; BFL, biceps femoris long head; BFS, biceps femoris short head; AM, adductor magnus.

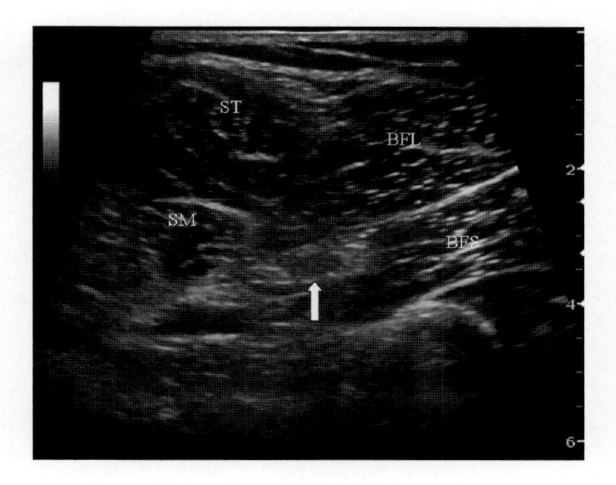

Figure 8.16. Sciatic nerve posterior mid thigh: a transverse ultrasound image. Note that the sciatic nerve does demonstrate anisotropy and can be made to appear artifactually hypoechoic as demonstrated here. Arrow, sciatic nerve; ST, semitendinosus; SM, semimembranosus; BFL, biceps femoris long head; BFS, biceps femoris short head.

identified at the level of the ischial tuberosity, the nerve can be followed distally into the hamstring compartment of the thigh. Bifurcation can occur anywhere from within the pelvis to the popliteal fossa, but it is more common distally in the proximal aspect of the popliteal fossa.

Imaging Protocols

There is no fixed imaging protocol for the thigh. Examination is tailored to the area of concern and the adjacent compartments. It is important to evaluate structures in their proximal and distal extensions to exclude referred symptoms.

References

1. Chau CLF, Griffith JF. Musculoskeletal infections: ultrasound appearances. Clin Radiol 2005;60:149–159.
2. Gray H. The Complete Gray's Anatomy, 16th ed., pp. 313–321. London: Longman, Green, and Co., 1905.
3. Gray H. The Complete Gray's Anatomy, 16th ed., pp. 540–558. London: Longman, Green, and Co., 1905.
4. Gray H. The Complete Gray's Anatomy, 16th ed., pp. 918–926. London: Longman, Green, and Co., 1905.
5. Bianchi S, Zwass A, Abdelwahab IF et al. Diagnosis of tears of the quadriceps tendon of the knee: Value of sonography. AJR 1994;162(5):1137–1140.
6. Weaver JS, Jacobson JA, Jamadar DA et al. Sonographic findings of adductor insertion avulsion syndrome with magnetic resonance imaging correlation. J Ultrasound Med 2003;22:403–407.
7. Bonaldi VM, Chhem RK, Drolet R et al. Iliotibial band friction syndrome: Sonographic findings. J Ultrasound Med 1998;17(4):257–260.
8. Choi Y, Lee S, Song B et al. Dynamic sonography of external snapping hip syndrome. J Ultrasound Med 2002;21:753–758.
9. Koulouris G, Connell D. Hamstring muscle complex: An imaging review. Radiographics 2005;25:571–586.

9

The Knee

Jon A. Jacobson

Ultrasound can effectively be used to evaluate many structures of the knee. The resolution of ultrasound is maximized when evaluating superficial structures. Therefore, evaluation of superficial structures such as the extensor mechanism of the knee, the medial collateral ligament, and joint recesses can be quite successful. Because resolution is generally decreased as the depth of the structure being evaluated increases, ultrasound is less effective for deep structures as well as intraarticular structures, such as cartilage or intrinsic knee ligaments.

There are several advantages of using ultrasound evaluation of the knee when compared to other imaging methods for particular indications. One advantage is the decreased cost when compared to magnetic resonance imaging (MRI) when evaluating for a focal soft tissue abnormality. In addition, there are advantages gained by patient interaction, enabling a detailed history and direct correlation with findings from the physical examination. Another important advantage of ultrasound is the ability to perform a dynamic evaluation. For example, a symptom that occurs only with a specific joint position, movement, or muscle contraction can be evaluated under ultrasound visualization. The color and power Doppler capabilities of ultrasound allow it to diagnose vascular abnormalities about the knee. Ultrasound can also directly guide a percutaneous aspiration or biopsy.

Imaging Indications

Indications for ultrasound of the knee vary depending on the experience and knowledge of the sonographer and availability of competing imaging methods. In general, ultrasound performs best in the evaluation of a superficial structure where there is a focused clinical question. One of the most common indications for ultrasound of the knee is to determine the cause of posterior knee or calf pain or mass, in particular, the presence of a Baker's or popliteal cyst. Ultrasound is helpful in that a Baker's cyst can be diagnosed or excluded, and complications of a Baker's cyst, such as rupture, can also be assessed. A ruptured Baker's cyst may produce a sterile cellulitis that extends into the ankle region. Ultrasound and color or power Doppler imaging can exclude deep venous thrombosis and popliteal aneurysm as causes for calf symptoms.

Another common indication for knee ultrasound involves the extensor mechanism of the knee and surrounding soft tissues and bursae.[1] For example, the specific question of a quadriceps or patellar tendon tear can be addressed with ultrasound. Other tendon problems, such as tendinosis, can also be diagnosed. Distention or inflammation of the adjacent bursa can easily be diagnosed, and ultrasound-guided percutaneous aspiration can be performed to exclude infection.

Although a knee joint effusion is typically suggested on a lateral radiograph, ultrasound can also be used for the evaluation of joint effusion and to help differentiate simple joint fluid, complex joint fluid, and synovitis. The use of color and power Doppler imaging to show hyperemia of tissue within the joint suggests synovitis, although other synovial proliferative disorders, such as pigmented villonodular synovitis, may appear similar. Ultrasound can guide percutaneous joint aspiration or synovial biopsy if indicated and can be used to evaluate other superficial soft tissue structures about the knee. For example, the medial collateral ligament, the pes anserinus, the iliotibial band, the lateral collateral ligament, the biceps femoris tendon, and the common peroneal nerve can all be visualized and assessed for abnormality. These structures are less commonly abnormal and a clinical history with specific clinical questions helps to guide ultrasound assessment.

The deep and intraarticular structures of the knee are more difficult to evaluate with ultrasound and MRI is usually considered the standard of care. For example, although ultrasound evaluation of the menisci, the cruciate ligaments, and the articular cartilage has been described in the literature, there are limitations in their assessment with ultrasound.[2] Nonetheless, ultrasound evaluation may be considered, but with consideration for MRI if ultrasound results are not definitive. Ultrasound is able to demonstrate ganglion cysts associated with the cruciate ligaments and meniscal cysts.

Technical Equipment

For superficial structures, linear array transducers of at least 10 MHz are used. Posterior knee evaluation typically requires 7- to 10-MHz transducers to evaluate the deeper structures, such as the menisci and cruciate ligaments.

Anatomy

Surface Anatomy

Several of the underlying anatomic structures of the knee can be visualized and palpated, depending on the patient's body habitus. Anterior to the distal femur, a small rounded bone, the patella, can be felt. It is partially movable. The quadriceps musculature can be identified as it tapers toward the superior aspect of the patella (Figure 9.1a). Distal to the patella, a strong tendinous band, the patellar tendon, can be easily palpated. It extends to the tibial tuberosity, a bony protuberance on the anterior aspect of the proximal tibia, and can be palpated and may be visible. The remaining structures about the knee are more difficult to identify because of their depth. However, on

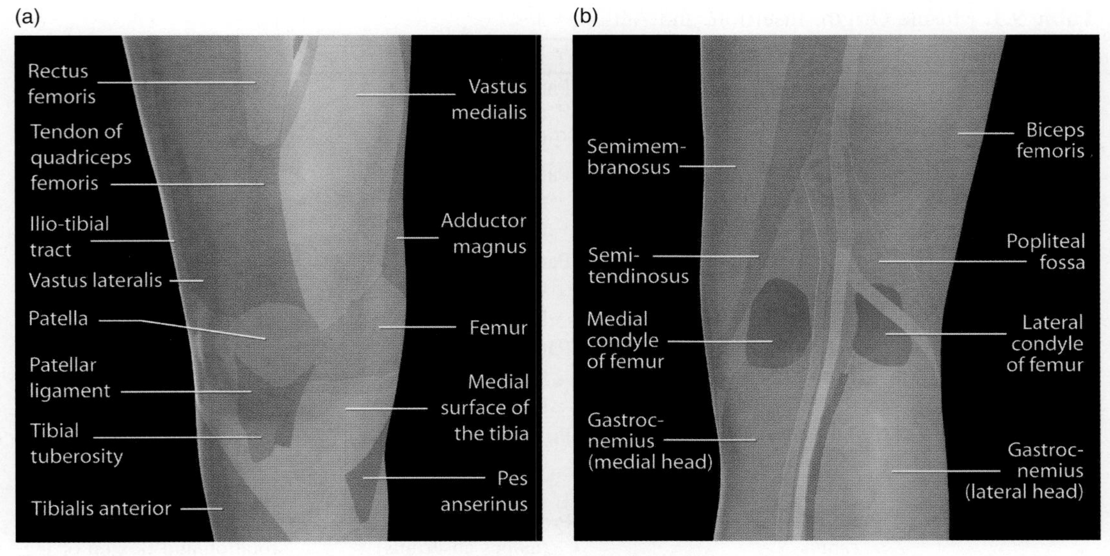

Figure 9.1. The surface anatomy of the knee: **(a)** anterior and **(b)** posterior views.

the lateral aspect of the knee the fibular head can be palpated distal to the knee joint and relatively posterior. The distal biceps femoris tendon may be identified as it extends to its attachment on the proximal fibula. The soft tissue anatomy of the posterior knee shows medial and lateral heads of the gastrocnemius muscle located relatively central as they taper to their origin at the distal femur. The medial and lateral margins of the proximal popliteal fossa are created by the visible and palpable semitendinous and biceps femoris tendons, respectively (Table 9.1).

Bones

The knee joint represents a hinge-like articulation between the distal femur and the proximal tibia. The articulating surfaces of the distal femur are composed of the medial and lateral femoral condyles, which articulate with the medial and lateral tibial plateaus (Figures 9.2a and b). The anterior surface of the distal femur also articulates with the patella, where the trochlear groove of the femur is in contact with the medial and lateral facets of the patella.

Ligaments

The knee joint is stabilized by various ligamentous structures, which extend from one bone to another (Table 9.2). Deep within the knee joint are the anterior cruciate and posterior cruciate ligaments (Figure 9.3d). They extend from the distal femur to the proximal tibia and are intracapsular but extrasynovial structures.

At the medial and lateral aspects of the knee are located the medial and lateral collateral ligaments, respectively. The medial collateral ligament complex consists of three layers[3] (Figures 9.3b and d and 9.4b). Layer 1, the most superficial layer, is the deep crural fascia and is not routinely evaluated at ultrasound. Layer 2 represents the tibial collateral ligament, which extends from the region of the adductor tubercle of the distal femur to the proximal tibial measuring 2–4 mm thick, 1–2 cm wide, and 12 cm long.[4] Layer 3, the

Table 9.1. Muscle Origin, Insertion, and Action.

Muscle/tendon	Origin	Insertion	Action
Rectus femoris	Ilium (anterior inferior iliac spine and acetabulum)	Patella and tibial tuberosity (via patellar tendon)	Extends leg, flexion of thigh
Vastus lateralis	Femur—-greater trochanter and lateral linea aspera	Patella and tibial tuberosity (via patellar tendon)	Extends leg
Vastus intermedius	Femur—-proximal shaft	Patella and tibial tuberosity (via patellar tendon)	Extends leg
Vastus medialis	Femur—-medial linea aspera and intertrochanteric line	Patella and tibial tuberosity (via patellar tendon)	Extends leg
Sartorius	Ilium (anterior superior iliac spine)	Proximal medial tibia (as pes anserinus)	Flexion of leg and thigh, abducts and external rotationof thigh
Gracilis	Pubis—- body and inferior ramus	Proximal medial tibia (as pes anserinus)	Adductor thigh, internal rotation and flexion of leg
Semitendinosus	Ischial tuberosity	Proximal medial l tibia (as pes anserinus)	Extends thigh, flexion of leg
Semimembranosus	Ischial tuberosity	Posterior medial tibial condyle (note: has multiple fibrous extensions)	Extends thigh, flexion of leg
Biceps femoris	Ischial tuberosity (long head) and linea aspera, supracondylar line femur (short head)	Fibula (long and short heads) and tibia (short head)	Extends thigh, flexion of leg
Popliteus	Femur—-lateral condyle	Proximal posterior tibia	Flexion and internal rotation of leg
Iliotibial tract	Tensor fasciae latae, fascia lata, gluteus maximus	Gerdy's tubercle Tibia	Stabilizer of knee

deepest layer, is a capsular ligament that connects the meniscus to the femur and tibia, called the meniscofemoral and meniscotibial ligaments, respectively. Layer 3 is a relatively weaker layer that tends to tear first with medial collateral ligament injury.[3]

The lateral collateral ligament is one of several structures that comprise the posterolateral corner of the knee (Figure 9.4c). The other components include the biceps femoris tendon, the popliteus tendon, the popliteofibular ligament, the fabellofibular ligament (when present), and the arcuate ligament.[5] Many of the structures are small and difficult to identify at imaging. The lateral collateral ligament extends from the lateral femur and attaches to the lateral surface of the proximal fibula with the distal biceps femoris tendon.[6] Deep to the lateral collateral ligament is located the popliteus tendon. A ligament extends from the popliteus tendon to the tip or styloid process of the fibula and is called the popliteofibular ligament.[6] When a fabella is present, a ligament extends from this structure to the fibula, called the fabellofibular ligament. Lastly, the arcuate ligament extends from the posterior joint capsule to insert on the styloid process of the fibula.[7]

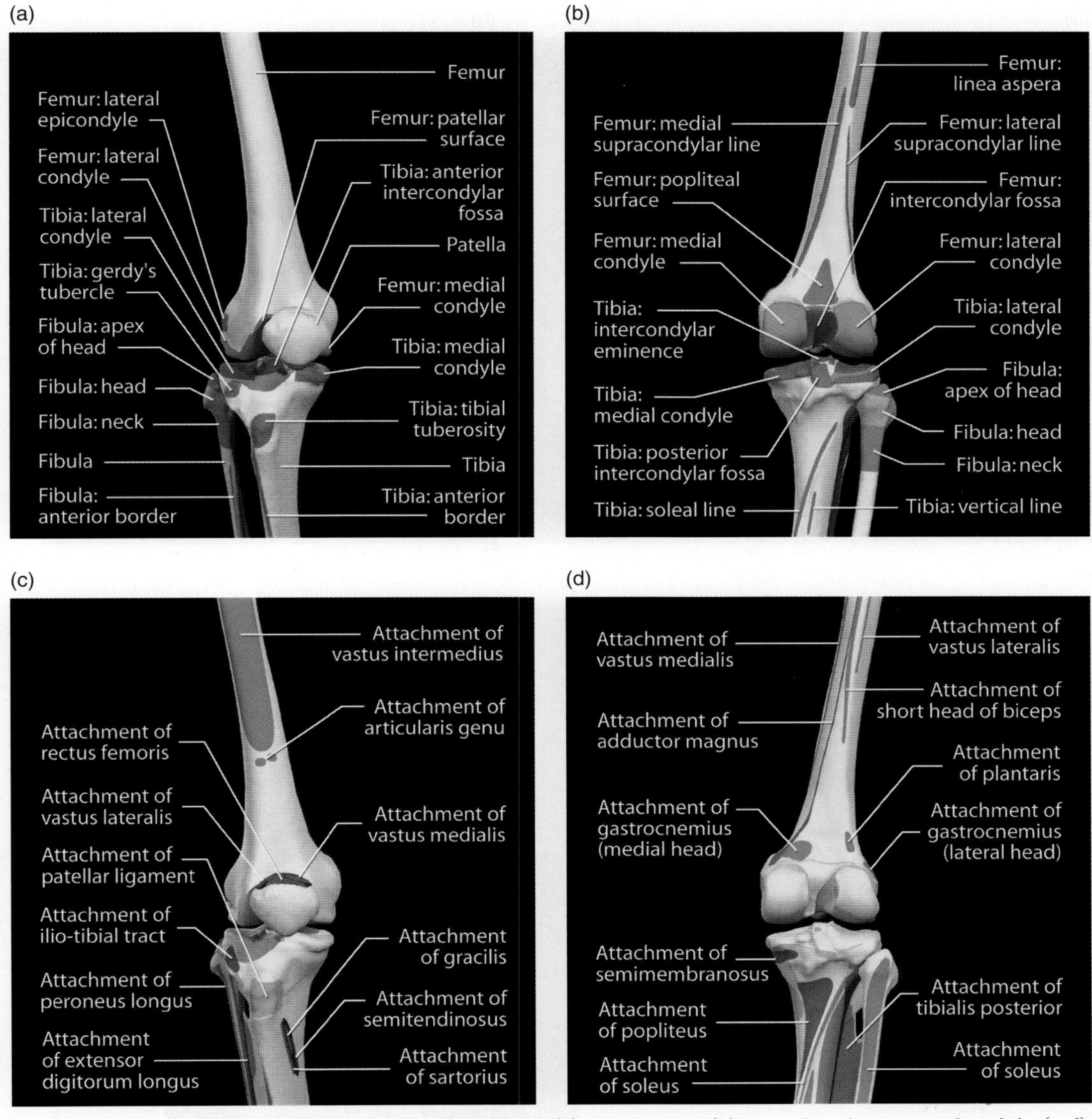

Figure 9.2. The important bony landmarks of the knee: **(a)** anterior and **(b)** posterior views; muscle origin (red) and insertion (blue) points of the **(c)** anterior and **(d)** posterior aspects of the knee joint.

Table 9.2. Ligaments.

Patellar ligament (or tendon)
Medial patellofemoral ligament (within medial patellar retinaculum)
Medial collateral ligament
Lateral collateral ligament
Popliteofibular ligament
Anterior cruciate ligament
Posterior cruciate ligament

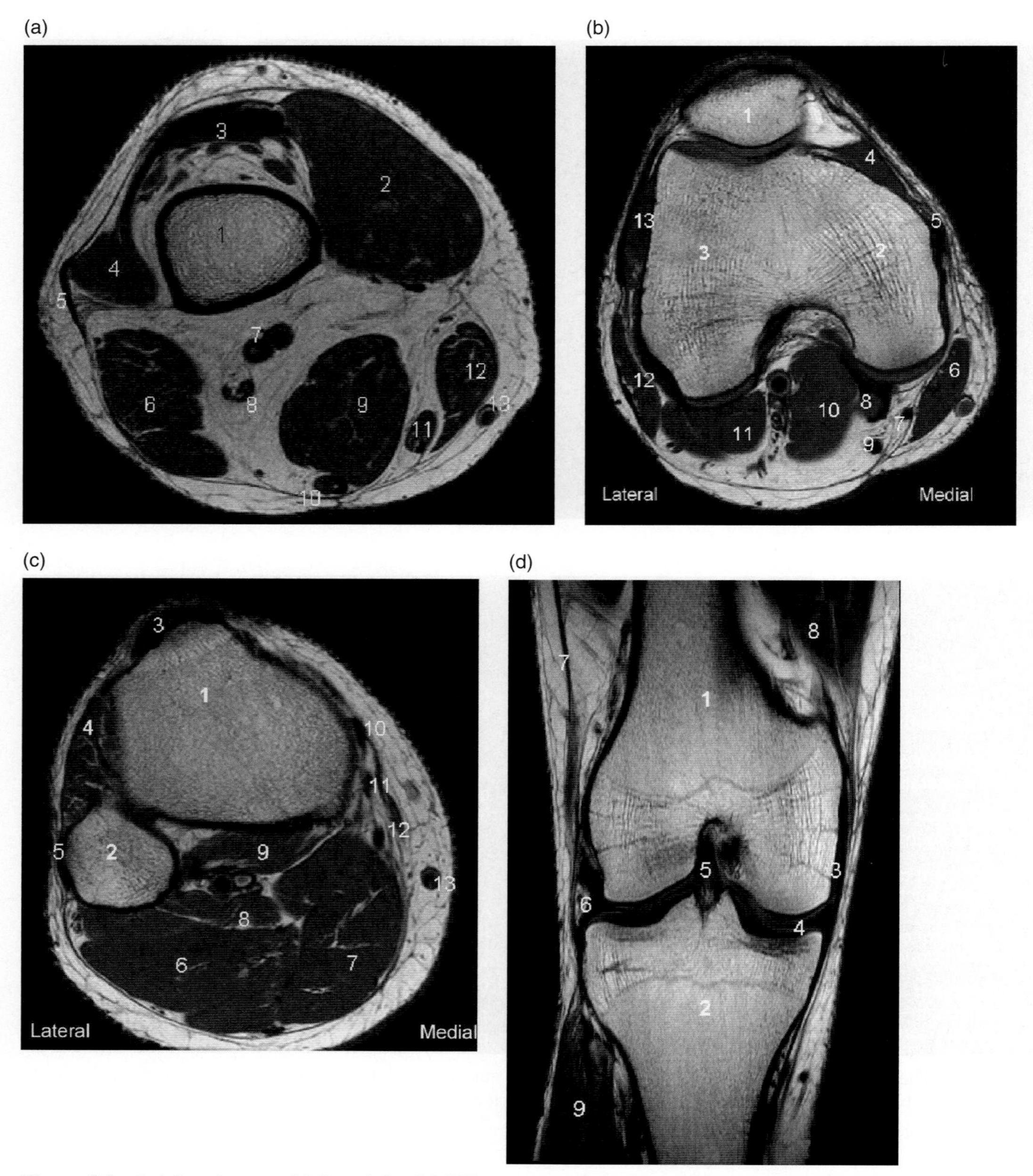

Figure 9.3. Axial and coronal T1-weighted MRI anatomy of the knee. (**a**) Axial above the level of the knee joint: 1–femur, 2–vastus medialis, 3–quadriceps tendon, 4–vastus lateralis, 5–iliotibial tract, 6–biceps femoris, 7–popliteal vessels, 8–sciatic nerve, 9–semimembranosus, 10–semitendinosus, 11–gracilis, 12–sartorius, 13–greater saphenous vein. (**b**) Axial at the level of the knee joint: 1–patella, 2–medial femoral condyle, 3–lateral femoral condyle, 4–vastus medialis, 5–medial collateral ligament, 6–sartorius, 7–gracilis, 8–semimembranosus, 9–semitendinosus, 10–medial head of gastrocnemius, 11–lateral head of gastrocnemius, 12–biceps femoris, 13–vastus lateralis.(**c**) Axial below the level of the knee joint: 1–tibia, 2–fibula, 3–patellar, 4–tibialis anterior, 5–biceps femoris, 6–gastrocnemius lateral head, 7–gastrocnemius medial head, 8–soleus, 9–popliteus, 10–sartorius, 11–gracilis, 12–semitendinosus, 13–greater saphenous vein. (**d**) Coronal of the knee joint: 1–femur, 2–tibia, 3–medial collateral ligament, 4–medial meniscus, 5–anterior cruciate ligament, 6–lateral meniscus, 7–iliotibial tract, 8–vastus medialis, 9–extensor digitorum longus.

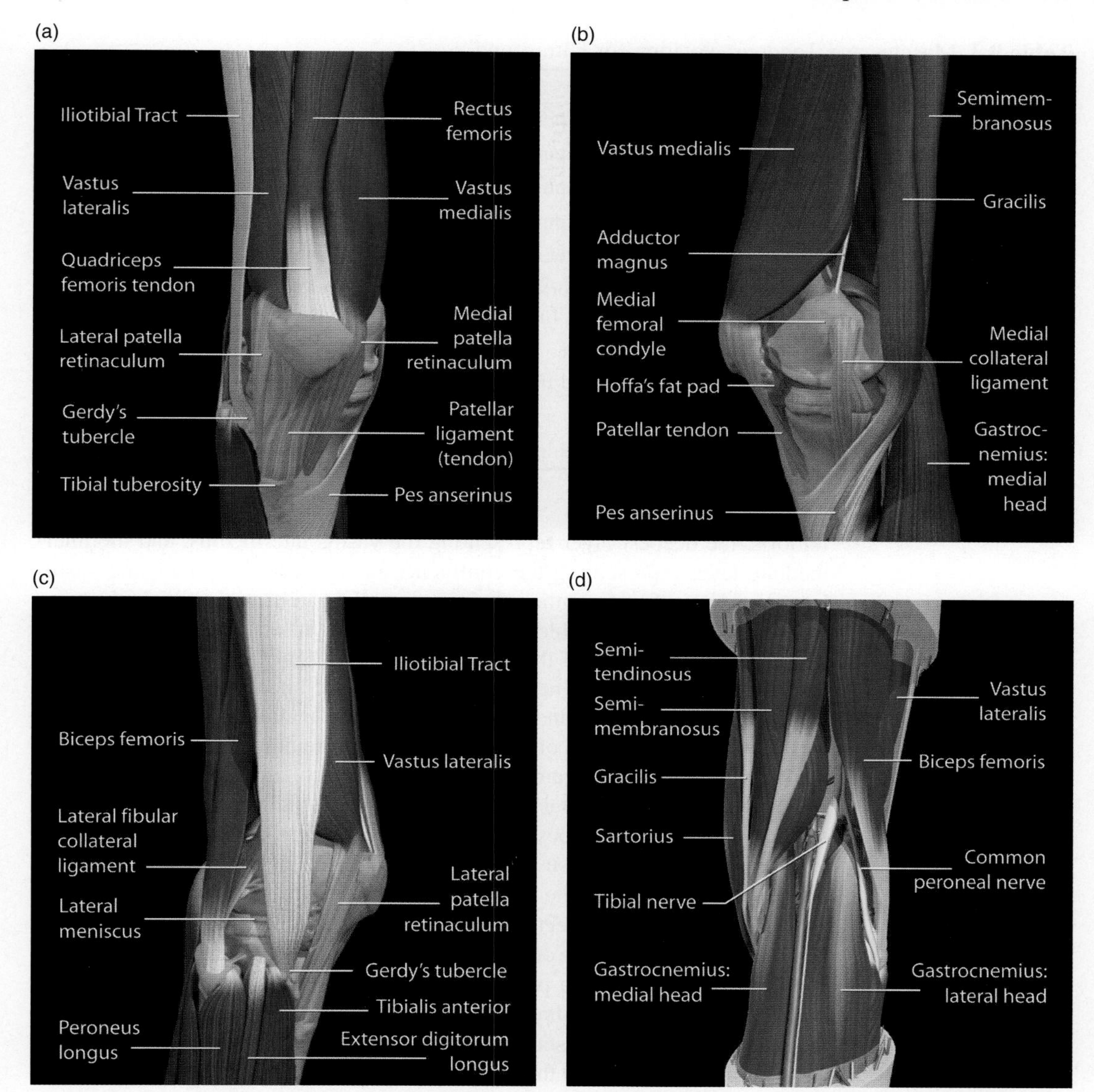

Figure 9.4. The muscles around the knee joint: **(a)** anterior, **(b)** medial, **(c)** lateral, and **(d)** posterior views.

Other ligaments about the knee include the medial patellofemoral ligament, which represents thickening of the deep layer of the medial patellar retinaculum (Figures 9.4a).[8] The medial patellofemoral ligament extends from the medial margin of the patella to the adductor tubercle of the distal femoral metaphysis.

Tendons and Muscles

The anterior thigh quadriceps muscles insert upon the superior pole of the patella (Figures 9.2, 9.3, and 9.4a and b). The distal quadriceps tendon has a trilaminar appearance, with the superficial layer representing the rectus

Table 9.3. Muscles and Tendons: Position for Ultrasound.

Muscle/tendon	Position examined
Rectus femoris	Minimal knee flexion (supine)
Vastus lateralis	Minimal knee flexion (supine)
Vastus intermedius	Minimal knee flexion (supine)
Vastus medialis	Minimal knee flexion (supine)
Sartorius Gracilis	Minimal knee flexion and external rotation of leg (supine)
Semitendinosus	Knee extension (prone) for proximal component and minimal knee flexion and external rotation of leg for pes anserinus (supine)
Semimembranosus	Knee extension (prone)
Biceps femoris	Minimal knee flexion and internal rotation of leg (supine)
Popliteus	Knee extension (prone)
Iliotibial tract	Minimal knee flexion and internal rotation of leg (supine)

femoris, the deepest layer representing the vastus intermedius, and the intermediate layer representing the confluence of the vastus medialis and vastus lateralis.[9] Extending from the inferior pole of the patella to the tibial tuberosity is the patellar tendon (Table 9.3).

At the medial aspect of the knee, the distal aspect of the adductor magnus inserts upon the adductor tubercle, a bone protuberance at the junction of the medial femoral condyle and the medial femoral metaphysis. Also attaching to the adductor tubercle of the femur are the femoral attachments of the medial patellofemoral ligament and the medial collateral ligament.[8] Superficial to the extreme distal aspect of the medial collateral ligament is the tibial attachment of the pes anserinus, which is composed of the sartorius, gracilis, and semitendinosus (Figure 9.4b). Just distal to the joint line at the posteromedial aspect of the proximal tibia inserts the semimembranosus.

At the anterolateral aspect of the knee, the distal aspect of the iliotibial tract inserts on Gerdy's tubercle of the proximal tibia (Figures 9.2c and 9.6a and c).[10] More posteriorly within a prominent groove or sulcus in the lateral femoral condyle is located the popliteus tendon (Figure 9.3c). This structure originates from the posterolateral distal femur and extends medial and inferior to insert on the tibia.[7] Attaching on the posterolateral aspect of the proximal fibula with the lateral collateral ligament is the biceps femoris, which has origins from the ischial tuberosity and femur. Some fibers of the short head of the biceps femoris also insert on the lateral tibia (Figures 9.2d and 9.4c).

Posterior to the knee, the medial and lateral heads of the gastrocnemius muscle are identified on either side of the popliteal artery, originating at the distal femoral metaphysis posteriorly (Figures 9.2c and d, 9.3a and b, and 9.4d). The semimembranosus and semitendinosus are identified medial to the medial gastrocnemius head.

Cartilage

Two forms of cartilage exist in the knee joint: hyaline cartilage and fibrocartilage. Hyaline cartilage, measuring 1–2 mm thick, covers the articulating surfaces of the distal femur, the proximal tibia, and the patella.[11] Fibrocartilage in the knee takes the form of the medial and lateral menisci, which are C-shaped and located between the femur and tibia. The meniscal root or meniscotibial ligaments attach the menisci to the tibia.

Joint Recesses

The knee joint has a number of joint recesses with the largest being the suprapatellar recess. The suprapatellar recess represents a normal communication between the joint cavity and the embryonic suprapatellar bursa; since this open communication exists, the term "recess" is used rather than "bursa." The suprapatellar recess extends proximal to the patella and deep to the quadriceps tendon where it is surrounded by the quadriceps fat pad anteriorly and the prefemoral fat pad posteriorly. A joint capsule does not exist at this location of the suprapatellar recess.[12] Anterior joint effusion will not only extend superiorly deep to the quadriceps tendon, but will also extend medially and laterally to the patella over the femoral condyles. Small anterior joint recesses are also seen extending anteriorly into Hoffa's infrapatellar fat pad, and a small joint recess is seen anterior to the lateral tibial plateau inferior to the anterior horn of the lateral meniscus. Another prominent joint recess represents the normal communication between the knee joint and the popliteus tendon sheath laterally. Here fluid can extend inferior, posterior, and medial from the popliteus groove of the lateral femoral condyle surrounding the popliteus tendon. Small joint recesses may also exist at the posterior knee about the posterior cruciate ligament, as well as adjacent to the medial and lateral gastrocnemius tendon origins. The medial gastrocnemius-semimembranosus bursa when communicating with the posterior knee joint effectively becomes a joint recess (see below).

Bursae

A commonly imaged bursa is the medial gastrocnemius-semimembranosus bursa located at the posterior medial knee[13] (Table 9.4). When this bursa is distended with the subjacent subgastrocnemius bursa, it is commonly termed a Baker's cyst. In approximately 50% of adults over the age of 50 years, the knee joint communicates with the medial gastrocnemius-semimembranosus bursa and subgastrocnemius bursa.[13] This is due to degeneration, thinning, and eventual perforation of the intervening joint capsule compounded by increased intraarticular joint pressures in the aging adult with a degenerative knee. The cause of a Baker's cyst in the adult is typically a joint effusion (many times due to internal derangement and osteoarthrosis), which fills the Baker's cyst through the communication. A Baker's cyst is a common

Table 9.4. Bursae.

Superficial infrapatellar bursa
Deep infrapatellar bursa
Medial collateral ligament bursa
Pes anserinus bursa
Semimembranosus-medial gastrocnemius bursa (with subgastrocnemius bursa)
Semimembranosus-tibial collateral ligament bursa
Prepatellar bursa
Medial and lateral gastrocnemius bursae

location for intraarticular bodies to reside. Several other bursae exist at the medial aspect of the knee. The semimembranosus-tibial collateral ligament has an inverted "U" shape and is located at the joint line.[14] Unlike a Baker's cyst, the semimembranosus-tibial collateral ligament bursa is located lateral to the semimembranosus and does not normally communicate with the knee joint. Another more inferior and anterior bursa at the medial knee is the pes anserinus bursa, located adjacent to the tendons of the pes anserinus at the proximal tibia. A small bursa may also exist between the superficial and deep layers of the medial collateral ligament.[15]

Several bursae exist about the anterior knee.[1] The largest is the prepatellar bursa located superficial to the patella and adjacent proximal patellar tendon. More distally, a superficial infrapatellar bursa is located superficial to the distal patellar tendon and tibial tuberosity. Another deep infrapatellar bursa is located between the patellar tendon and the proximal tibia. Small bursa may also be found deep to the medial and lateral gastrocnemius tendon origins at the distal and posterior femur.

Nerves

The sciatic nerve divides into its two terminal branches—the tibial and common peroneal nerves—in the posterior aspect of the lower third of the thigh (Figures 9.1b, 9.3a, and 9.4d). The tibial nerve continues into the popliteal fossa adjacent to the popliteal artery and vein. The common peroneal nerve courses laterally from its origin to the biceps tendon within the popliteal fossa. It crosses the lateral head of the gastrocnemius and the head of the fibula to wind anteriorly around the neck of the fibula. Between the fibula and peroneus longus, it divides into the anterior tibial and superficial peroneal nerves. These nerves are reviewed in greater detail in Chapter 12.

Technique

Ultrasound examination of the knee will follow a sequence: anterior, medial, lateral, and posterior. At each location, a checklist of structures will be followed to guide imaging evaluation. A standardized examination, such as described below, is advocated. This will ensure completeness, and will make it possible to develop an efficient sonographic examination. In addition, becoming comfortable with the sonographic appearances of normal structures also serves to improve imaging skills. A thorough examination will also address the possibility of referred symptoms. At the completion of the standardized ultrasound examination, it is critical to focus the ultrasound examination at the site of any focal signs or symptoms. This will ensure that the patient's most important complaints are addressed. In addition, this will often lead the sonographic evaluation to pathology involving a structure that is not routinely evaluated during the standardized examination.

For evaluation of the anterior knee, the patient is lying supine. A rolled up towel or sponge is placed under the knee to slightly flex it. This tightens the extensor mechanism of the knee and reduces anisotropy of the quadriceps and patellar tendons. To evaluate the medial and lateral aspects, the patient is asked to turn partway to one side or the other to gain access. For posterior evaluation, the patient is asked to lie prone. Liberal transmission gel is used

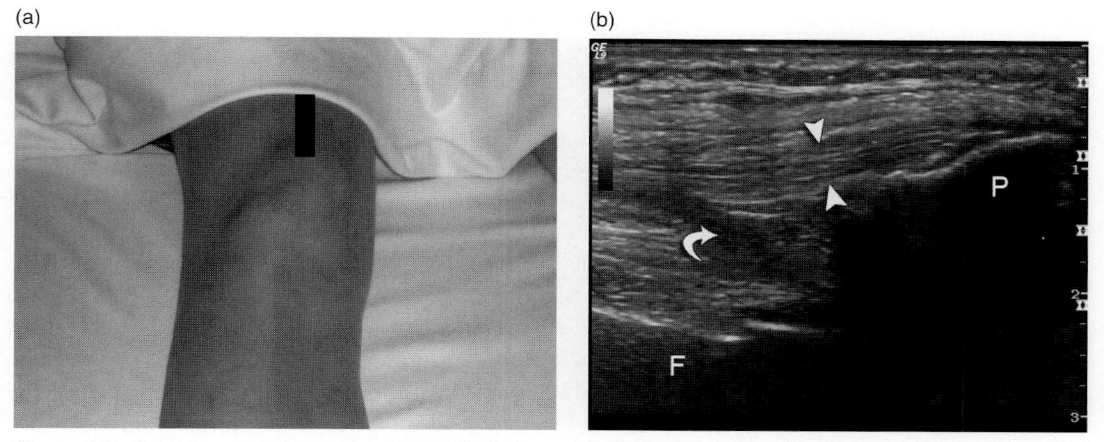

Figure 9.5. Quadriceps tendon and suprapatellar recess. **(a)** Transducer placement in the sagittal plane (black box) over the anterior knee shows **(b)** the quadriceps tendon (arrowheads) and collapsed suprapatellar recess (curved arrow). P, patella; F, femur.

rather than a standoff pad. When holding the transducer, the edge of the hand or the fifth finger is in contact with the patient for stabilization of the transducer and to allow fine controlled adjustments in the transducer position.

Anterior Knee Evaluation

Sonographic evaluation in the sagittal plane superior to the patella evaluates the distal quadriceps tendon and the suprapatellar recess (Figure 9.5a). A normal tendon is hyperechoic and fibrillar. The three individual layers of the distal quadriceps tendon are often difficult to visualize as separate structures, but rather they are seen as one continuous structure (Figure 9.5b). The normally collapsed suprapatellar recess may not be visualized or is seen as a thin hypoechoic structure extending superiorly from between the patella and femur. The transducer is then moved inferiorly (Figure 9.6) to evaluate the

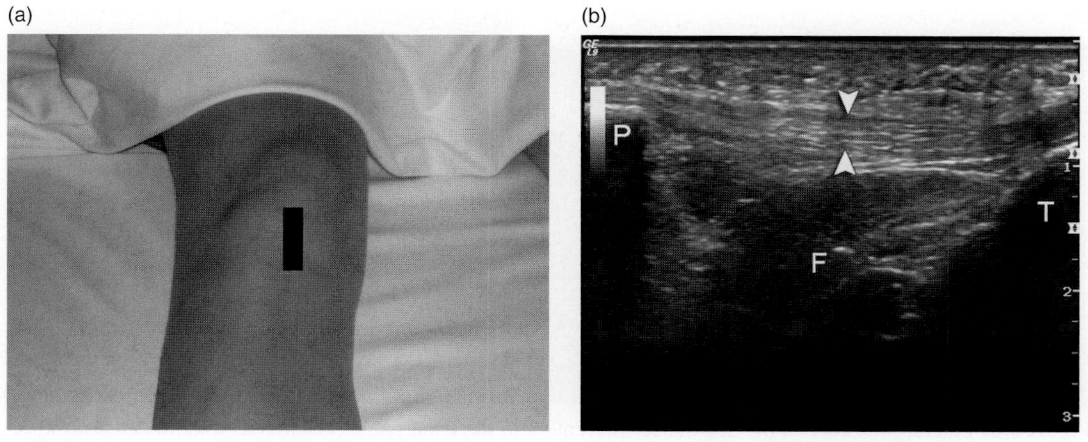

Figure 9.6. Patellar tendon. **(a)** Transducer placement in the sagittal plane (black box) over the anterior knee shows **(b)** the patellar tendon (arrowheads). P, patella; T, tibia; F, Hoffa's fat pad.

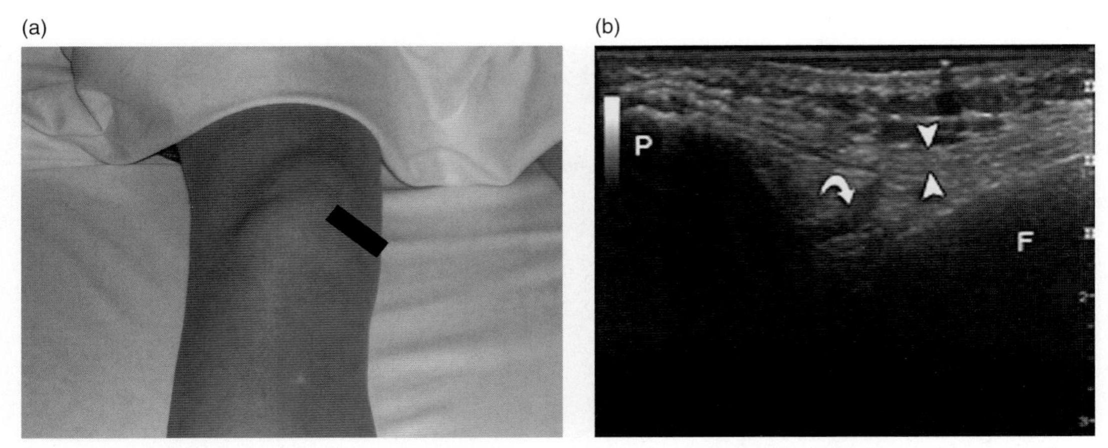

Figure 9.7. Medial joint recess. **(a)** Transducer placement in the axial plane (black box) over the anterior knee shows **(b)** the patellar retinaculum (arrowheads) and collapsed medial joint recess (curved arrow). P, patella; F, femur.

patellar tendon and any anterior knee bursae. It is important to float the transducer on a thick layer of gel as even a small amount of pressure can displace fluid in a superficial bursa out of view. The transducer is then turned 90° or transverse to the knee to evaluate the medial and lateral joint recesses superficial to the femur and adjacent to the patella (Figures 9.7a and 9.8a). The collapsed joint recesses will appear as a thin hypoechoic area extending away from the patellofemoral articulation (Figures 9.7b and 9.8b). The imaging planes described above are the key imaging planes; orthogonal imaging is always carried out, in particular, to accurately characterize and measure any visualized pathology. It is also important to image the surface of the patella for fracture (Figure 9.9). The hyaline articular cartilage of the trochlea can be visualized as a thin hypoechoic layer over the anterior femur with the knee flexed (Figure 9.10).

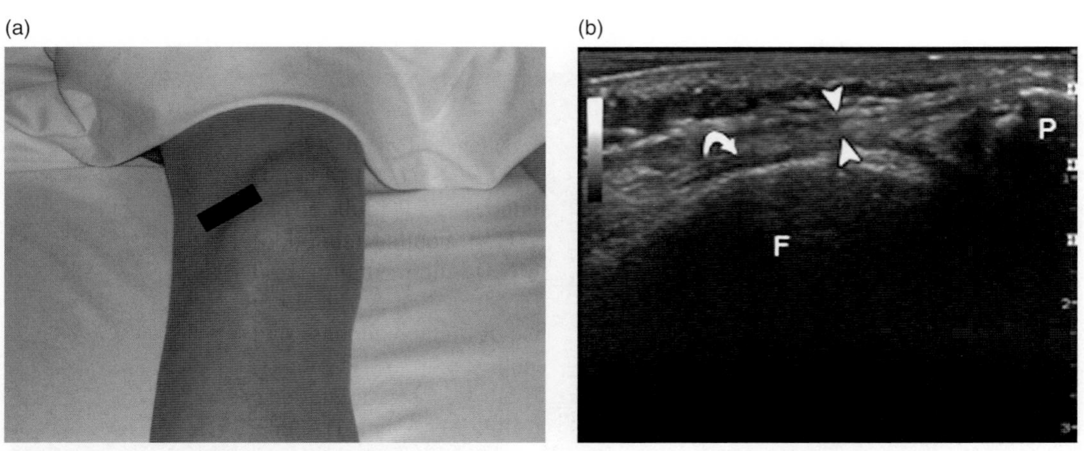

Figure 9.8. Lateral joint recess. **(a)** Transducer placement in the axial plane (black box) over the anterior knee shows **(b)** the patellar retinaculum (arrowheads) and collapsed lateral joint recess (curved arrow). P, patella; F, femur.

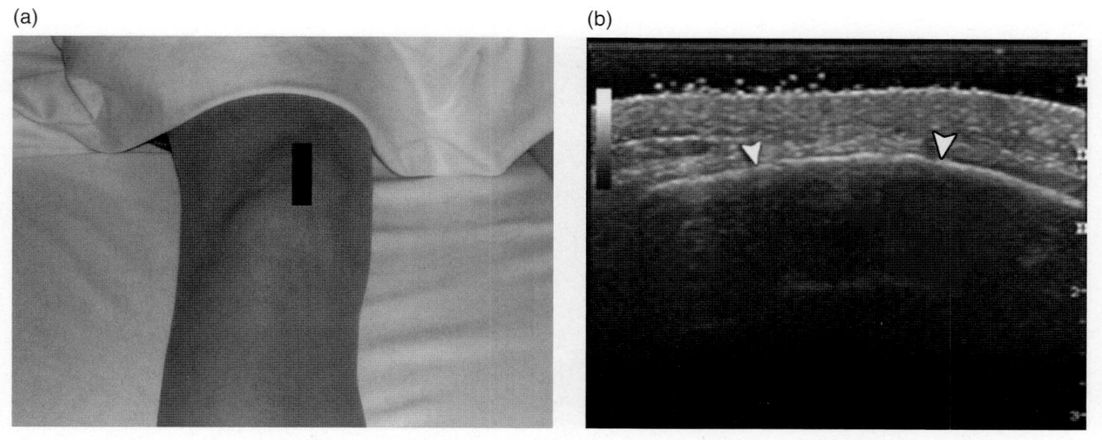

Figure 9.9. Patella. **(a)** Transducer placement in the sagittal plane (black box) over the anterior knee shows **(b)** the normal smooth echogenic cortex of the patella (arrowheads).

> **Insider Information 9.1**
>
> - Slight knee flexion reduces quadriceps tendon anisotropy.
> - Minimal joint effusion will be suprapatellar with knee flexion and on each side of the patella in knee extension.
> - Float the transducer on a layer of gel in the evaluation for anterior bursae.

Medial Knee Evaluation

Sonographic determination in the coronal plane at the level of the knee joint evaluates the medial collateral ligament and the body of the medial meniscus (Figure 9.11). The deep and thin meniscofemoral and meniscotibial ligaments

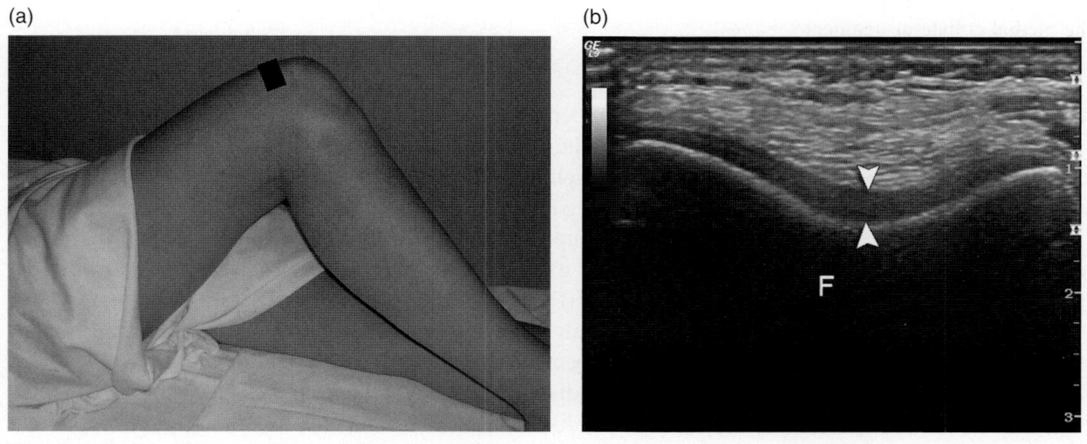

Figure 9.10. Trochlear cartilage of the femur. **(a)** Transducer placement in the axial plane in knee flexion (black box) shows **(b)** hypoechoic hyaline cartilage (arrowheads) of the trochlea (T).

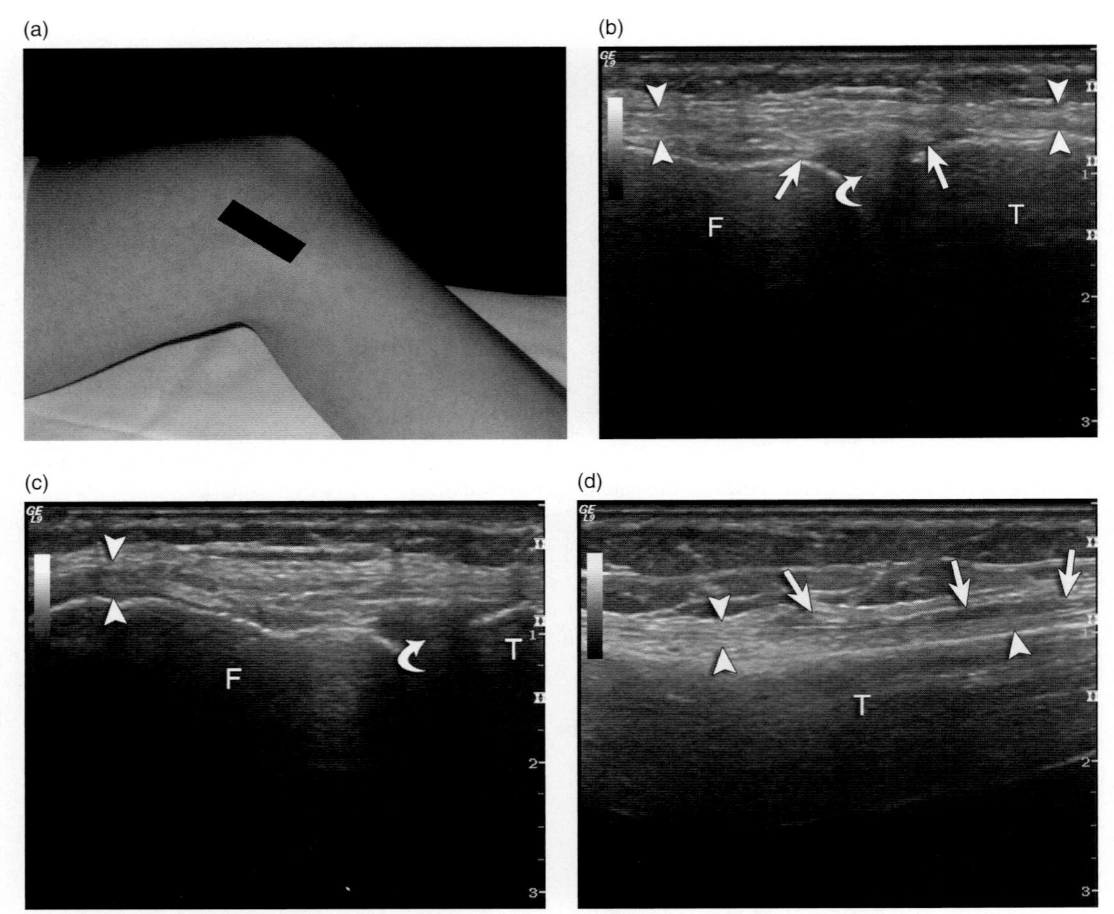

Figure 9.11. Medial collateral ligament and medial meniscus (body). **(a)** Transducer placement in the coronal plane (black box) over the medial knee shows **(b)** the superficial layer (arrowheads) and deep layer (arrows) of the medial collateral ligament. Curved arrow, body of the medial meniscus. T, tibia. **(c)** Imaging proximal to the joint shows proximal attachment of the medial collateral ligament (arrowheads). F, femur; curved arrow, body of medial meniscus; T, tibia. **(d)** Imaging distal to the joint shows distal attachment of the medial collateral ligament (arrowheads). T, tibia. Note: (arrows) pes anserinus tendons (sartorius, gracilis, semitendinosus) superficial to the medial collateral ligament.

can be seen as thin hyperechoic and compact fibrillar structures extending from the meniscus to the femur and tibia, respectively. The fibrocartilage meniscus appears hyperechoic and triangular between the femur and the tibia.[2] It is important to optimize imaging with proper transducer frequency and focal zone placement to attempt complete evaluation of the meniscus, including the tip of the meniscus extending deep from the transducer. Superficial to the meniscus is the superficial layer of the medial collateral ligament, which appears hyperechoic with compact fibrillar architecture several millimeters thick. The proximal aspect of the medial collateral ligament attaches at the adductor tubercle of the distal femur, several centimeters proximal to the joint line (Figure 9.11c). The distal aspect of the medial collateral ligament extends quite distally over the tibia to attach near the tibial metaphysis-diaphysis junction (Figure 9.11d). This superficial layer of the medial collateral ligament

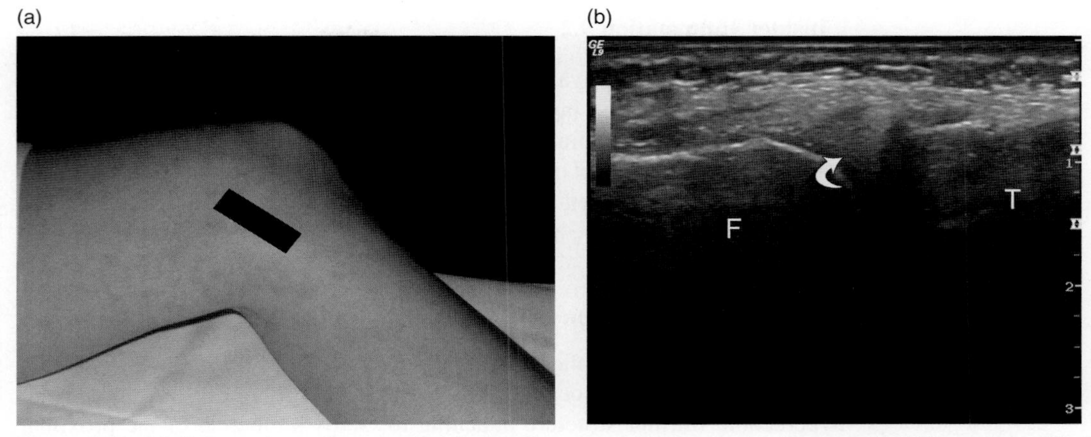

Figure 9.12. Medial meniscus (anterior horn). **(a)** Transducer placement in the coronal-oblique plane (black box) over the anteromedial knee shows **(b)** hyperechoic, triangle-shaped anterior horn of the medial meniscus (curved arrow). F, femur; T, tibia; Fb, fibula.

is between 1 and 2 cm wide in the anteroposterior dimension, so it is important to sweep the transducer from anterior to posterior and to image in the orthogonal plane to ensure complete evaluation.

With the transducer again positioned over the body of the medial meniscus, it is moved anteriorly to visualize the anterior horn of the medial meniscus (Figure 9.12). Lastly, the transducer is moved back over the medial collateral ligament, and then over the extreme distal attachment on the tibia. At this location, the three tendons of the pes anserinus—the sartorius, gracilis, and semitendinosus—are seen as small oval structures superficial to the medial collateral ligament (Figure 9.11d). The transducer can be rotated 45° angled posteriorly and superiorly to elongate the individual tendons of the pes anserinus (Figure 9.13). This area is also assessed for a pes anserine bursitis.

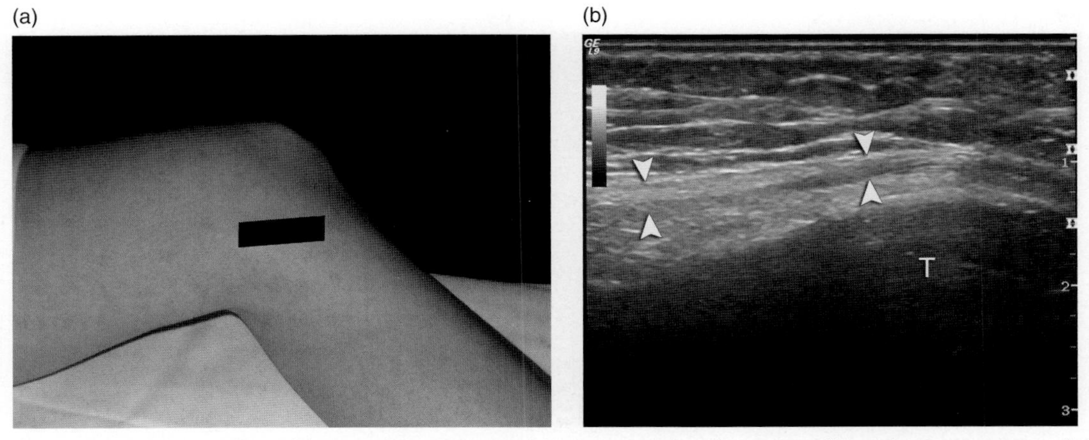

Figure 9.13. Pes anserinus. **(a)** Transducer placement in the coronal-oblique plane (black box) over the medial knee shows **(b)** the sartorius (arrowheads). T, tibia.

Insider Information 9.2

- It is important to evaluate the entire extent of the medial collateral ligament superficial layer, which is several centimeters anteroposterior and extends longitudinally up to 5 cm beyond the knee joint.
- The most distal aspect of the medial collateral ligament superficial layer is a key landmark in identification of the pes anserinus tendons distally.

Lateral Knee Evaluation

Imaging begins in the oblique sagittal plane just lateral to the patellar tendon (Figure 9.14a). At this location, the iliotibial tract is seen as a thin and flat hyperechoic fibrillar structure attaching to Gerdy's tubercle of the proximal tibia (Figure 9.14).[5] It is important to assess this structure proximally over the distal femur where abnormalities related to iliotibial band friction syndrome occur. Next, the transducer is moved posteriorly over the distal femur to visualize a prominent groove in the lateral femoral condyle (Figure 9.15). This is an important landmark as the lateral collateral ligament attaches just proximal to this groove, which contains the popliteus tendon.[5] The distal aspect of the transducer is then rotated posteriorly with the proximal aspect stationary on the femur (Figure 9.15). This position brings the fibula into view and elongates the lateral collateral ligament, which appears as a uniform hyperechoic and thin compact fibrillar structure.[5] The distal aspect of the lateral collateral ligament may appear slightly thickened and heterogeneous near the proximal fibular attachment due to the adjacent biceps femoris tendon and possible anisotropy. With the distal aspect of the transducer now fixed on the fibula, the proximal aspect of the transducer is rotated posteriorly to bring the transducer into the coronal plane (Figure 9.16). This position elongates the biceps femoris tendon (Figure 9.16).[5] More proximal evaluation will show the hypoechoic biceps femoris muscle fibers tapering to its tendon. By moving the transducer just posterior to the biceps femoris, the common peroneal nerve

(a)

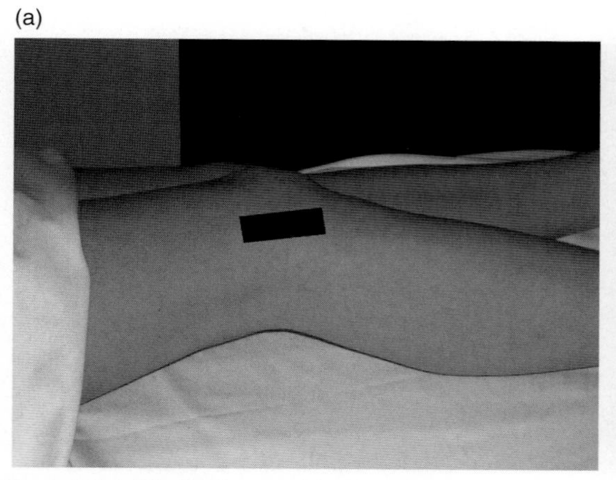

(b)

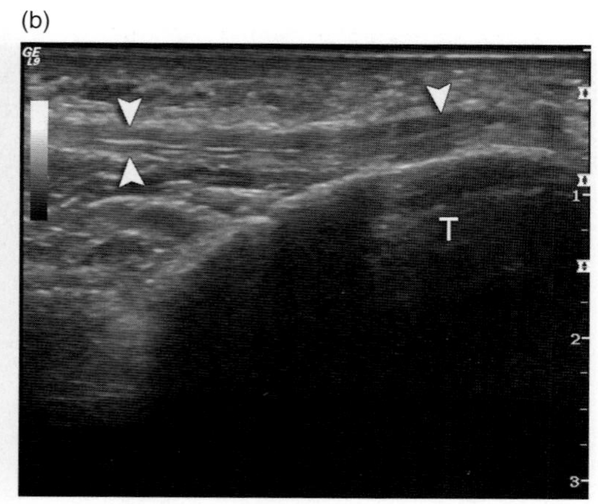

Figure 9.14. Iliotibial tract. **(a)** Transducer placement in the sagittal-oblique plane (black box) over the anterolateral knee shows **(b)** the iliotibial tract (arrowheads). T, tibia.

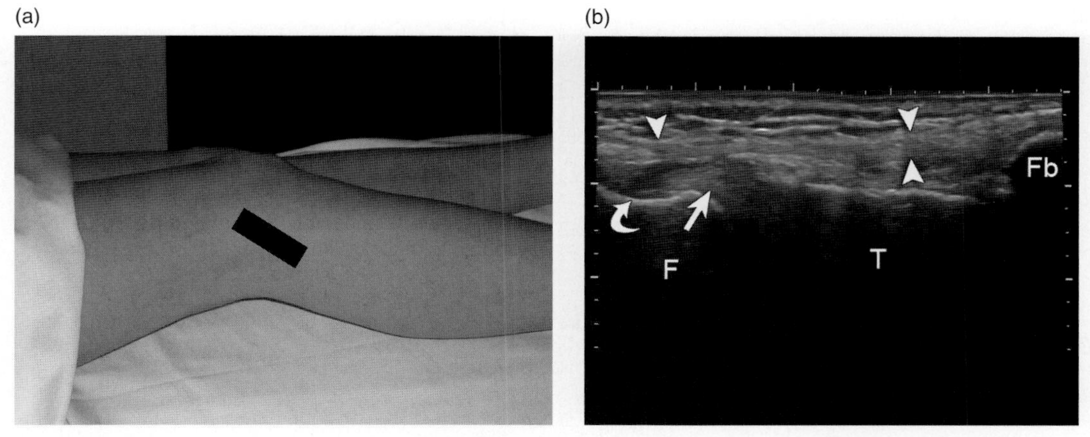

Figure 9.15. Lateral collateral ligament. **(a)** Transducer placement in the coronal-oblique plane (black box) over the lateral knee shows **(b)** the lateral collateral ligament (arrowheads), which extends over a groove (curved arrow) in the femur (F) and the popliteus tendon (arrow). T, tibia; Fb, fibula.

is identified by its hypoechoic nerve fascicles surrounded by hyperechoic connective tissue and fat (Figure 9.17). Each of the previously cited structures can be assessed in the orthogonal planes by rotating the transducer 90° to characterize and measure pathology (Figure 9.18).

Other structures of the lateral knee are more difficult to completely evaluate. While the proximal aspect of the popliteus tendon is easily identified in a groove in the lateral femoral condyle as described previously, its continual curved course around the lateral knee and its deep location posterior to the knee make evaluation difficult but not impossible (Figure 9.19).[5] The smaller structures of the posterolateral corner prove very difficult to visualize. The popliteofibular ligament appears as a compact hyperechoic structure extending from the popliteus tendon to the tip of the fibula (Figure 9.19c).[5] The

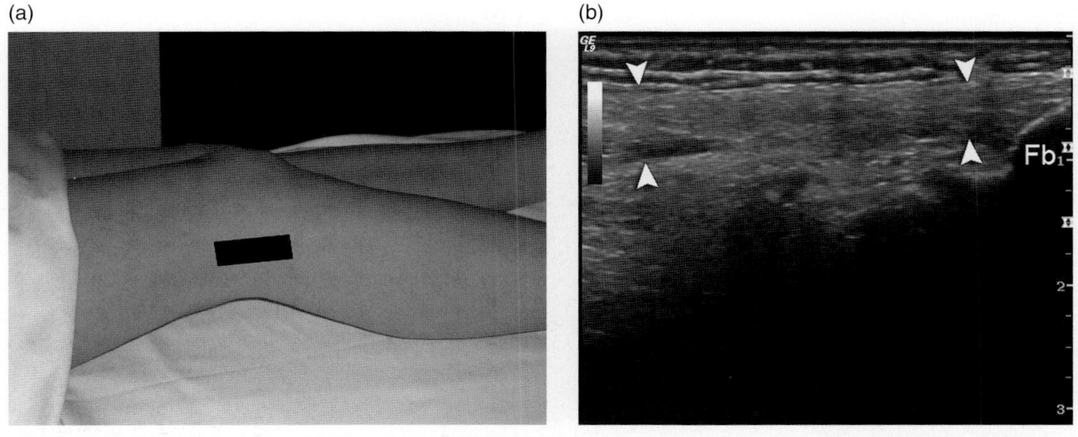

Figure 9.16. Biceps femoris. **(a)** Transducer placement in the coronal plane (black box) over the posterolateral knee shows **(b)** the hypoechoic muscle and hyperechoic tendon of the biceps femoris (arrowheads). F, femur; Fb, fibula.

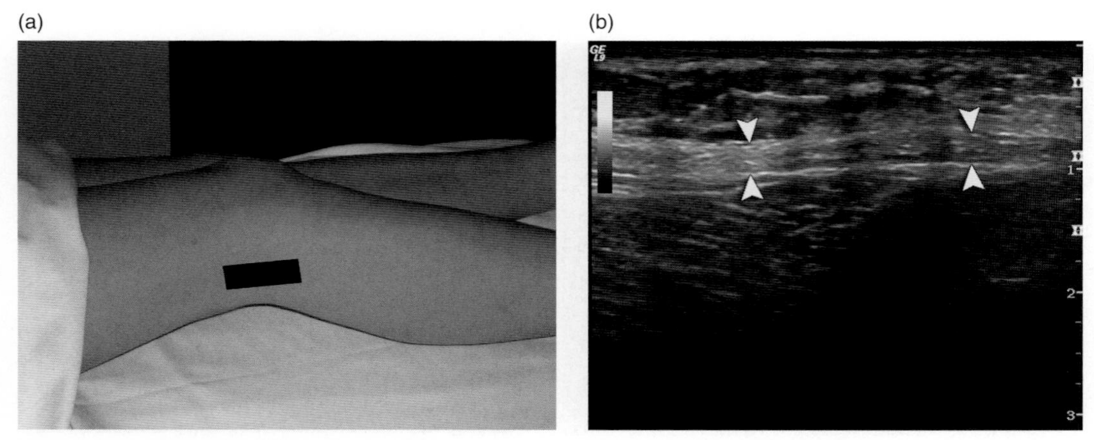

Figure 9.17. Common peroneal nerve. (a) Transducer placement in the coronal plane (black box) posterior to the biceps femoris shows (b) the predominantly hypoechoic common peroneal nerve (arrowheads).

fabellofibular ligament and arcuate ligament are quite thin and are difficult to assess. The body and anterior horn of the lateral meniscus appear hyperechoic and triangle-shaped.

Insider Information 9.3

- Bone landmarks are the key for orientation in the evaluation of the lateral knee.
- The normal lateral collateral ligament may have a wavy appearance if the knee is in valgus angulation; place the knee over the contralateral tibia to straighten the lateral collateral ligament.
- The normal body of the lateral meniscus often appears heterogeneous.

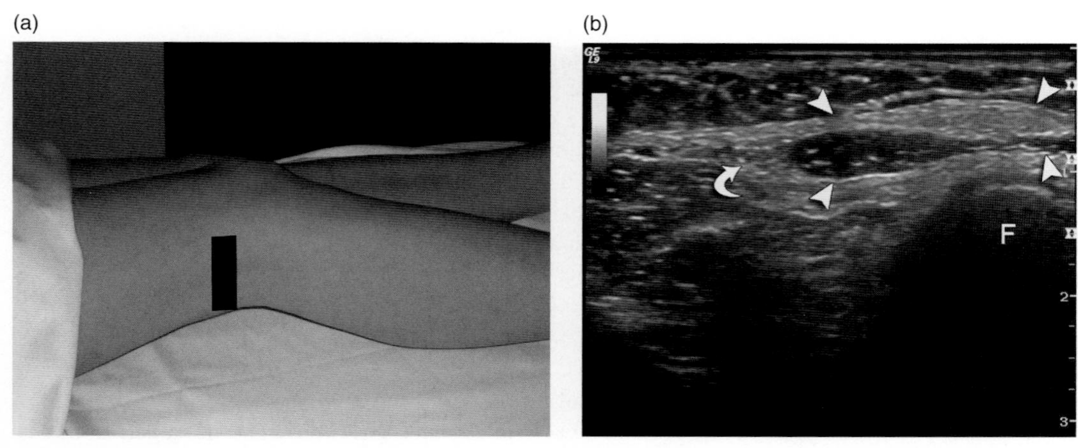

Figure 9.18. Common peroneal nerve and biceps femoris. (a) Transducer placement in the axial plane (black box) over the posterolateral knee shows (b) the honeycomb appearance of the common peroneal nerve (curved arrow) and the hypoechoic muscle and hyperechoic tendon of the biceps femoris (arrowheads). F, fibula.

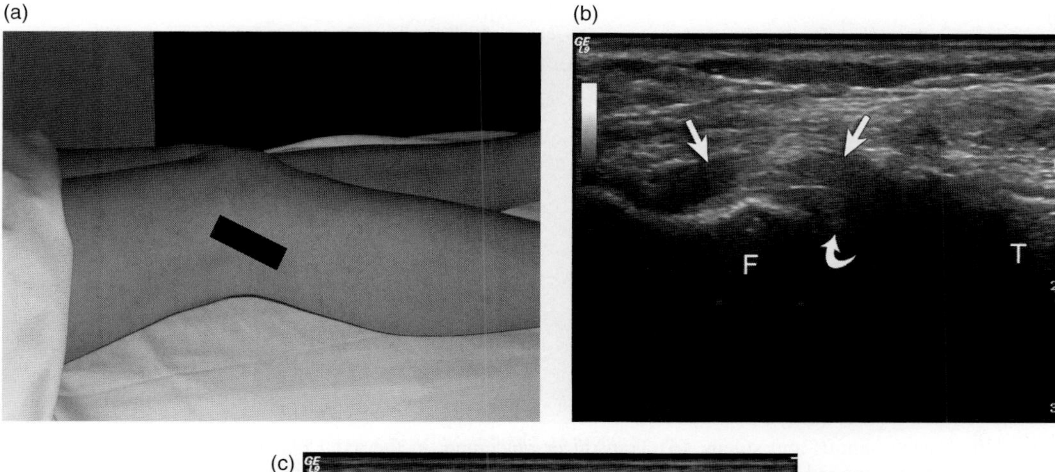

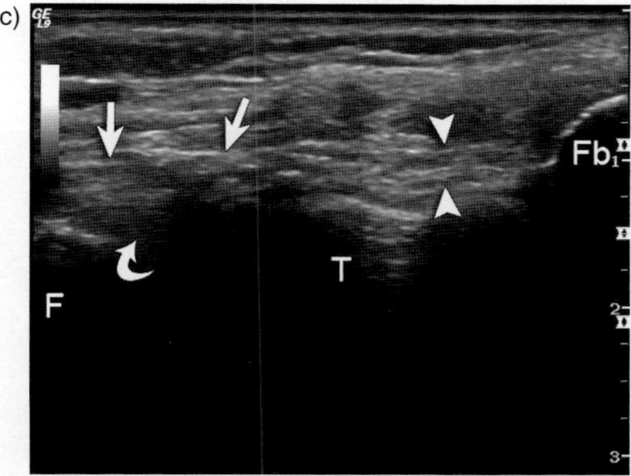

Figure 9.19. Popliteus tendon and popliteofibular ligament. **(a)** Transducer placement in the coronal-oblique plane (black box) over the posterolateral knee shows **(b)** the popliteus tendon (arrows) (curved arrow, lateral meniscus; F, femur; T, tibia). **(c)** Imaging between the popliteus tendon (arrows) and the fibula (Fb) shows the popliteofibular ligament (arrowheads). F, femur; T, tibia; curved arrow, lateral meniscus.

Posterior Knee Evaluation

Posterior knee evaluation begins with an assessment for a Baker's cyst. While identification of a large Baker's cyst is not difficult, it is important to recognize the normal anatomic landmarks in the absence of a Baker's cyst to exclude pathology. This can be quickly accomplished by beginning scanning in the transverse plane over the mid calf (Figure 9.20).[13] This starting point is used as the anatomy is simple, with the medial and lateral heads of the gastrocnemius muscle identified superficial to the soleus muscle (Figure 9.20). The transducer is then moved over the medial aspect of the medial gastrocnemius muscle head and proximally toward the knee joint. Approaching the knee joint, the semimembranosus tendon can be seen just lateral to the medial head of the gastrocnemius tendon and muscle (Figure 9.21).[13] This is where a Baker's cyst extends from the posterior knee joint. Due to the oblique course of the semimembranosus and medial gastrocnemius head tendons relative to each other, it is common for one of the tendons to appear hypoechoic and the other to appear hyperechoic due to anisotropy.[13] It is also important not to mistake the hypoechoic appearance of the semimembranosus tendon due to

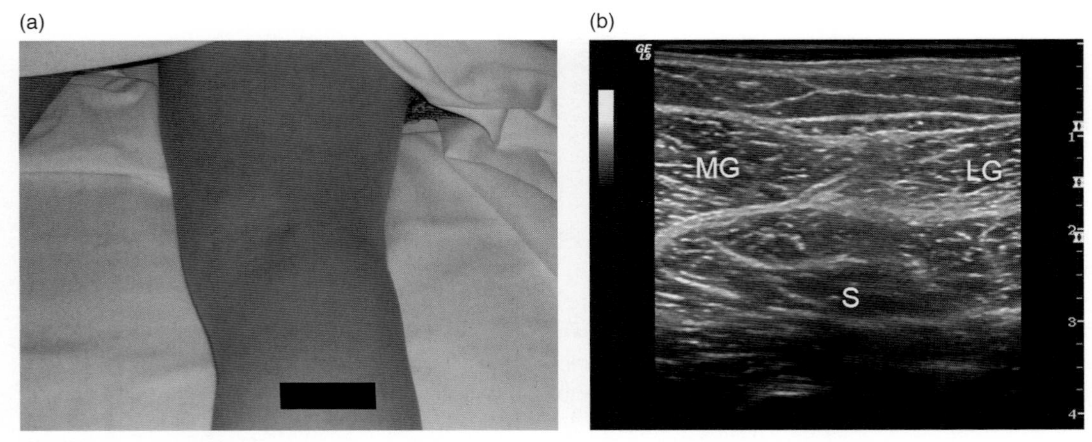

Figure 9.20. Gastrocnemius and soleus. **(a)** Transducer placement in the axial plane (black box) over the calf midline shows **(b)** the medial head (MG) and lateral head (LG) of the gastrocnemius superficial to the soleus (S).

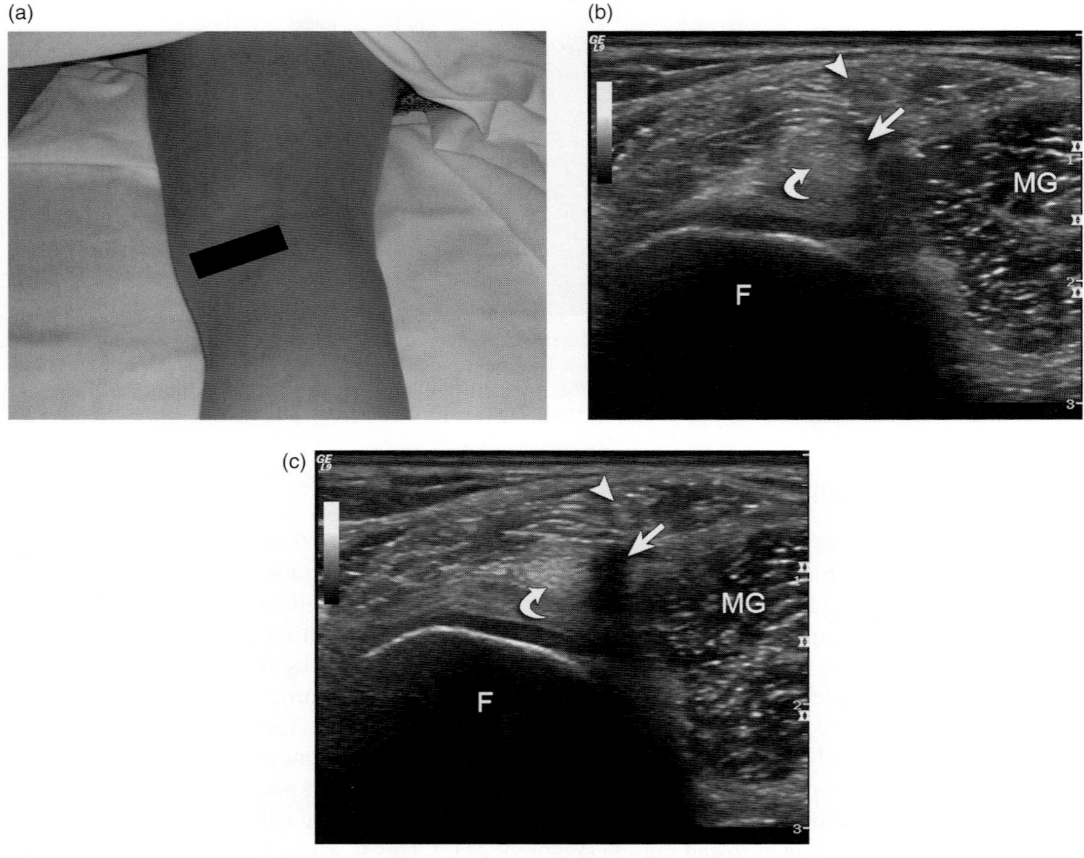

Figure 9.21. Medial head of the gastrocnemius and semimembranosus. **(a)** Transducer placement in the axial plane (black box) over the Posteromedial knee shows **(b)** the medial head of the gastrocnemius tendon (arrow) and muscle (MG), semimembranosus tendon (curved arrow), and semitendinosus (arrowhead). Note the hypoechoic cartilage over the medial femoral condyle (F). **(c)** Slight angulation of the transducer along the long axis of the medial head of the gastrocnemius shows the hypoechoic appearance of the medial head gastrocnemius tendon (arrow) due to anisotropy, which may simulate fluid in a Baker's cyst.

anisotropy as a small hypoechoic Baker's cyst (Figure 9.21c).[13] If a Baker's cyst is identified, imaging in the sagittal plane can assess the sagittal extent of the Baker's cyst, and evaluate its distal aspect for rupture superficial to the medial gastrocnemius muscle. Superficial to the semimembranosus tendon is found the smaller semitendinosus tendon.

The transducer is then turned to the sagittal plane over the medial knee at the joint line to visualize the posterior horn of the medial meniscus, appearing hyperechoic and triangular (Figure 9.22). This area of the meniscus is important to evaluate, as it is the most common site for meniscal tears, which appear as an anechoic or hypoechoic cleft. The transducer is moved from medial to lateral to ensure complete evaluation. If the transducer is moved medial toward the body of the medial meniscus, it is not uncommon to visualize the tibial attachment of the semimembranosus tendon as an oval hypoechoic structure due to anisotropy (Figure 9.22b). It is important not to mistake this appearance for a meniscal cyst.

The transducer is then moved over the midline of the posterior knee to visualize the posterior cruciate ligament.[16] One helpful landmark is the characteristic bone contours of the tibial plateau at the posterior cruciate ligament attachment. The transducer is then rotated slightly to elongate the posterior cruciate ligament (Figure 9.23). One pitfall is the artifactual hypoechoic appearance of the posterior cruciate ligament due to its oblique course. This can be minimized by rocking the transducer in the longitudinal plane relative to the ligament, or by using beam-steering if this is an option on the ultrasound equipment. The posterior cruciate ligament is considered abnormal if it is greater than 10 mm in thickness.[16] The posterior recess of the knee about the posterior cruciate ligament is also assessed for pathology, including cruciate ganglion cysts. Orthogonal imaging is used to characterize and measure pathological processes.

The transducer remains in the sagittal plane and is moved laterally over the lateral meniscus. The lateral aspect of the posterior horn of the lateral meniscus is problematic in that the popliteus tendon courses at its posterior border with

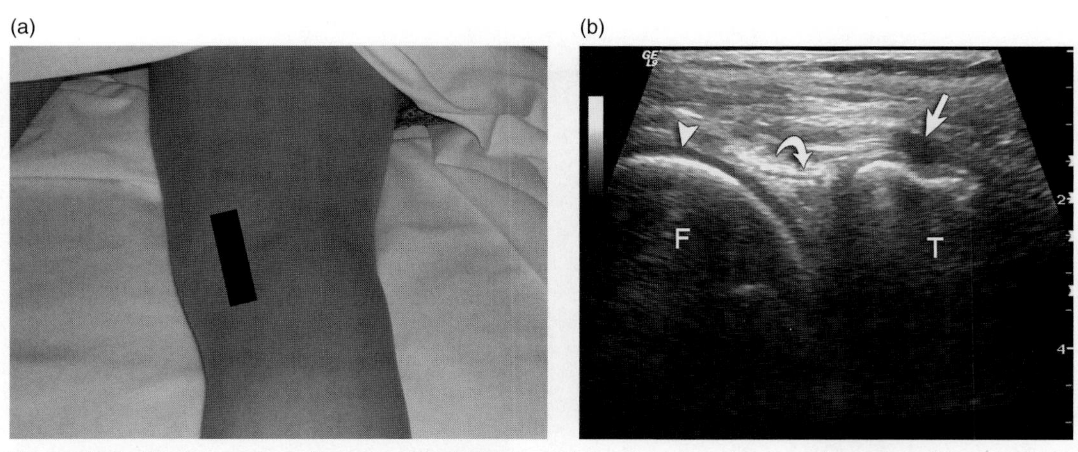

Figure 9.22. Medial meniscus (posterior horn). **(a)** Transducer placement in the sagittal plane (black box) over the posteromedial knee shows **(b)** the hyperechoic and triangle-shaped posterior horn of the medial meniscus (curved arrow). Note the semimembranosus tendon (arrow) and femoral hyaline cartilage (arrowhead). F, femur; T, tibia.

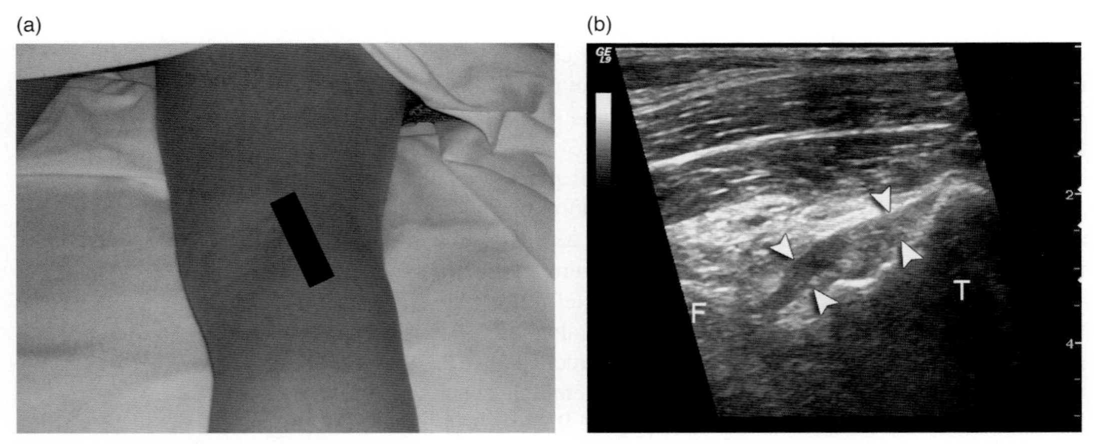

Figure 9.23. Posterior cruciate ligament. **(a)** Transducer placement in the sagittal-oblique plane (black box) over the posterior knee shows **(b)** the posterior cruciate ligament (arrowheads). F, femur; T, tibia. Note the use of beam-steering to obtain a more perpendicular orientation to the posterior cruciate ligament to minimize anisotropy.

the popliteus recess. This normal appearance may easily be confused with a meniscal tear (Figure 9.24). For this reason, ultrasound is least effective in the evaluation of the posterior horn of the lateral meniscus.

Lastly, the transducer is moved back over the midline of the posterior knee and is rotated into the transverse plane (Figure 9.25a). Between the characteristic bone contours of the posterior femoral condyles is located the intercondylar notch. This space is normally hyperechoic, from the hyperechoic anterior cruciate ligament and the adjacent hyperechoic fat (Figure 9.25b). An anterior cruciate ligament tear will appear as an abnormal hypoechoic area in the lateral aspect of the intercondylar notch.[17] Also in the transverse plane, the popliteal vasculature can be assessed with gray-scale and color Doppler imaging.

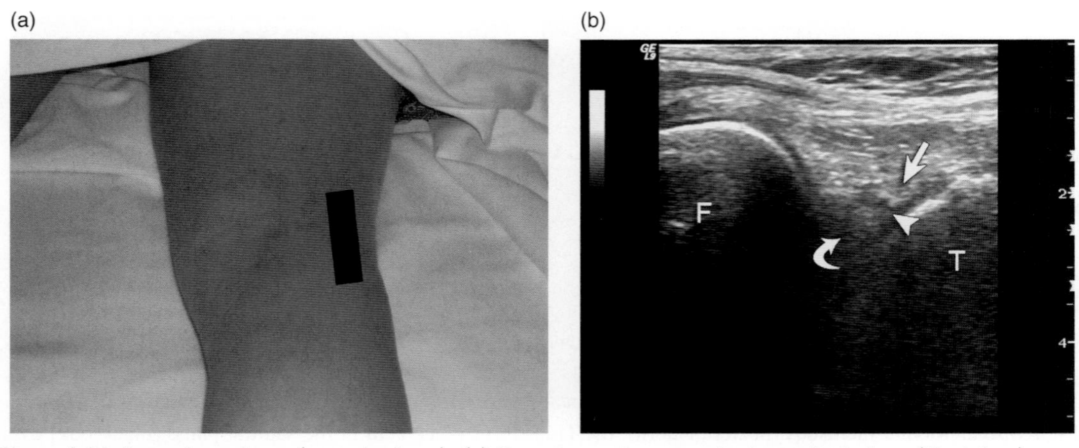

Figure 9.24. Lateral meniscus (posterior horn). **(a)** Transducer placement in the sagittal plane (black box) over the posterolateral knee shows **(b)** the hyperechoic cleft (arrowhead) between the triangle-shaped posterior horn of the lateral meniscus (curved arrow) and popliteus tendon (arrow). F, femur; T, tibia.

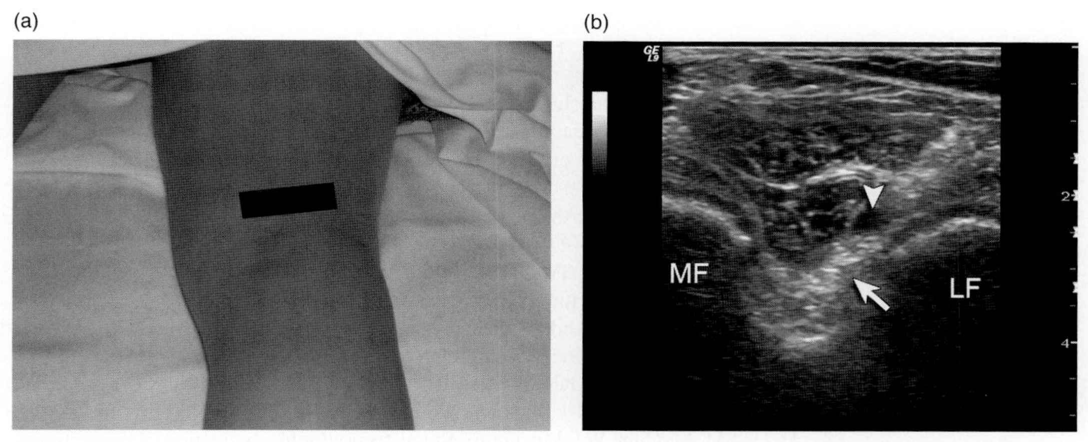

Figure 9.25. Anterior cruciate ligament. **(a)** Transducer placement in the axial plane (black box) over the posterior knee shows **(b)** the hyperechoic anterior cruciate ligament (arrow) in the lateral aspect of the intercondylar notch. LF, lateral femoral condyle; MF, medial femoral condyle; arrowhead, popliteal artery.

Imaging Protocols

As described previously, a standardized approach to sonographic evaluation of the knee will ensure a complete and efficient examination. If a standardized sequence is followed with every patient, with individual structures assessed using a checklist, evaluation can be completed in a short period of time. It is, however, important to focus the evaluation at the end of the examination, as the patient will often lead to pathology—perhaps a pathology not routinely evaluated.

There are two situations in which only a targeted approach may be considered. One is with a busy ultrasound practice, in order to increase patient throughput. However, this is not optimal, as important pathology may be overlooked and ultrasound will be viewed as a limited examination. The other situation in which a targeted approach is considered is when first learning ultrasound of the knee. In this setting, time may not allow an entire examination of the knee with every patient. An ultrasound examination may then be targeted to the area of symptoms. However, as one's technique becomes faster and more efficient, it is important to begin adding other components of the complete examination, resulting, over time, in a complete standardized and efficient knee ultrasound examination (see Appendix).

References

1. Friedman L, Finlay K, Popovich T et al. Sonographic findings in patients with anterior knee pain. J Clin Ultrasound 2003;31(2):85–97.
2. Azzoni R, Cabitza P. Is there a role for sonography in the diagnosis of tears of the knee menisci? J Clin Ultrasound 2002;30(8):472–476.
3. Schweitzer ME, Tran D, Deely DM et al. Medial collateral ligament injuries: Evaluation of multiple signs, prevalence and location of associated bone bruises, and assessment with MR imaging. Radiology 1995;194(3):825–829.
4. De Maeseneer M, Van Roy F, Lenchik L et al. Three layers of the medial capsular and supporting structures of the knee: MR imaging-anatomic correlation. Radiographics 2000;20(Spec No):S83–S89.

5. Sekiya JK, Jacobson JA, Wojtys EM. Sonographic imaging of the posterolateral structures of the knee: Findings in human cadavers. Arthroscopy 2002;18(8): 872–881.
6. Huang GS, Yu JS, Munshi M, et al. Avulsion fracture of the head of the fibula (the "arcuate" sign): MR imaging findings predictive of injuries to the posterolateral ligaments and posterior cruciate ligament. AJR 2003;180(2):381–387.
7. Munshi M, Pretterklieber ML, Kwak S et al. MR imaging, MR arthrography, and specimen correlation of the posterolateral corner of the knee: An anatomic study. AJR 2003;180(4):1095–1101.
8. Starok M, Lenchik L, Trudell D et al. Normal patellar retinaculum: MR and sonographic imaging with cadaveric correlation. AJR 1997;168(6):1493–1499.
9. Bianchi S, Zwass A, Abdelwahab IF et al. Diagnosis of tears of the quadriceps tendon of the knee: Value of sonography. AJR 1994;162(5):1137–1140.
10. Bonaldi VM, Chhem RK, Drolet R et al. Iliotibial band friction syndrome: Sonographic findings. J Ultrasound Med 1998;17(4):257–260.
11. Aisen AM, McCune WJ, MacGuire A et al. Sonographic evaluation of the cartilage of the knee. Radiology 1984;153(3):781–784.
12. Roth C, Jacobson J, Jamadar D et al. Quadriceps fat pad signal intensity and enlargement on MRI: Prevalence and associated findings. AJR 2004;182(6): 1383–1387.
13. Ward EE, Jacobson JA, Fessell DP et al. Sonographic detection of Baker's cysts: Comparison with MR imaging. AJR 2001;176(2):373–380.
14. Rothstein CP, Laorr A, Helms CA et al. Semimembranosus-tibial collateral ligament bursitis: MR imaging findings. AJR 1996;166(4):875–877.
15. De Maeseneer M, Shahabpour M, Van Roy F et al. MR imaging of the medial collateral ligament bursa: Findings in patients and anatomic data derived from cadavers. AJR 2001;177(4):911–917.
16. Cho KH, Lee DC, Chhem RK et al. Normal and acutely torn posterior cruciate ligament of the knee at US evaluation: Preliminary experience. Radiology 2001;219(2):375–380.
17. Ptasznik R, Feller J, Bartlett J et al. The value of sonography in the diagnosis of traumatic rupture of the anterior cruciate ligament of the knee. AJR 1995;164(6):1461–1463.

10

The Leg

John O'Neill

The leg is commonly imaged as an extension of an examination from the adjacent joints when symptoms or pathology extend proximally or distally. The leg, which extends between the knee and ankle joints, is highly suited to ultrasound evaluation given the superficial nature of its structures. Ultrasound has the advantage over other imaging modalities in that it can localize the site of symptoms and then trace the pathology proximally or distally in real time as required. Magnetic resonance imaging (MRI), for example, may require changing the imaging field of view and coils. In addition, ultrasound will allow a dynamic assessment, e.g., in the evaluation of an intermittent muscle hernia or tendon subluxation. Ultrasound, however, can be limited as resolution decreases with depth, whereas MRI will provide excellent imaging of deeper structures, e.g., the deep posterior compartment. Although ultrasound and MRI are often viewed as competing imaging modalities, they are more often complementary in a musculoskeletal imaging center.

Imaging Indications

The Achilles tendon is the commonest tendon evaluated in the leg. It has a wide range of pathologies including tendonosis, partial thickness, full thickness, and complete tears. Associated paratendonitis, peritendonitis, enthesopathy, retroachillean, and retrocalcaneal bursitis may occur. Anatomical variation in the calcaneus (Haglund deformity) may be related to Achilles tendon pathology. When assessing the Achilles tendon, the full tendon should be evaluated from the musculotendinous junction to insertion. This may reveal pathology extending into or from the parent muscle bellies.

Muscles may be affected by hematomas and by partial, interstitial, or complete posttraumatic tears. A muscle hernia may be only intermittent and may require dynamic evaluation with alternate contracture and relaxation of the parent muscle. Intramuscular masses can be assessed for cystic versus solid components, intralesional and perilesional flow on Doppler, and dynamic changes with contracture of the muscle, including changes in hemodynamics and the relationship to surrounding neurovascular bundles. In addition, ultrasound can guide biopsy to the most appropriate solid component and avoid significant perilesional and intralesional vessels. In general, all biopsies should be performed in consultation with a surgeon and should avoid routes through adjacent compartments.

The nerves of the leg can be readily assessed, particularly when those that are relatively superficial (as in the common peroneal nerve at the fibular head and the posterior tibial nerve behind the medial malleolus) for neuropathy, entrapment, and primary lesions such as neuromas. The tibia and fibula, except for their posterior surfaces, are quite superficial and can be assessed throughout their length for pathology, including stress fractures and periosteal reactions.

Technical Review

The choice of ultrasound transducer will depend on the region being evaluated and the habitus of the patient. In general, the transducer is chosen that will offer the highest resolution at the depth of the structure being evaluated. This may be a linear multifrequency 9- to 15-MHz transducer for superficial structures; deep structures, e.g., the deep group within the posterior compartment, may require a curvilinear 2.5- to 5-MHz transducer. Knowledge of ultrasound equipment is essential for optimal examination. As always, structures are evaluated with the transducer perpendicular to the anatomy and in orthogonal planes.

Anatomy

The leg extends between the knee and ankle joint. It is composed of two bones—the tibia and fibula, and three muscle compartments—anterior, peroneal, and posterior. The latter is subdivided into a superficial and a deep compartment. We will begin with surface anatomy, which is an important adjunct to a full ultrasound study, allowing the examiner to identify important anatomical landmarks. The individual anatomical components of the leg will then be reviewed.

Surface Anatomy

The anterior and medial surfaces of the tibia are subcutaneous and can be palpated throughout their length.[1] The anterior border of the tibia forms the shin. The medial border continues distally to form the medial malleolus. On the anterior aspect of the proximal tibia is a bony prominence, the tibial tuberosity, which is the site of attachment for the patellar tendon (Figure 10.1a). The latter extends from the inferior pole of the patella and is easily palpable as a tight soft tissue band overlying the anterior aspect of the knee joint. The tibia articulates with the femoral condyles with its own medial and lateral plateaus or condyles. The fibular head is lateral and slightly posterior to the tibia below the level of the knee joint and is palpated as a bony prominence. In thin patients, the common peroneal nerve can be felt wrapping around the neck of the fibula as a rounded cord. Posteriorly, at the level of the knee joint, lies the popliteal fossa, which has been described in detail in Chapter 9 (Figure 10.1c). At the lower end of the popliteal fossa is a small depression between the medial and lateral heads of the gastrocnemius.

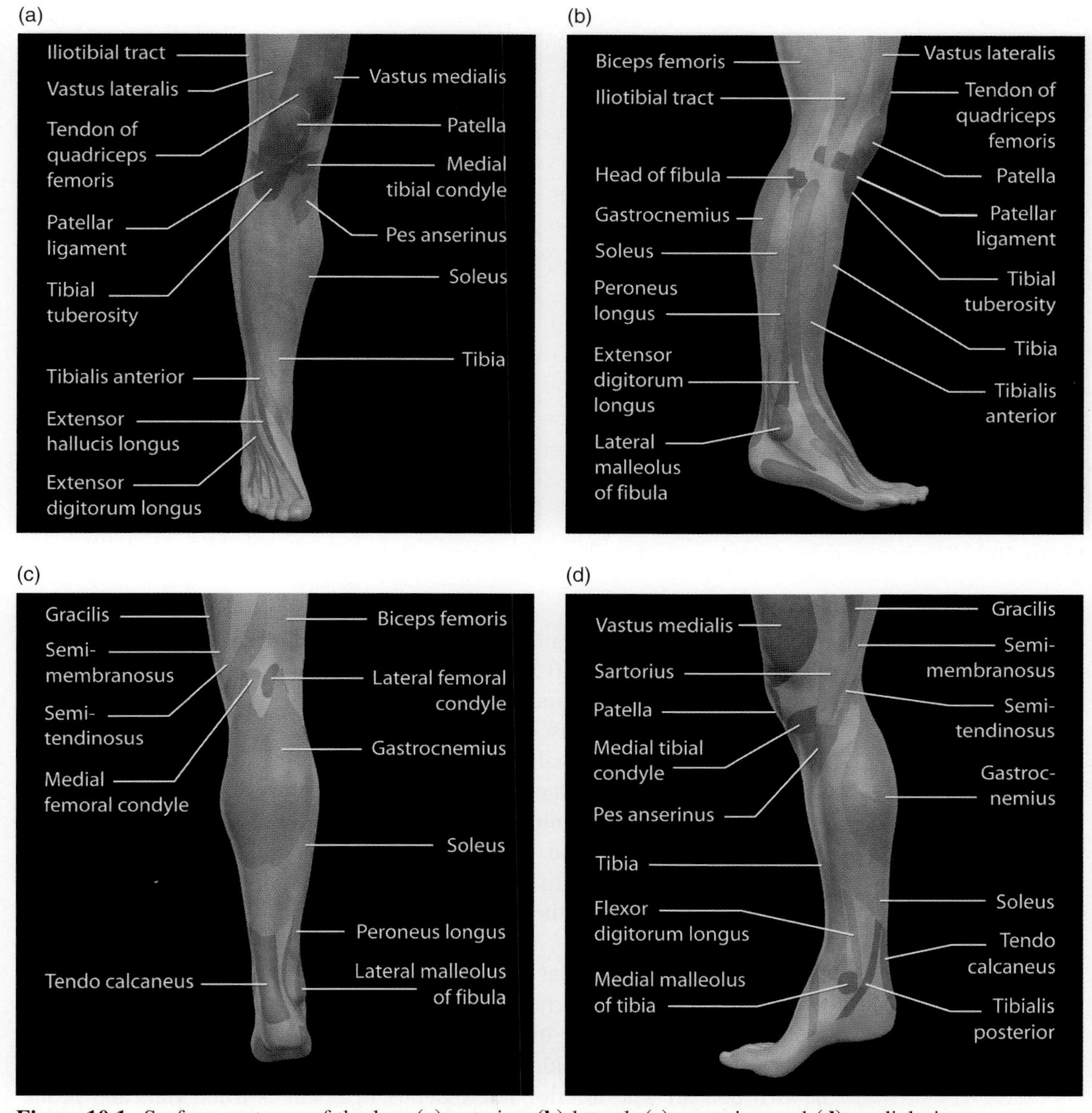

Figure 10.1. Surface anatomy of the leg: **(a)** anterior, **(b)** lateral, **(c)** posterior, and **(d)** medial views.

Distally, at the level of the ankle joint, the medial and lateral malleoli are well-defined, bony prominences on the medial and lateral surfaces, respectively (Figure 10.1b and d). Posteriorly the thick soft tissue band of the Achilles tendon is easily palpable to its calcaneal insertion (Figure 10.1c). The surface anatomy of the ankle is reviewed in Chapter 11.

Bones

The tibia is the medial and larger of the two bones within the leg and is the primary weight bearer. The shaft is triangular in cross-section and has three surfaces: medial, lateral, and posterior, and three borders: medial, lateral, and

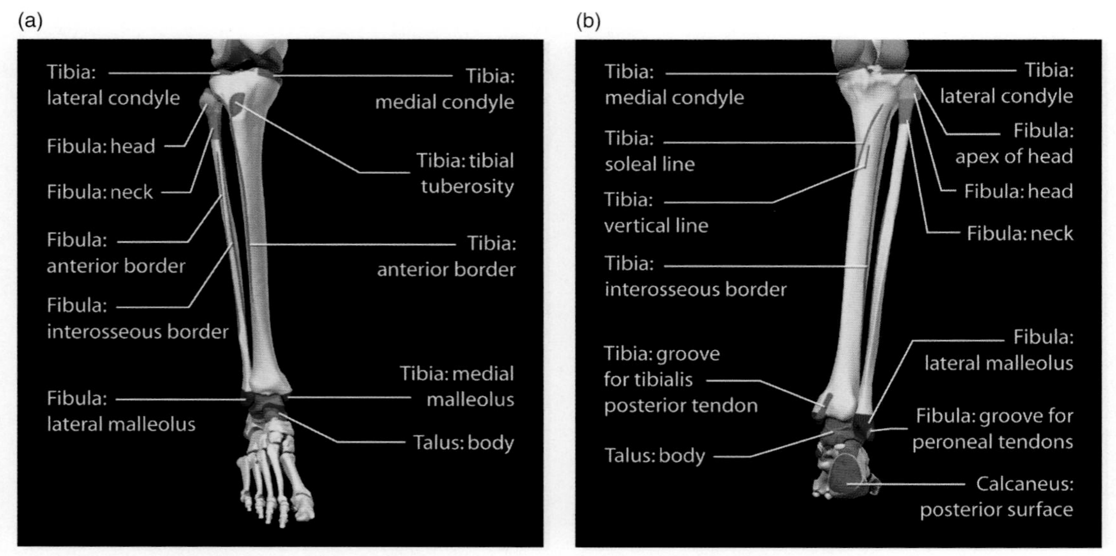

Figure 10.2. The important bony landmarks of the leg: (**a**) anterior and (**b**) posterior views.

anterior.[1] It has proximal and distal expansions for articulating with the knee and ankle joints (Figure 10.2); these are detailed in their relevant chapters.

The fibula is a comparatively slender bone that serves primarily as a site of attachment for muscles, ligaments, and tendons. It has four surfaces and borders. The proximal tibiofibular articulation is an arthrodial joint, which allows a gliding motion.[1] The synovium and capsule of this joint may occasionally communicate posteriorly with the knee joint. The joint is surrounded by the capsular ligament and the anterior superior and posterior superior ligaments; these extend superomedially from the fibula to the tibia. The posterior aspect of the joint is covered by the popliteus tendon and muscle.

The inferior tibiofibular articulation is predominantly a syndesmosis between the roughened surfaces of the convex medial aspect of the fibula and the concave lateral aspect of the tibia. Inferior to the syndesmosis are small contact facets covered with articular cartilage with direct contact between the two bones.[2] The inferior interosseous ligament is triangular, and is the distal continuation of the interosseous membrane that forms the apex of the ligament. The fibers pass inferolaterally from the tibia to the fibula with occasional fibers running transversely or anterosuperiorly.

Interosseous Membrane

The interosseous membrane is a thin aponeurotic membrane arising from the lateral border or interosseous crest of the tibia to the anteromedial surface of the fibula. The fibers are predominantly oriented in a downward and outward direction with fibers occasionally traveling in the opposite direction (Figure 10.3). It begins just inferior to the head of the fibula and has a concave upper margin for the passage of the anterior tibial vessels. Inferiorly, the anterior peroneal vessels transverse the membrane. The interosseous membrane continues as the inferior interosseous ligament. It functions as a

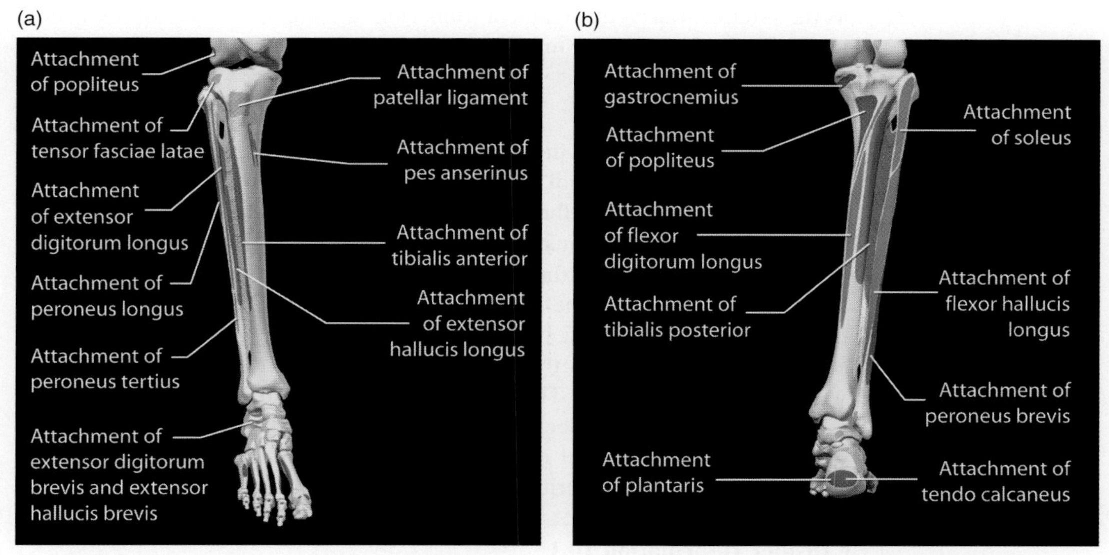

Figure 10.3. The important muscle origin (red) and insertion (blue) points of the muscles of the leg: **(a)** anterior and **(b)** posterior views.

stabilizer between the tibia and fibula, the site of muscular attachment, and separates the lateral compartment from the deep posterior compartment.[1]

Ligaments

The anterior inferior tibiofibular ligament has three components, separated by up to 2 mm, which run obliquely laterally and inferiorly from the anterior aspect of the tibia to the fibula above the level of the ankle joint (Table 10.1). It is triangular in shape with a broader attachment to the fibula.[1] It is a continuation from the anterior fibers of the interosseous tibiofibular ligament from which it is separated by 2 mm. The upper part of the ligament is short and narrow. The middle part passes from the anterior tubercles of the tibia and fibula and is longer and wider. The lower part is long, narrow, and thin.

The posterior inferior tibiofibular ligament is similar in shape, but has a more horizontal orientation than the anterior tibiofibular ligament. It lies in close relation to the posterior-inferior margin of the interosseous ligament. The upper part of this ligament attaches to the posterior tubercle of the tibia and fibula. The inferior portion of this ligament, which has also been described

Table 10.1. Tibiofibular Ligaments.

Proximal tibiofibular joint
Anterior superior tibiofibular
Posterior superior tibiofibular
Distal tibiofibular joint
Anterior inferior tibiofibular
Posterior inferior tibiofibular
Transverse (inferior) tibiofibular
Inferior interosseous

as the inferior transverse ligament, runs from the medial surface of the lateral malleolus to the posterior-inferior aspect of the tibia.

Fascia

The deep fascia encloses the muscles of the leg except over the superficial surface of the tibia where it is attached to its medial and anterior borders. It is continuous above with the deep fascia of the thigh and inferiorly with the annular ligaments of the ankle. Its deep surface, on its outer aspect, gives off two intermuscular septae that enclose the peroneal or lateral compartment.[3] Posteriorly, it gives off the deep transverse fascia of the leg, which divides the posterior compartment into superficial and deep compartments. Smaller septae are given off from the deep fascia to enclose the individual muscles within the compartments. The interosseous membrane separates the anterior compartment from the deep posterior compartment. Knowledge of these compartments is important in any interventional procedures, such as biopsy, so as to preserve the integrity of adjacent compartments

Insider Information 10.1
The leg has three main muscle compartments: the anterior, lateral, and posterior compartments. The posterior compartment is divided into superficial and deep compartments. Knowledge of these different compartments is important in any interventional procedures, such as biopsy, so as not to violate the integrity of adjacent compartments.

Muscles and Tendons

The leg has three main muscle compartments: the anterior, lateral, and posterior compartments; the posterior is divided into superficial and deep compartments.[3] The individual muscles are outlined in Table 10.2, which details their origin, insertion, and action. The evaluation of the popliteus is included in Chapter 9; the distal tendons of the remaining muscles, excluding the superficial component of the posterior compartment, are reviewed in Chapter 11.

The anterior compartment contains the tibialis anterior, extensor hallucis longus, extensor digitorum longus, and peroneus tertius (Figures 10.3, 10.4, and 10.5). The tibialis anterior is anteromedial within the compartment and has a large muscular belly and a long tendon. The extensor hallucis longus is a thin muscle between the tibialis anterior and the extensor digitorum longus. The latter is a penniform muscle on the lateral aspect of the anterior compartment. The peroneus tertius is part of the extensor digitorum longus and arises in the distal aspect of the leg and passes through the same canal within the annular ligament. It is occasionally absent.

The lateral compartment contains the peroneus brevis and longus. The peroneus longus is superficial and larger and has a longer tendon, as its name implies, than the deeper brevis, which allows for clear distinction of the peroneal tendons in the supramalleolar region (Figures 10.3 and 10.4). Occasionally the peroneus quadratus tendon, an accessory muscle, is present. It usually arises from the peroneus brevis and inserts into the calcaneus, but is quite variable in origin and insertion, as is the position of its musculotendinous junction.[4]

Table 10.2. Muscles and Compartments of the Leg.

Muscle	Origin	Insertion	Main action
Anterior compartment			
Tibialis anterior	Lateral proximal shaft tibia, interosseous membrane	Medial cuneiform, base of first metatarsal	Dorsiflexion and inversion of foot
Extensor hallucis longus	Anterior fibula and interosseous membrane	Base of distal phalanx of great toe	Dorsiflexion and extension of great toe
Extensor digitorum longus	Lateral tibial condyle, anterior shaft fibula, and interosseous membrane	Base of middle and distal phalanges of second to fifth toes	Dorsiflexion and extension of second to fifth toes
Peroneus tertius	Lower third of the anterior surface of the fibula and interosseous membrane	Dorsal base of fifth metatarsal	Dorsiflexion and eversion of foot
Lateral compartment			
Peroneus longus	Head and proximal lateral shaft of fibula	Medial cuneiform and plantar aspect of base of first metatarsal	Eversion and plantar flexion of foot
Peroneus brevis	Distal lateral shaft of fibula	Base of fifth metatarsal	Eversion and plantar flexion of foot
Posterior compartment	**Superficial group**		
Gastrocnemius	Lateral and medial heads from lateral and medial femoral condyles, respectively	Posterior calcaneus (via the Achilles tendon)	Plantar flexion of foot
Soleus	Posterior head of fibula and adjacent proximal shaft, soleal line of tibia	Posterior calcaneus (via the Achilles tendon)	Plantar flexion of foot
Plantaris	Lateral femoral supracondylar line	Posterior calcaneus, medial to Achilles insertion	Plantar flexion of foot
Posterior compartment	**Deep group**		
Tibialis posterior	Posterior aspects of the interosseous membrane, tibia and fibula	Navicular tuberosity and fibrous expansions to the cuboid, cuneiforms, bases of second to fourth metatarsals	Plantar flexion and inversion of foot
Flexor digitorum longus	Posterior shaft of tibia	Bases of distal phalanges second to fifth toes	Plantar flexion of second to fifth toes
Flexor hallucis longus	Posterior fibula lower two-thirds	Base of distal phalanx of great toe	Plantar flexion of great toe
Popliteus	Popliteal groove of lateral femoral condyle	Posterior proximal shaft of tibia	Flexion of knee and internal rotation of tibia

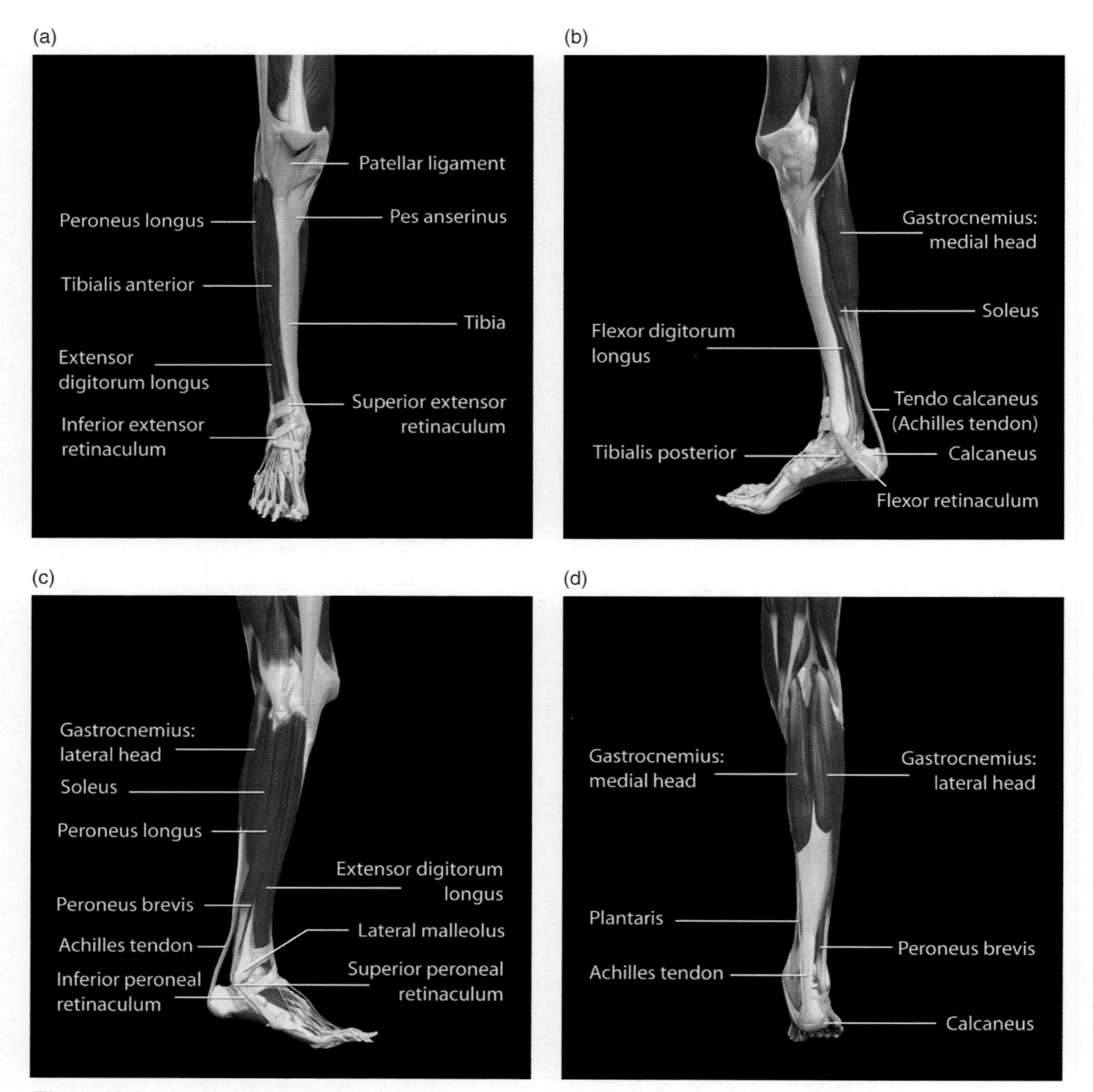

Figure 10.4. Muscles of the thigh: (**a**) anterior, (**b**) medial, (**c**) lateral, and (**d**) posterior views.

The posterior compartment is composed of a superficial and deep group of muscles (Figures 10.3, 10.4, and 10.5). The superficial group contains the gastrocnemius muscle, the plantaris, and the soleus. The gastrocnemius is the largest and most superficial muscle of the calf, arising from two heads: the lateral and the larger medial head. The soleus is deep to the gastrocnemius. It is a broad flat muscle, resembling a sole fish, hence its name. Within the midcalf, the Achilles tendon (AT) is formed by the union of the two heads of the gastrocnemius muscle and the soleus tendons. The AT fibers spiral to their insertion, with the posterior fibers from the gastrocnemius passing medial to lateral, creating a wavelike contour anteriorly. The AT has a crescent shape with a slightly concave anterior surface, although in 10% of normal tendons

(a)

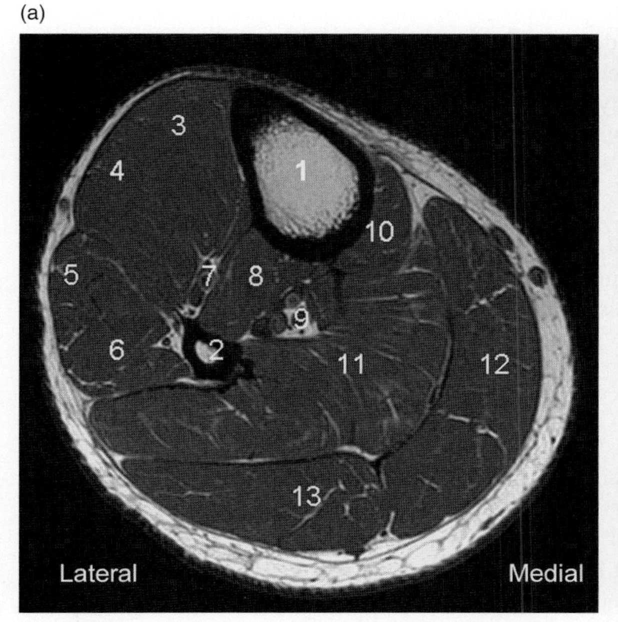

(b)

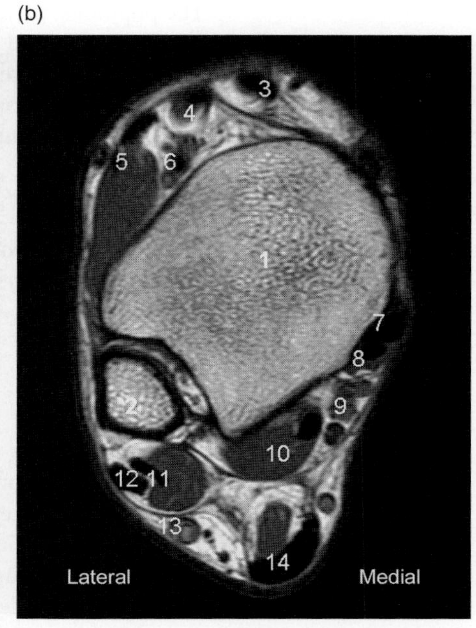

Figure 10.5. Axial T1-weighted MRI anatomy. **(a)** Axial image of the upper leg: 1–tibia, 2–fibula, 3–tibialis anterior, 4–extensor hallucis longus, 5–extensor digitorum longus, 6–peroneus longus and brevis, 7–anterior tibial vessels and deep peroneal nerve, 8–tibialis posterior, 9–posterior tibial vessels and tibial nerve, 10–flexor digitorum longus, 11–soleus, 12–medial head of gastrocnemius, 13–lateral head of gastrocnemius. **(b)** Axial above level of ankle joint: 1–tibia, 2–fibula, 3–tibialis anterior tendon, 4–extensor hallucis longus tendon, 5–extensor digitorum longus, 6–anterior tibial vessels and deep peroneal nerve, 7–tibialis posterior tendon, 8–flexor digitorum longus tendon, 9–posterior tibial vessels and tibial nerve, 10–flexor hallucis longus, 11–peroneus brevis, 12–peroneus longus, 13–lesser saphenous vein and sural nerve, 14–Achilles tendon.

it may be rounded. It is enclosed by the paratenon, a connective tissue layer analogous to synovium. Approximately 2–6 cm from its insertion is a zone of decreased vascular supply that is less resilient to repetitive microtrauma. It inserts by way of an enthesis into the posterior calcaneus.

The plantaris has a small muscle belly and a long thin tendon that crosses from the lateral to medial aspect of the calf, between the soleus and gastrocnemius muscles, and inserts on the posterior calcaneus, medial to the AT. It may normally be absent. Its presence and integrity should be carefully assessed for incomplete tears of the AT, as it may appear in these circumstances to be a remnant of a large full-thickness tear of the AT.

Insider Information 10.2

The Achilles tendon fibers spiral to their insertion, with the posterior fibers from the gastrocnemius passing medial to lateral, creating a wavelike contour on ultrasound.

An accessory soleus may occur as a normal anatomical variation. It may not present clinically until early adulthood when hypertrophy of the muscle may cause symptoms. It typically arises from the anterior surface of the soleus, tibia, or fibula and attaches either to the AT or calcaneus.[5,6]

The popliteus, tibialis posterior, flexor digitorum longus, and flexor hallucis longus comprise the deep group of the posterior compartment. The flexor hallucis longus is the more superficial and largest of these muscles and is separated posteriorly from the soleus by the deep transverse fascia. The flexor digitorum longus has a small muscle belly that gradually increases in size distally.

Insider Information 10.3
Common accessory muscles include the peroneus quadratus, the accessory soleus, and the accessory flexor digitorum longus.

Nerves

The two terminal branches of the sciatic nerve, the tibial nerve and the common peroneal nerve, arise in the posterior aspect of the lower third of the thigh.[7,8] The tibial nerve is the larger of the two and maintains the path of its parent, traveling into the popliteal fossa adjacent to the popliteal artery and vein. It passes deep to the soleus, becoming the posterior tibial nerve, to enter the posterior deep compartment, initially related to the posterior aspect of the tibialis posterior and then the posterior surface of the tibia distally (Figure 10.5). It is accompanied by the posterior tibial artery and vein. It passes posterior to the lateral malleolus, lateral to the artery and under the flexor retinaculum to divide into the medial and lateral plantar nerves. It supplies all the muscles within the posterior compartment, gives articular branches to the knee and ankle joints as well as cutaneous branches, the sural nerve to the calf and posterior leg, and the medial calcaneal branch to supply the medial surface of the heel.

The common peroneal nerve courses laterally from its origin toward the biceps femoris tendon within the popliteal fossa. It crosses the lateral head of the gastrocnemius and the head of the fibula to wind anteriorly around the neck of the fibula. Between the fibula and peroneus longus, it divides into the anterior tibial and superficial peroneal nerves.

The anterior tibial nerve passes deep to the extensor digitorum longus and descends with the anterior tibial artery into the anterior compartment. At the level of the ankle joint, it lies lateral to the artery and divides into its terminal branches: the external and internal nerves. It supplies the muscles of the anterior compartment. The superficial peroneal nerve descends between the peroneus longus and brevis, which it supplies, and pierces the deep fascia in the lower third of the leg, dividing into internal and external cutaneous branches.

Bursae

The retrocalcaneal bursa is a horseshoe-shaped structure between the postero-superior aspect of the calcaneus, Kager's fat pad, and the AT posteriorly. It may normally be mildly distended with fluid measuring less than 1 mm in anteroposterior diameter.[9] A subcutaneous bursa, the retroachillean bursa, can develop posterior to the AT and is always abnormal. Bursae of the ankle and knee are detailed in their respective chapters.

Technique

The examination of the leg is usually focused on a specific clinical problem; a pertinent clinical history is thus very important. Knowledge of the different compartments is important, as pathology within a compartment may arise from any component of that compartment and present with similar clinical complaints. Technique will initially be described for the assessment of individual muscle compartments. In addition to static examination, muscles and tendons should be evaluated while in a contracted and relaxed state for a full dynamic assessment. This movement can be important in assessing and identifying pathologies, including the full extent of a tear and intermittent muscle hernias. Table 10.3 summarizes the ultrasound position for the different muscle compartments.

Anterior Compartment

The patient lies supine on a couch, with the knee flexed to 45° and the plantar aspect of the foot flat on the couch. The anterior compartment contains the tibialis anterior, extensor hallucis longus, extensor digitorum longus, and peroneus tertius. Locate by palpation the tibial tuberosity on the anterior and superior aspect of the tibia. Place the transducer in a transverse plane to the tibia and move the transducer slowly laterally (Figure 10.6). The first structure seen is the tibialis anterior (TA) at the level of its musculotendinous junction. The TA is anteromedial within the compartment and has a large muscular belly and a long tendon. Once identified, it can be followed proximally and distally. The extensor digitorum longus (EDL) is a penniform muscle on the lateral aspect of the TA (Figure 10.7).

The extensor hallucis longus (EHL) is a thin muscle between the TA and EDL, but does not arise until the mid leg and is identified by moving the transducer in the transverse plane distally, after having identified the TA and EDL (Figure 10.8). The peroneus tertius is part of the EDL that arises in the distal aspect of the leg and passes through the same canal under the annular

Table 10.3. Ultrasound Position in the Evaluation of Muscle Compartments.

Muscle	Position examined
Anterior compartment	
Tibialis anterior	Patient supine, knee flexed, and plantar aspect of foot flat on table
Extensor hallucis longus	
Digitorum longus peroneus tertius	
Lateral compartment	
Peroneus longus	Patient supine, knee flexed, and plantar aspect of foot flat on table with mild inversion.
Peroneus brevis	
Posterior compartment	**Deep group**
Tibialis posterior	Patient supine, knee flexed, and plantar aspect of foot flat on table
Flexor digitorum longus	
Flexor hallucis longus	
Popliteus	Patient prone, leg extended
Posterior compartment	**Superficial group**
Gastrocnemius	Patient prone with foot dorsiflexed, hanging over table end
Soleus	
Plantaris	

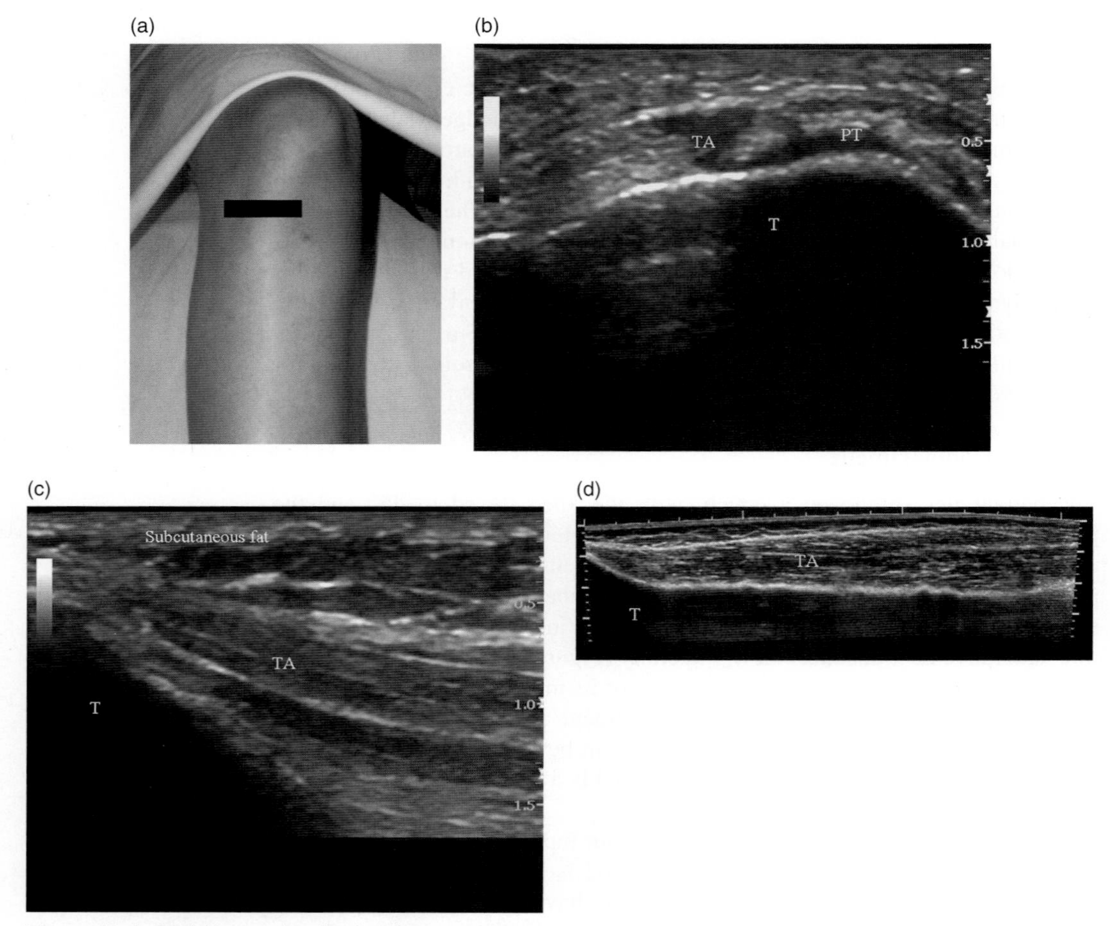

Figure 10.6. Tibialis anterior (TA). **(a)** Transducer position at the level of the tibial tuberosity and the tibialis anterior origin, with **(b)** corresponding transverse and **(c)** longitudinal ultrasound images. **(d)** Longitudinal extended field of view. PT, patellar tendon; T, tibia.

ligament. It is occasionally absent. It may be easier to identify its distal tendon where it inserts onto the fifth metatarsal shaft and to trace it proximally.

> **Insider Information 10.4**
> For a full dynamic assessment, muscles and tendons are evaluated while in a contracted and relaxed state. This dynamic motion can be important in assessing pathologies, including the full extent of a tear and intermittent muscle hernias.

Lateral Compartment

The patient remains in the same position as for the anterior compartment and inverts the foot. Placing a pillow between both knees may increase patient comfort. The lateral compartment contains the peroneus longus (PL) and peroneus brevis (PB). The PL can be identified by first palpating the lateral aspect of the head of the fibula. Place the transducer in a transverse plane with

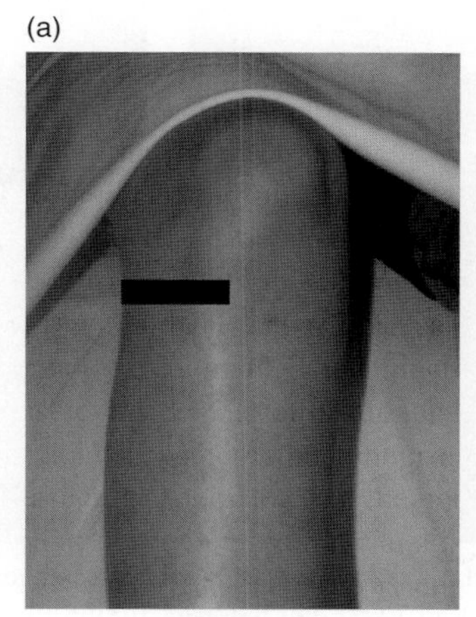

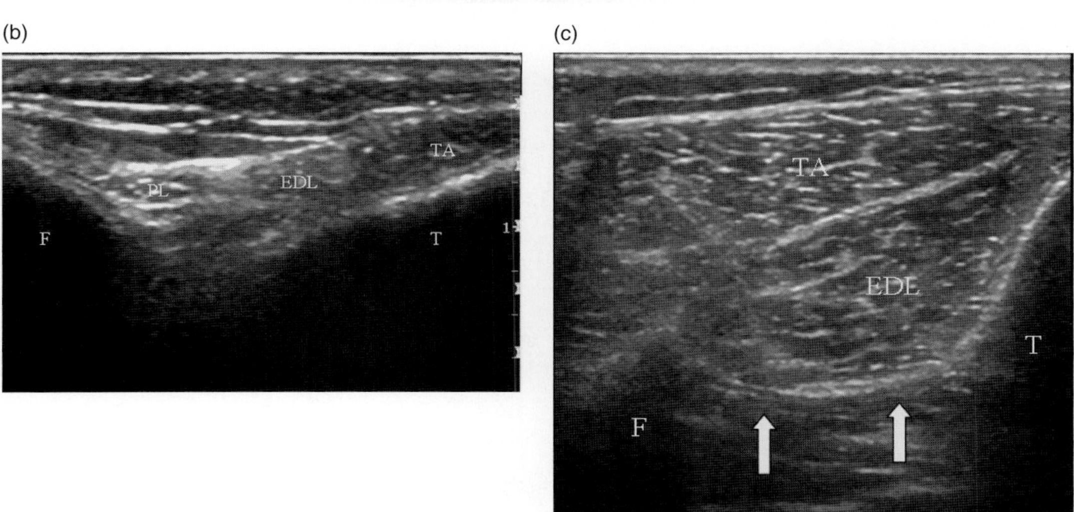

Figure 10.7. Proximal anterior compartment. **(a)** Transducer position at the level of the tibial tuberosity and **(b)** a corresponding transverse ultrasound image. **(c)** Anterior compartment level of the mid leg demonstrating the interosseous membrane. F, fibula; T, tibia; TA, tibialis anterior; EDL, extensor digitorum longus; PL, peroneus longus; arrow, interosseous membrane.

respect to the fibula. The cortex is identified as a continuous hyperechoic line. Directly superficial to the cortex is the PL tendon (Figures 10.7 and 10.9). As its name implies, the PL has a long tendon that arises at the level of the mid shaft of the fibula. Deep to the musculotendinous junction of the PL is the origin of the PB, whose musculotendinous junction is just proximal to the ankle and allows for easy differentiation of the tendons (Figure 10.10). The PB tendon lies on the medial aspect of its parent muscle belly.

Posterior Compartment

The patient lies prone, legs straight, with the feet projecting over the end of the couch. The posterior compartment is divided into deep and superficial groups. The superficial group contains the medial and lateral gastrocnemius, the soleus, and the plantaris muscles. All, except the plantaris, insert via the AT.

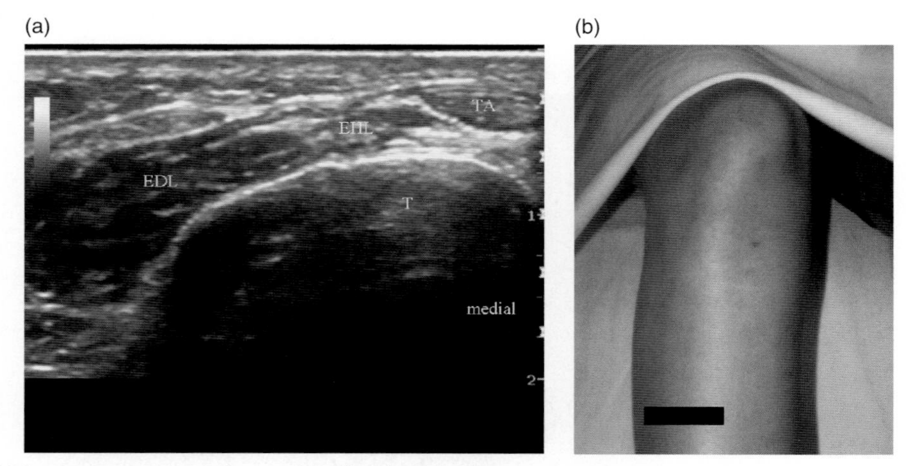

Figure 10.8. Extensor hallucis longus (EHL). **(a)** Transverse ultrasound image of the mid-leg demonstrating the relationship of the EHL to the tibialis anterior (TA) and extensor digitorum longus (EDL) within the anterior compartment and **(b)** a corresponding transducer position. T, tibia.

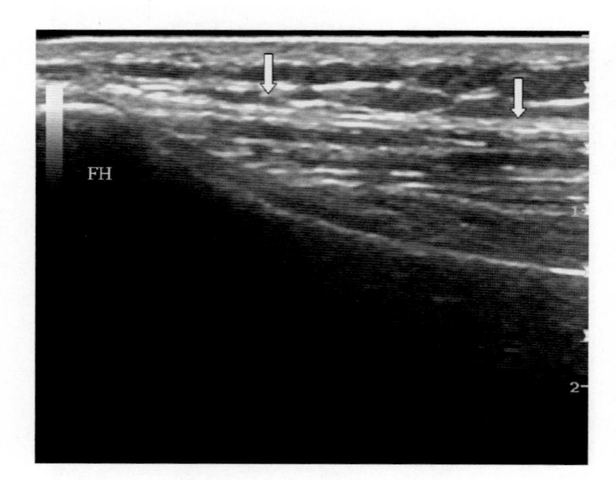

Figure 10.9. A longitudinal ultrasound image of the origin of the peroneus longus from the head and proximal shaft of the fibula. Peroneus longus (arrows); FH, fibular head.

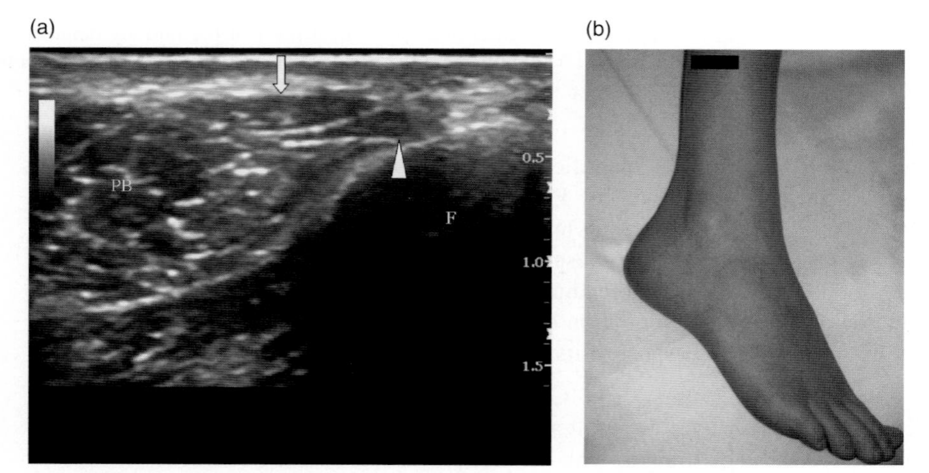

Figure 10.10. Peroneus brevis and longus. **(a)** Transverse ultrasound image of the anterolateral aspect of the junction of the mid and distal leg, demonstrating the musculotendinous junction of the peroneus longus (arrow), the peroneus brevis muscle (PB) (arrowhead) abutting the cortical surface of the fibula (F) and **(b)** a corresponding transducer position.

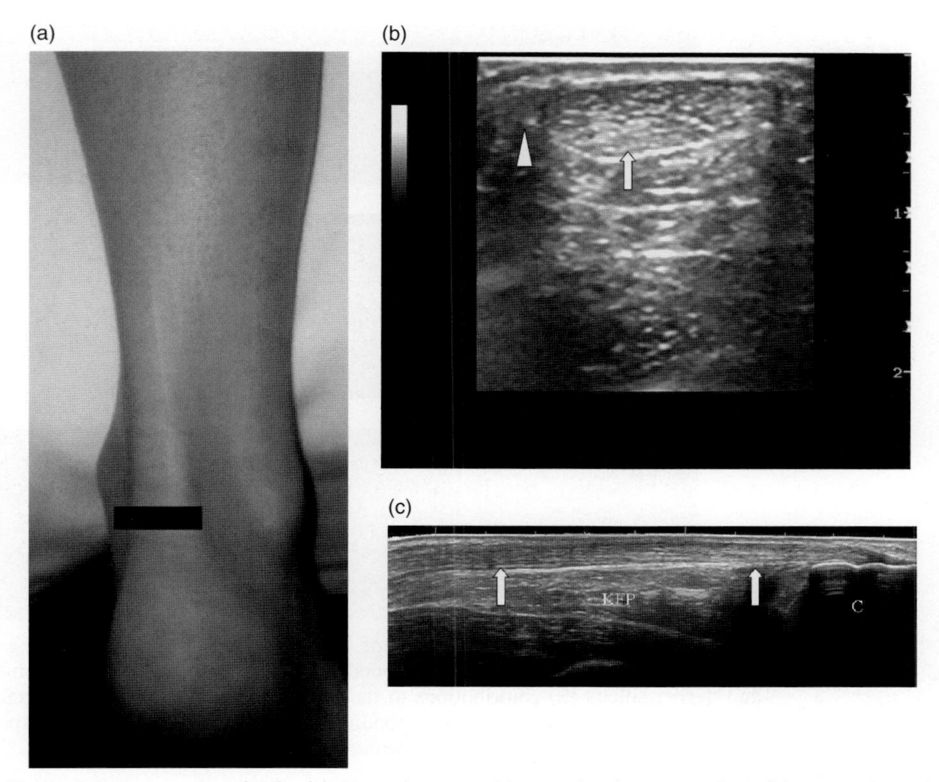

Figure 10.11. Achilles tendon (AT). **(a)** Transducer position and a corresponding **(b)** transverse ultrasound image of the AT (arrows) and adjacent plantaris tendon (arrowhead) medially. The paratenon is identified as the thin hyperechoic rim surrounding the AT. **(c)** Longitudinal extended field of view of the AT. C, calcaneus; KFP, Kager's fat pad.

The AT is first palpated as a soft tissue band in the midline of the lower calf. Place the transducer in a transverse plane on the AT (Figure 10.11a). It has a wavelike contour, due to the oblique nature of its fibers, which is appreciated by moving the transducer over the length of the tendon. The hyperechoic thin rim surrounding the tendon represents the paratenon. Deep to the paratenon lies Kagar's fat pad. Once fully evaluated in the transverse plane, the AT tendon is assessed in the longitudinal plane from insertion to origin (Figure 10.11). The contributions from the medial and lateral gastrocnemius and the deeper muscle of the soleus are then evaluated (Figure 10.12).[10] Dynamic assessment of the AT with alternate plantar and dorsiflexion of the foot should be performed. AT pathology is often bilateral and it is standard protocol in our center to evaluate the contralateral AT, even if asymptomatic. The plantaris, when present, has a thin short muscle between the gastrocnemius and soleus muscles. The tendon is easier to identify distally at the medial border of the AT and followed proximally (Figure 10.11). In the presence of a complete AT rupture it is important to identify the plantaris correctly and not to mistake its fibers for residual intact fibers of the AT.

The deep group can be more difficult to identify and may require the use of a lower frequency linear or possibly a curvilinear probe. It contains the

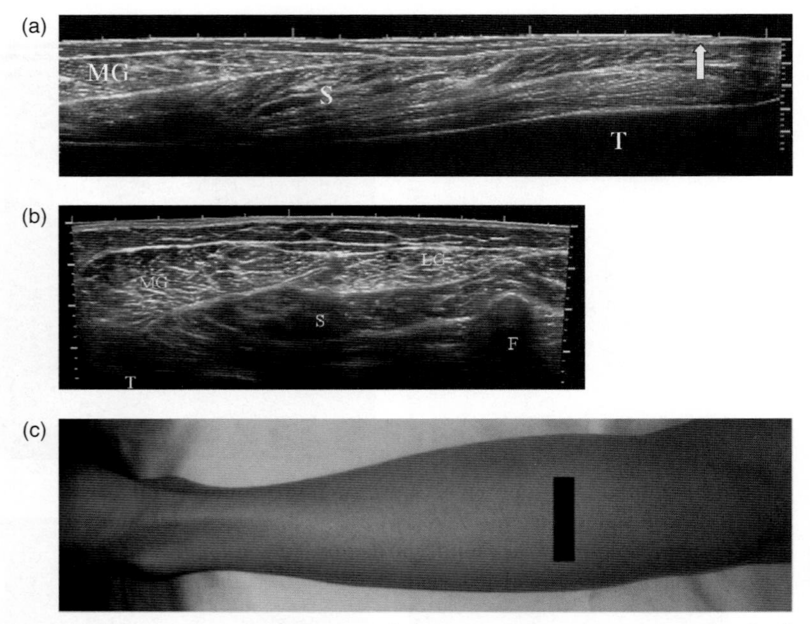

Figure 10.12. Posterior compartment of the superficial group. **(a)** A longitudinal extended field of view (EFOV) ultrasound image of the medial gastrocnemius (MG) and deeper soleus (S) contributions to the Achilles tendon (arrow). **(b)** A transverse EFOV ultrasound image and corresponding **(c)** transducer position of the proximal leg. T, tibia; F, fibula; LG, lateral gastrocnemius.

tibialis posterior (TP), flexor digitorum longus (FDL), and flexor hallucis longus (FHL). Evaluation can begin at the level of the ankle joint where the tendons pass behind the medial malleolus, in that order (Figures 10.13 and 10.14). The examination of the malleolar region is reviewed in detail in Chapter 11. Once the individual tendons are identified, they can be traced proximally into the calf.

Insider Information 10.5
Identification of muscles within a compartment can be difficult in uncommonly imaged areas. It is often easier to identify the appropriate tendon at a fixed point, e.g., the site of insertion or a fibroosseous tunnel, and then trace it proximally.

Interosseous Membrane and Ligaments

The interosseous membrane is identified by palpating the tibial tuberosity and placing the probe in a transverse orientation. The transducer is then slowly moved laterally until the hyperechoic surface of the fibula is seen in the same image as the tibia. The interosseous membrane is identified as a thin, hyperechoic line arising from the lateral border of the tibia to the anteromedial surface of the fibula with fibers oriented in a downward and

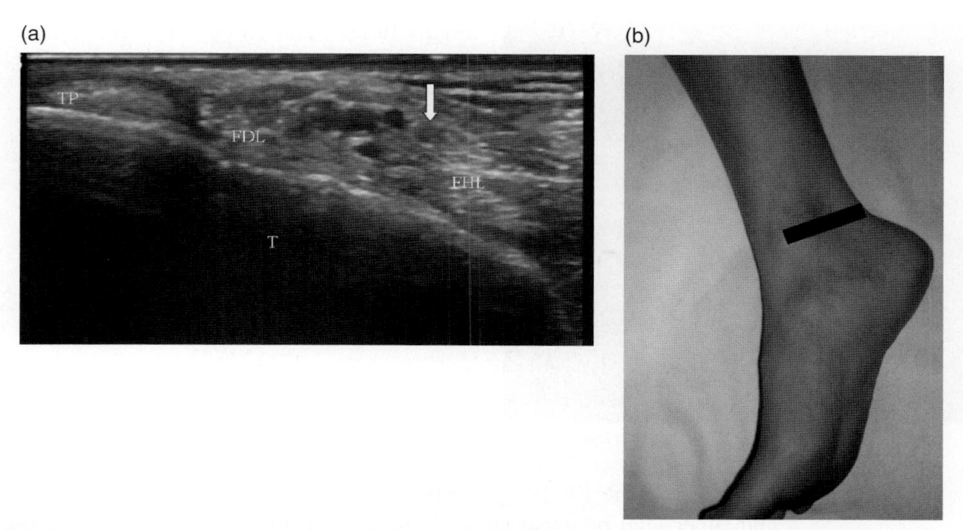

Figure 10.13. (**a**) Transverse ultrasound of the tendons in the deep posterior compartment of the leg at the level of the medial malleolus and (**b**) a corresponding transducer position. TP, tibialis posterior; FDL, flexor digitorum longus; arrow, posterior tibial nerve; FHL, flexor hallucis longus; T, tibia.

outward direction (Figure 10.7). It begins just inferior to the head of the fibula and has a concave upper margin for the passage of the anterior tibial vessels, which can be identified with power Doppler. It continues as the inferior interosseous ligament. The anterior and posterior inferior talofibular ligaments are reviewed in detail in Chapter 11.

Nerves

The common peroneal nerve is one of the two terminal branches of the sciatic nerve. It courses laterally from its midline origin to the posteromedial border of the biceps femoris tendon. The latter is palpated as a tense, soft tissue structure that forms the lateral margin of the posterior knee compartment. Place the transducer on the tendon transversely with the patient in a prone position and leg extended. The mixed hyperechoic pattern of the nerve is easily recognizable adjacent to the fibrillar pattern of the tendon (Figure 10.15). The common peroneal nerve winds around the hyperechoic neck of the fibula

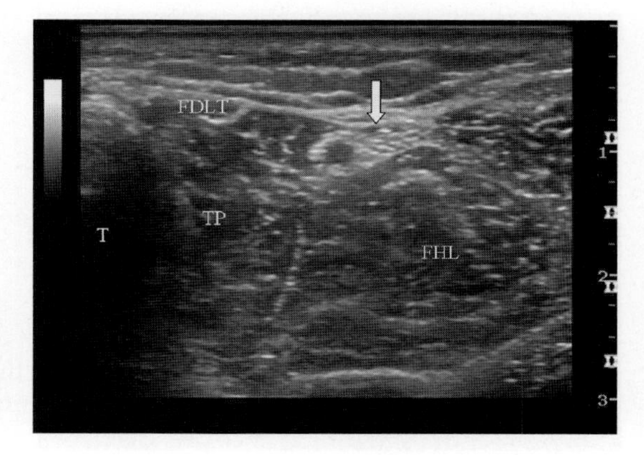

Figure 10.14. Transverse ultrasound of the tendons in the deep posterior compartment of the distal leg, proximal to Figure 10.13. TP, tibialis posterior; FDLT, flexor digitorum longus tendon; arrow, posterior tibial nerve; FHL, flexor hallucis longus; T, tibia.

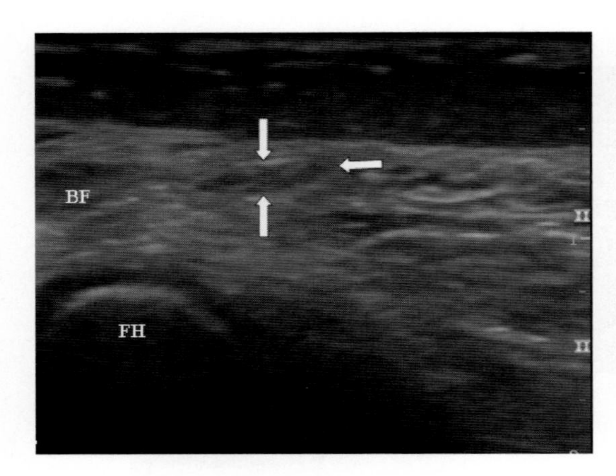

Figure 10.15. Common peroneal nerve (arrows) just proximal to the fibular head (FH) and medial to the biceps femoris (BF) tendon.

and between the fibula and peroneus longus, dividing into the anterior tibial and superficial peroneal nerves. The former dives deep between the muscles of the anterior compartment and is difficult to evaluate distally. The superficial peroneal nerve, once visualized proximally, can often be traced distally between the peroneal muscles and extensor digitorum longus.[8] It is often easier to first evaluate the nerves in the transverse plane.

Place the transducer in a transverse plane in the mid-popliteal fossa. The tibial nerve can be identified adjacent to the popliteal vessels (Figure 10.16). It passes deep to the soleus to enter the posterior deep compartment, accompanied by the posterior tibial artery and vein. The vessels can be easier to trace distally with power Doppler. The posterior tibial nerve passes deep to the medial retinaculum at the level of the ankle joint.

Bursae: Retrocalcaneal and Retroachillean

The retrocalcaneal bursa is located by palpating the distal AT and placing the transducer in a longitudinal plane. Anterior to the distal AT and just proximal to the hyperechoic cortical line of the calcaneus, a small anechoic structure with hyperechoic margins is easily seen; this is the retrocalcaneal bursa (Figure 10.17). The retroachillean bursa lies posterior to the AT and is always pathological, usually arising due to friction between footwear and the AT.

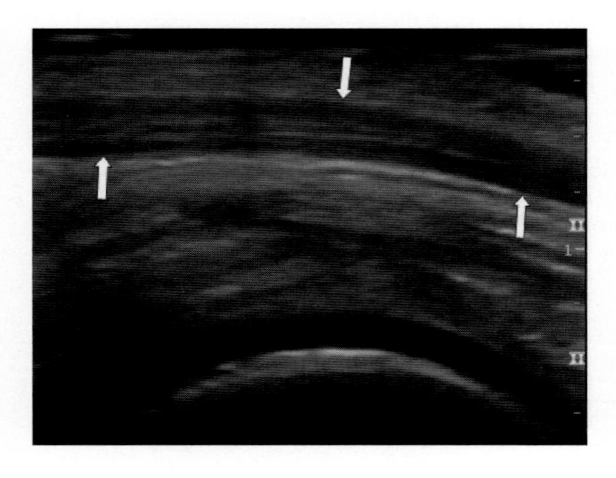

Figure 10.16. Tibial nerve (arrows). Longitudinal ultrasound image at the level of the popliteal fossa. Note that the tibial nerve changes from a relatively superficial structure in the proximal popliteal fossa to a deeper plane in the distal aspect of the fossa.

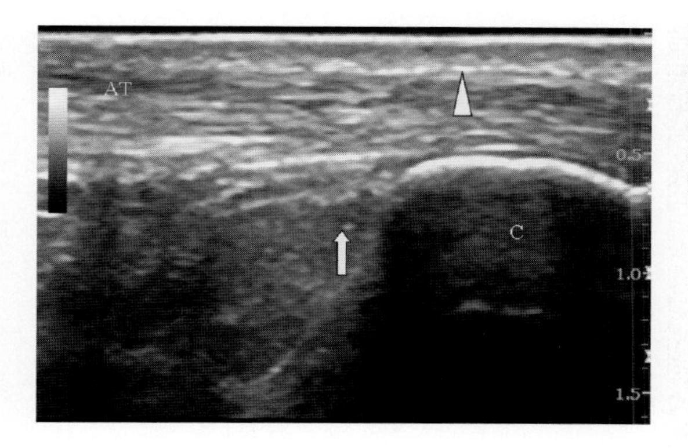

Figure 10.17. Retrocalcaneal bursa (RB). Longitudinal ultrasound at the site of insertion of the Achilles tendon (AT) into the calcaneus (C). The RB is not distended in this case; its expected site is marked with an arrow and the potential retroachillean bursa site is marked with an arrowhead.

Imaging Protocols

As in most musculoskeletal evaluations outside of joints there is no standardized protocol. The examination is tailored to the area of concern and the adjacent compartments. By reviewing the technique as described previously a structured approach can be utilized for evaluation of individual compartments, noting that it is important to evaluate adjacent structures that may cause referred symptoms.

References

1. Gray H. The Complete Gray's Anatomy, 16th ed., pp. 402–416. London: Longman, Green, and Co., 1905.
2. Bartonicek J. Anatomy of the tibiofibular syndesmosis and its clinical relevance. Surg Radiol Anat 2003;25(5–6):379–386.
3. Gray H. The Complete Gray's Anatomy, 16th ed., pp. 558–566. London: Longman, Green, and Co., 1905.
4. Chepuri NB, Jacobson JA, Fessell DP et al. Sonographic appearance of the peroneus quadratus muscle: Correlation with MR imaging appearance in seven patients. Radiology 2001;218(2):415–419.
5. Buschmann WR, Cheung Y, Jahss MH. Magnetic resonance imaging of anomalous leg muscles: Accessory soleus, peroneus quartus and the flexor digitorum longus accessories. Foot Ankle 1991;218(2):415–419.
6. Lorentzon R, Wirell S. Anatomic variations of the accessory soleus muscle. Acta Radiol 1987;28:627–629.
7. Gray H. The Complete Gray's Anatomy, 16th ed., pp. 926–930. London: Longman, Green, and Co., 1905.
8. Gruber H, Kovacs P. Sonographic anatomy of the peripheral nervous system. In Peer S, Bodner G (eds.). High Resolution Sonography of the Peripheral Nervous System, 1st ed., pp. 28–32. New York: Springer, 2003.
9. Bottger B, Schweitzer M, K El-Noueam et al. MR imaging of the normal and abnormal retrocalcaneal bursae. AJR 1998;170(5):1239–1241.
10. Astrom M, Gentz C-F, Nilsson P. Imaging in chronic Achilles tendinopathy: A comparison of ultrasonography, magnetic resonance imaging and surgical findings in 27 histologically verified cases. Skeletal Radiol 1996;25:615–620.

11

The Ankle and Foot

John O'Neill and Aaron Glickman

The ankle and foot are mostly superficial structures and thus are particularly suitable for ultrasound evaluation. Direct patient contact allows accurate identification of the site of symptoms and allows a pertinent history to be obtained. Ultrasound also offers real-time comparison with the contralateral side. In addition, the dynamic nature of ultrasound may allow visualization of intermittent pathology, such as tendon subluxation and impingement. The internal vascularity of pathology—e.g., synovitis—can be assessed with Doppler without resorting to intravenous contrast injection. Magnetic resonance imaging (MRI) also has many inherent advantages including the imaging of deeper soft tissue structures, bones, and joints, and it is less operator dependent. MRI and ultrasonography are, however, complementary imaging techniques and the choice of modality will often depend upon local expertise, accessibility, and cost.

Imaging Indications

Assessment of tendon pathology, particularly the posteromedial and posterolateral compartments, is the commonest indication at our imaging center. Tendonopathy, tenosynovitis, and partial, interstitial, and complete tendon tears can be evaluated, as well as dynamic studies for intermittent subluxation, dislocations, and impingement.[1–5]

Rheumatological referrals—for tenosynovitis, erosions, joint effusion, and synovial proliferation—are now the second commonest group for which we image. Studies may be performed to diagnose or confirm the presence of disease as well as to assess progression or absence thereof, including response to treatment. The metatarsophalangeal, ankle, and talonavicular joints are the commonest joints studied in this regard. Diagnostic joint aspirations and injections are also commonplace in this group of patients.[6] Joints may also be evaluated for loose bodies, synovial pathology including synovial osteochondromatosis and pigmented villonodular synovitis (PVNS).

Ligament injuries, often diagnosed clinically, can be confirmed and the full extent of injury assessed.[7,8] The plantar fascia is a common source of symptoms on the plantar aspect of the foot with plantar fasciitis and fibromas being the commonest pathology. Pathology affecting the internal muscles of the foot is uncommon. Nerve entrapment is most often seen affecting the posterior tibial nerve in tarsal tunnel syndrome. Soft tissue masses include cystic lesions such as ganglions, synovial cysts, hematomas, soft tissue abscess, giant cell tumors, and hemangiomas, as well as nerve sheath tumors including Morton's neuroma, sarcomas, myxomas, pseudoaneurysm, and anomalous musculature.[9–11] These lesions can be assessed for location, extent, changes on passive and active movement, cystic and solid components, and internal and adjacent vascularity.

Foreign bodies are evaluated for site, depth, number, local anatomy, and reactions including abscess formation, and can be localized for surgical removal. Interventional procedures can be performed under direct ultrasound guidance allowing accurate placement of the needle tip for aspirations, injections, or soft tissue biopsy.[6]

Technical Review

The ankle and foot are best assessed using a high-resolution, multifrequency, linear 9- to 15-MHz transducer. This will offer excellent resolution while providing good depth penetration for the majority of patients. Very superficial structures including ligaments and retinaculae can be assessed with a linear hockey stick probe; this probe is particularly useful if there is limited anatomical contact surface for the transducer. Use of liberal amounts of coupling gel alleviates the need for stand-off pads, which are now rarely required given the advances in transducer technology. As always, structures should be evaluated in orthogonal planes, with the transducer perpendicular to the structure under evaluation, to eliminate anisotropy, and in static and dynamic modes when relevant. For unfamiliar regions, comparison with the contralateral side and a thorough knowledge of local anatomy and its ultrasound appearance are essential.

Anatomy

Surface Anatomy

The medial and lateral malleoli are palpated at the distal end of the tibia and fibula, respectively (Chapter 10, Figure 10.1). The sustentaculum tali, a bony shelf extending from the medial calcaneus, is palpable 2 cm distal to the medial malleolus.[12] The tendons of the anterior ankle and foot are palpable and become clearly visible when the toes and forefoot are flexed against resistance.[12] The extensor tendon group, from medial to lateral, includes the tibialis anterior, the extensor hallucis longus, the extensor digitorum, and the peroneus tertius, e.g., the tibialis anterior is visible as it passes anterior to the ankle joint just lateral to the anterior edge of the medial malleolus to its distal attachment on the medial cuneiform (Chapter 10, Figure 10.1). The dorsalis pedis artery, the continuation of the anterior tibial artery, is palpable, with some variability, as it crosses the ankle medially between the tibialis anterior and extensor hallucis tendons. The extensor digitorum brevis is the prominent, palpable, fleshy mass along the dorsolateral aspect of the midfoot. It becomes prominent on resisted dorsiflexion.

The posteromedial tendon group includes, from anterior to posterior, the tibialis posterior, the flexor digitorum longus, and the flexor hallucis longus. The latter tendon lies deep and is usually not palpable. The posterior tibial artery pulsations can be felt just behind the flexor digitorum tendon. The posterolateral tendon group, peroneus longus and brevis, can be palpated posterior to the lateral malleolus. Of the posterior tendon group, the Achilles tendon is readily visualized and palpable as a thick noncompressible soft tissue band, extending in the midline from the mid-calf distally to its insertion on the posterior surface of the calcaneus (Chapter 10, Figure 10.1).

On the sole of the foot, the tuberosity of the navicular bone is palpable medially, 3 cm distal to the sustentaculum tali. The abductor digiti minimi tendon runs along the lateral aspect of the sole of the foot lying fairly superficial, making it easily palpable. Along the medial aspect of the sole of the foot, the abductor hallucis muscle is both palpable and visible as a prominent bulge at the concave surface.[12]

Bones and Joints

The ankle joint proper, also referred to as the talocrural joint, largely comprises the tibia and talar dome. The medial and lateral aspect of the joint is stabilized by the medial malleolus of the tibia and the lateral malleolus of the distal fibula (Figure 11.1). This is a synovial joint within the spectrum of a hinge joint, with the axis of rotation being predominantly between the extremes of plantar flexion and dorsiflexion. The capsule of the ankle joint is attached to the margins of the articulating surfaces of the tibia, talus, and fibula. Exceptions include the capsule anteriorly where it attaches, distal to the cartilage, along the talar neck and the posterosuperior capsule, which attaches to the posterior tibiofibular ligament.[13]

The bones of the foot are made up of the tarsus, metatarsals, and phalanges (Figure 11.1). The tarsus is divided into a total of seven bones subdivided into proximal and distal articular rows. The proximal row includes the talus and calcaneus and the distal row includes the medial, intermediate, and lateral cuneiforms and the cuboid. The navicular, regarded as separate from the described rows, lies between the talus and medial cuneiform along the medial surface of the foot.[13] Only the calcaneus and the metatarsal heads rest upon the ground. The calcaneus, the largest of the tarsal bones, articulates directly with the talus and cuboid bones. Along the upper and medial surface there is a bony shelf, the sustentaculum tali, which serves as a roof for the flexor hallucis longus tendon. The lateral calcaneal surface is almost vertical and flat aside from a small crest, the peroneal trochlea, from which extends the inferior peroneal retinaculum, under which travel the inframalleolar components of the peroneal tendons.[13] The calcaneofibular ligament attaches just posterior to this tubercle.

The talus rests between the distal tibia and the calcaneus. It has a prominent body leading anteriorly into the neck and head. The convex articular surface along the superior surface of the body is called the trochlea. Behind the trochlea is the posterior process, which is grooved in the midline to accommodate the flexor hallucis longus tendon. This process is commonly seen unfused, in which case it is referred to as the os trigonum.

The cuboid is somewhat conical and has a notch on its lateral border for the peroneus longus tendon. The navicular bone, on the medial surface, has

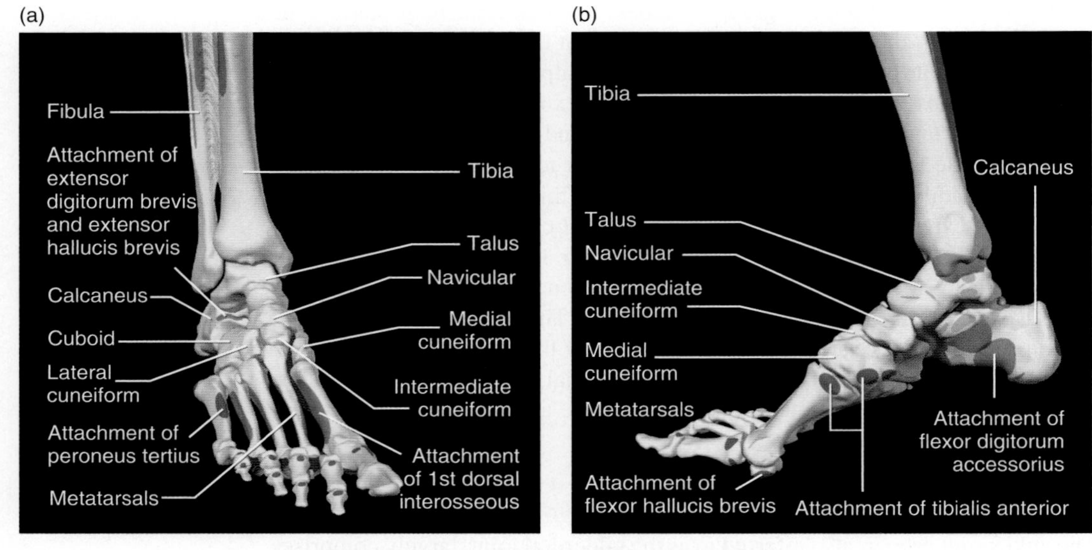

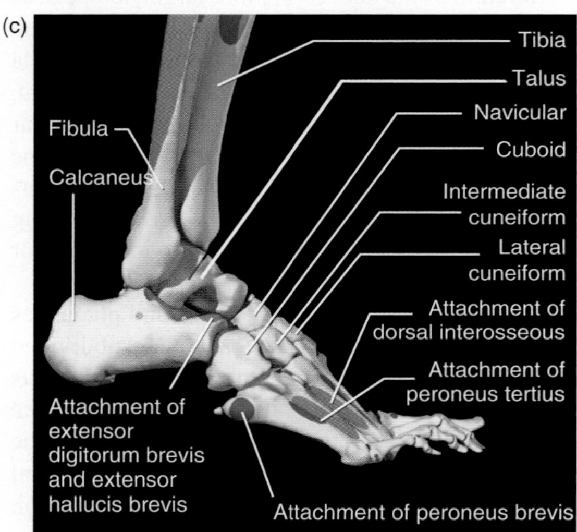

Figure 11.1. The important bony landmarks and muscle origin (red) and insertion (blue) points of the muscles and bones around the ankle: (**a**) anterior, (**b**) medial, and (**c**) lateral views.

a posteriorly projecting process for insertion of part of the tibialis posterior tendon. There are three cuneiform bones in the distal tarsal row. The medial is the largest and the intermediate is the smallest. They articulate distally with the bases of the metatarsals and proximally with the navicular. The peroneus longus inserts into a tubercle along the anteroinferior surface of the medial cuneiform.

There are five metatarsal bones; the first is the largest. The first metatarsal articulates predominantly with the medial cuneiform and, to a much lesser degree, with the second metatarsal. The metatarsal heads are joined by transverse ligaments. The base of the fifth metatarsal has a prominent tubercle for insertion of the peroneus brevis tendon (Figure 11.1c). The first digit, as in the hand, contains only two phalanges, while there are three for the second through fifth digits. The metatarsophalangeal and interphalangeal joints are strengthened by collateral ligaments.[13]

Muscles and Tendons

The tendons about the ankle are divided into anterior, posterolateral, posteromedial, and posterior groups. The tendons of the plantar and dorsal surfaces will be discussed separately. Table 11.1 details the origins, insertions, and actions of the individual muscles and tendons.

The anterior, or extensor, group is contained within the space bounded by the deep fascia anteriorly and posteriorly by the interosseous membrane (Figures 11.1a, 11.2 and 11.3). From medial to lateral lie the tibialis anterior, extensor hallucis longus, extensor digitorum longus, and peroneus tertius. The anterior tibial artery and vein and deep peroneal nerve are also found within this space. The tibialis anterior descends within its synovial sheath deep to the superior and inferior retinaculae to insert onto the medial and inferior surfaces of the medial cuneiform and the base of the first metatarsal (Figures 11.1b and 11.2b). The extensor hallucis longus tendon also passes deep to the retinaculae and extends just medial to the tibialis anterior, but proceeds more distally to insert into the dorsal surface of the base of the first distal phalanx (Figure 11.2a).

The extensor digitorum longus passes deep to the superior extensor retinaculum. By the time it extends deep to the inferior retinaculum, it has acquired its synovial sheath in common with the peroneus tertius. This sheath is enclosed in a distinct loop of the inferior extensor retinaculum. Distal to the retinaculum it splits into four tendons that travel superficial to the extensor digitorum brevis to insert onto the second through fifth digits with the same configuration seen at the extensor digitorum tendons in the hands. At the proximal phalanx, the tendon divides into central, medial, and lateral slips. The central slip inserts onto the base of the middle phalanx with the lateral and medial slips inserting into the distal phalanx after coalescing with the interossei and lumbricals.[13,14] The peroneus tertius is the most lateral of the anterior extensor group (Figure 11.2a).

The extensor digitorum brevis is considered separate from the described extensor tendons, as it is the only one to originate and insert in the foot (Figure 11.2a). As it courses obliquely along the dorsum of the foot, it gives separate tendons to each of the medial four toes. The tendon slip extending to the great toe is considered separate—the extensor hallucis brevis. It inserts into the base of the proximal phalanx, whereas those to the second through fourth digits travel to the distal phalanx after coalescing with the extensor digitorum brevis as part of the dorsal extensor expansion via a configuration similar to that seen in the hand.[13]

Insider Information 11.1

Regarding the medial aspect of the ankle joint as the epicenter, the anterior extensors progress anteriorly following the mnemonic Tom (tibialis anterior) Hates (extensor hallucis longus) Dick (extensor digitorum longus). The flexors are arranged posteriorly as Tom (tibialis posterior), Dick (flexor digitorum longus), and Harry (flexor hallucis longus).

Table 11.1. Ankle and Foot Muscles and Tendons[a].

Muscle	Origin	Insertion	Main action
Anterior compartment			
Tibialis anterior	Lateral proximal shaft of the tibia, interosseous membrane	Medial cuneiform, base of the first metatarsal	Dorsiflexion and inversion of the foot
Extensor hallucis longus	Anterior fibula and interosseous membrane	Base of the distal phalanx of the great toe	Dorsiflexion and extension of the great toe
Extensor digitorum longus	Lateral tibial condyle, anterior shaft of the fibula and interosseous membrane	Base of the middle and distal phalanges of the second to fifth toes	Dorsiflexion and extension of the second to fifth toes
Peroneus tertius	Lower third of the anterior surface of the fibula and interosseous membrane	Dorsal base of the fifth metatarsal	Dorsiflexion and eversion of the foot
Lateral compartment			
Peroneus longus	Head and proximal lateral shaft of the fibula	Medial cuneiform and plantar aspect of the base of the first metatarsal	Eversion and plantar flexion of the foot
Peroneus brevis	Distal lateral shaft of the fibula	Base of the fifth metatarsal	Eversion and plantar flexion of the foot
Posterior compartment	**Superficial group**		
Gastrocnemius	Lateral and medial heads from the lateral and medial femoral condyles, respectively	Via the Achilles tendon onto the posterior calcaneus	Plantar flexion of the foot
Soleus	Posterior head of the fibula and adjacent proximal shaft, soleal line tibia	Via the Achilles tendon onto the posterior calcaneus	Plantar flexion of the foot
Plantaris	Lateral femoral supracondylar line	Posterior calcaneus, medial to Achilles insertion	Plantar flexion of the foot
Posterior compartment	**Deep group**		
Tibialis posterior	Posterior aspects of the interosseous membrane, tibia, and fibula	Navicular tuberosity and fibrous expansions to the cuboid, cuneiforms, second to fourth metatarsal bases	Plantar flexion and inversion of the foot
Flexor digitorum longus	Posterior shaft of the tibia	Bases of the distal phalanges of the second to fifth toes	Plantar flexion of the second to fifth toes
Flexor hallucis longus	Posterior fibula lower two thirds	Base of the distal phalanx of the great toe	Plantar flexion of the great toe

Popliteus	Popliteal groove of the lateral femoral condyle	Posterior proximal shaft of the tibia	Flexion of the knee and internal rotation of the tibia
Sole of the foot	**First layer**		
Flexor digitorum brevis	Medial process of calcaneus and deep plantar aponeurosis	Middle phalanx of the second through fifth toes	Toe flexion
Abductor hallucis	Medial process of calcaneus and flexor retinaculum	Medial proximal phalanx of the great toe	Great toe abduction
Abductor digiti minimi	Medial and lateral processes of the calcaneus	Lateral aspect of the base of the fifth proximal phalanx	Abduction of the little toe
Sole of the foot	**Second layer**		
Flexor hallucis longus	See above		
Flexor digitorum longus	See above		
Flexor accesorius	Medial and lateral heads from the calcaneus	Into tendon of the flexor digitorum longus	Flexion of the lateral four toes
Lumbrical muscles	From tendons of the flexor digitorum longus	Into extensor expansions at the medial base of the lateral four MTP joints	Assist in MTP flexion and IPJ extension
Sole of the foot	**Third layer**		
Flexor hallucis brevis	Medial head: cuboid and lateral cuneiform Lateral head: medial and intermediate cuneiforms	Medial and lateral tendons to base of the first proximal phalanx	Flexion of the first MTP
Adductor hallucis	Dominant oblique head from bases of the second to fourth metatarsals	Blends with lateral head of the flexor hallucis brevis	Adducts the hallus and flexes at the MTPJ
Flexor digiti minimi brevis	Base of the fifth metatarsal	Base of the fifth proximal phalanx	Flexion of the fifth MTPJ
Sole of the foot	**fourth layer**		
Interossei	Metatarsal heads	Lateral base of the proximal phalanx	Abducts the toe
Tibialis posterior	See above		
Peroneus longus	See above		

[a]MTP, metatarsophalangeal; IPJ, interphalangeal joint; MTPJ, metatarsophalangeal joint.

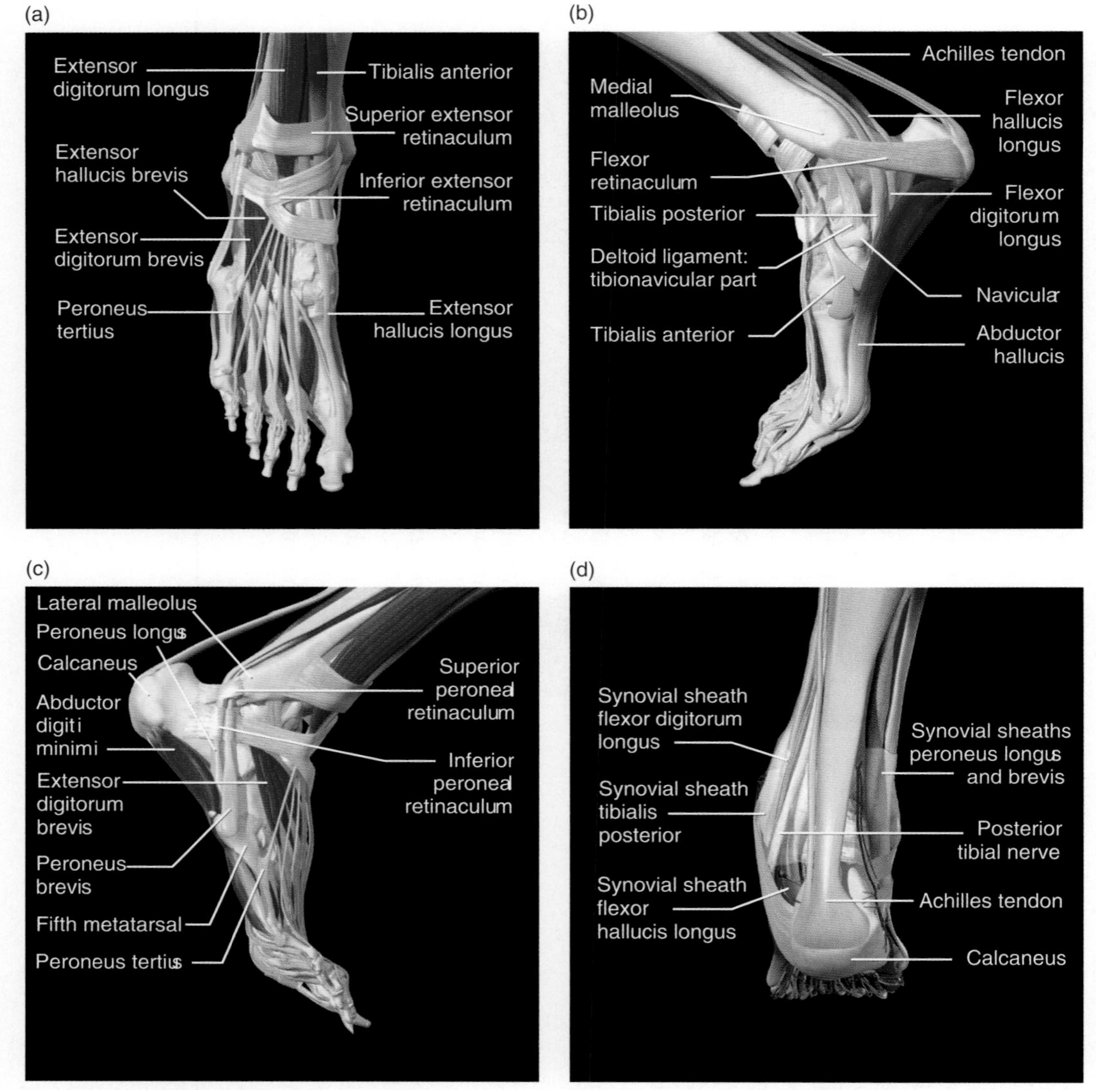

Figure 11.2. The muscles, tendons, and retinaculae around the ankle joint: **(a)** anterior, **(b)** medial, **(c)** lateral, and **(d)** posterior views.

The posteromedial group of tendons lie at the level of the medial malleolus (Figures 11.1b,11.2b and d, and 11.3). From anteromedial to posteromedial, they are the tibialis posterior, flexor digitorum longus, and flexor hallucis longus. This order of tendons is known as Tom, Dick, and Harry. They are each enclosed within their own synovial sheath deep to the flexor retinaculum.

The tibialis posterior tendon passes, in its inframalleolar component, just cranial to the medial aspect of the sustentaculum tali, superficial to the deltoid ligament. It mainly inserts onto the tuberosity of the navicular. It also sends slips to the plantar surfaces of all of the cuneiforms, the sustentaculum tali, the cuboid, and the second through fourth metatarsals.[12,13] A small, internal

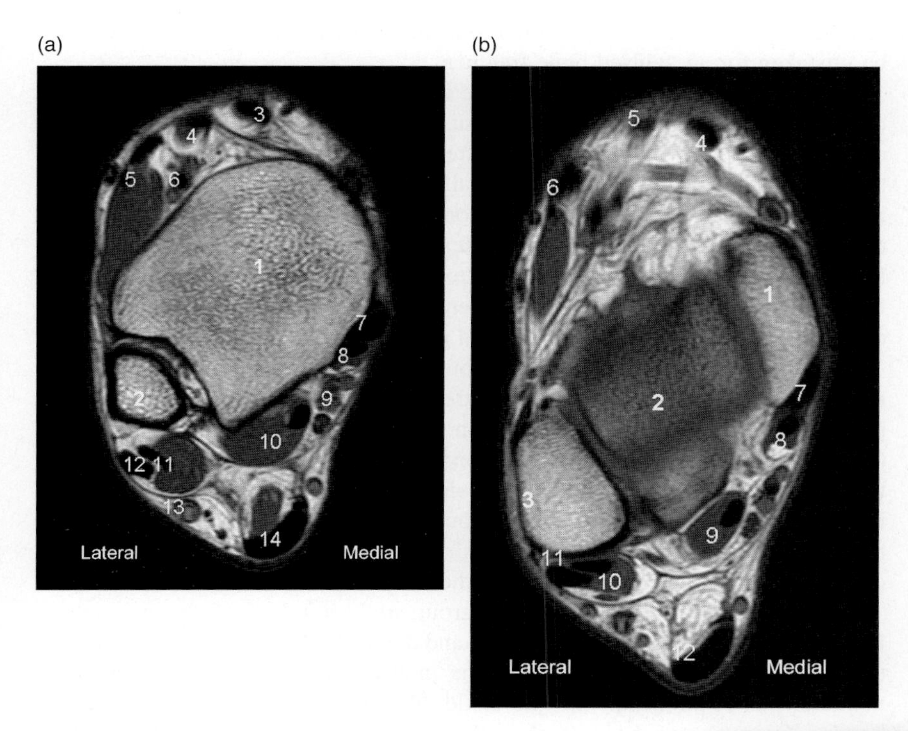

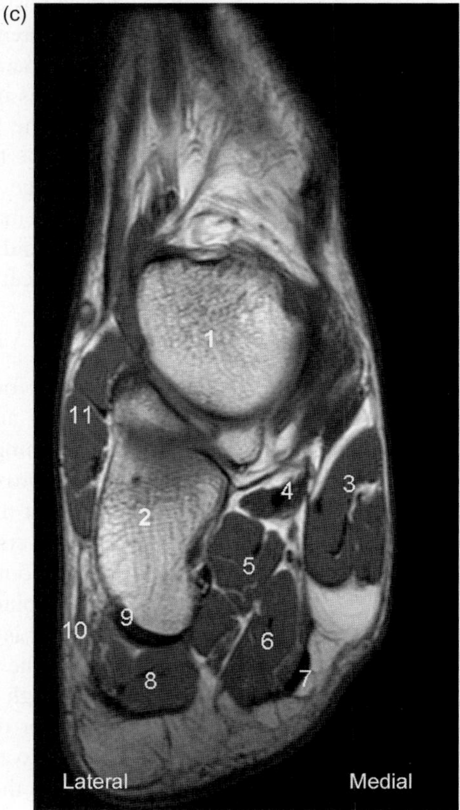

Figure 11.3. T1-weighted MRI anatomy. (**a**) Axial above the level of the ankle joint. 1–tibia, 2–fibula, 3–tibialis anterior tendon, 4–extensor hallucis longus tendon, 5–extensor digitorum longus, 6–anterior tibial vessels and deep peroneal nerve, 7–tibialis posterior tendon, 8–flexor digitorum longus tendon, 9–posterior tibial vessels and tibial nerve, 10–flexor hallucis longus, 11–peroneus brevis, 12–peroneus longus, 13–lesser saphenous vein and sural nerve, 14–Achilles tendon. (**b**) Axial at the level of the ankle joint. 1–tibia, 2–talar dome, 3–fibula, 4–tibialis anterior, 5–extensor hallucis longus, 6–extensor digitorum longus, 7–tibialis posterior, 8–flexor digitorum longus, 9–flexor hallucis longus, 10–peroneus brevis, 11–peroneus longus, 12–Achilles tendon. (**c**) Coronal of the ankle joint. 1–talus, 2–cuboid, 3–abductor hallucis, 4–flexor digitorum longus, 5–quadratus plantae, 6–flexor digitorum brevis, 7–plantar aponeurosis, 8–abductor digiti minimi, 9–peroneus longus, 10–peroneus brevis, 11–extensor digitorum brevis.

ossicle may be present just proximal to its navicular insertion; this should not be mistaken for an avulsed bone fragment.

The inframalleolar component of the flexor digitorum longus, at the level of the medial aspect of the calcaneal sustentaculum tali, courses to the sole of the foot (Figure 11.4c). At the posteromedial plantar surface, it crosses the superficial surface of the flexor hallucis longus tendon. It then divides into four distinct tendons for the second through fifth digits. The medial two receive contributions from the flexor hallucis longus. Proximally all four receive contributions from the flexor accessories muscle and distally from fibers of the lumbricals. They then perforate the tendons of the flexor digitorum brevis to insert into the distal phalanges.

The flexor hallucis longus tendon courses along a groove at the posterior margin of the talus; it travels under the sustentaculum tali directly to the plantar surface of the foot inserting on the distal phalanx of the first digit (Figure 11.4c). It forms a bowstring along the arched medial plantar foot. The tendon is crossed superficially on the sole of the foot by the flexor digitorum longus to which it contributes tendinous slips as described. Note that the tendon sheath is often in continuity with the tibiotalar joint. A small amount of fluid within the proximal aspect of the sheath is thus acceptable.

The tendons of the posterolateral group are composed of the peroneus longus and brevis (Figures 11.1c, 11.2c and d, and 11.3). The peroneus longus tendon lies behind the peroneus brevis in the lower leg, and the tendons maintain this relationship into the ankle. The wide tendon of the peroneus brevis courses posterior to and abuts the lateral malleolus. Both tendons then course into the lateral foot adjacent to the calcaneus, separated by the peroneal trochlea. They share a common tendon sheath to the trochlea, at which point the sheath divides in two. The brevis courses above the trochlea to insert into the tubercle at the base of the fifth metatarsal. The peroneus longus tendon courses below the trochlea into the sole of the foot where it lies adjacent to the posterior ridge of the groove on the plantar surface of the cuboid bone. The tendon here most often contains a sesamoid bone that articulates with a facet on the cuboid.[1] Inferiorly, it courses along the sole of the foot to insert at the lateral aspect of the base of the first metatarsal and medial cuneiform.

Sole of the Foot

The sole of the foot has extremely thick subcutaneous tissue with fibrous bands extending and anchoring it to the plantar aponeurosis. The plantar aponeurosis is composed of dense bands arranged largely along the long axis of the foot. Its proximal origin is the medial process of the calcaneus, after which it fans out dividing into five bands, one to each toe, attaching to the superficial transverse metatarsal ligament (Figure 11.4a).[13] The muscles along the sole of the foot are divided into four distinct layers with the first layer just deep to the plantar aponeurosis.[13]

The first layer is composed of three short muscles lying side by side. The most central is the flexor digitorum brevis, which gives off four tendons to the second through fifth toes (Figures 11.3c, 11.4a). Its arrangement parallels that of the flexor digitorum superficialis of the palm of the hand, dividing and inserting into the sides of the middle phalanx of each digit. The most medial muscle is the abductor hallucis. The abductor digit minimi runs along the lateral aspect of the sole of the foot.

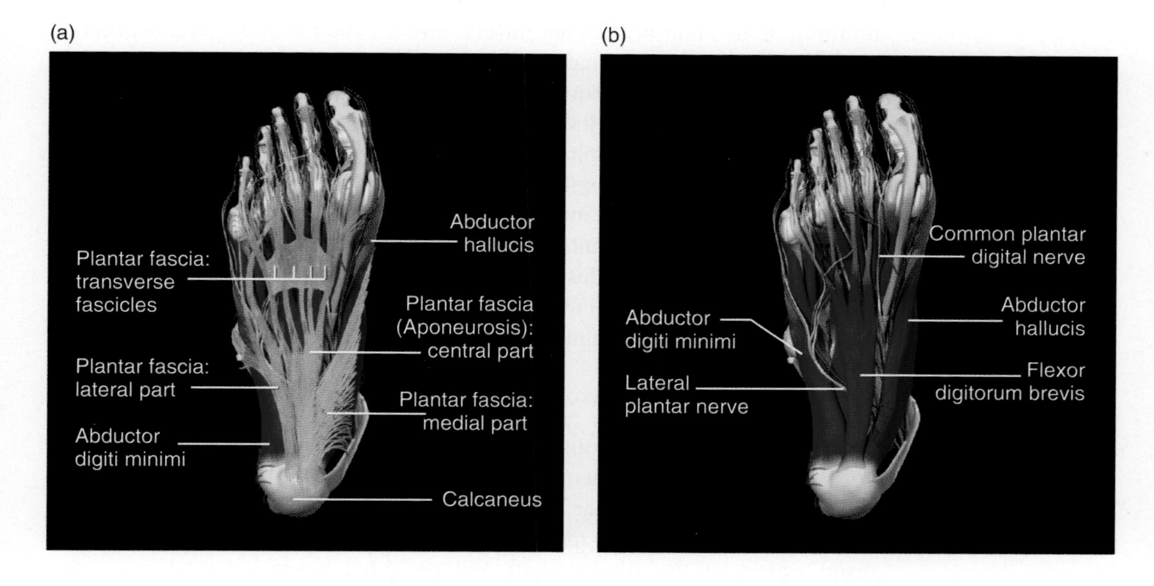

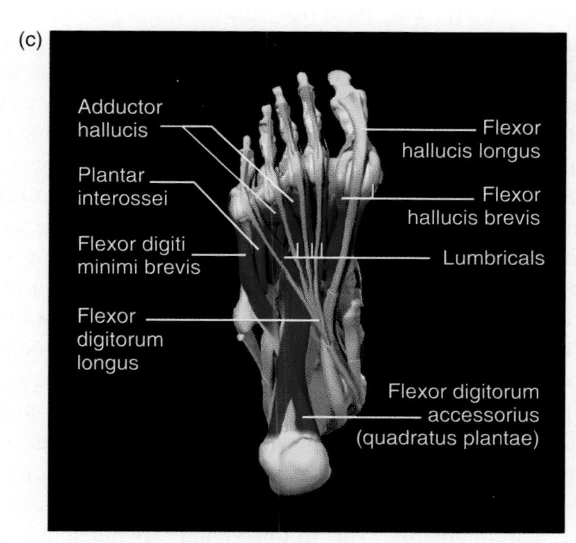

Figure 11.4. The muscles and tendons on the sole of the foot: **(a)** demonstrating plantar fascia, **(b)** layer one, and **(c)** post removal layer one.

The second layer includes the long flexor tendons (Figures 11.3c and 11.4c). These include the tendon of flexor hallucis longus and flexor digitorum longus, which were described earlier in this chapter. The flexor accessorius has two heads that converge at the muscle belly and insert into the tendon of flexor digitorum longus. The lumbricals originate from the tendons of the flexor digitorum longus. They run distally along the medial aspect of the four lateral toes inserting into the extensor expansions at the base of the metatarsophalangeal joint.

The third layer is composed of three short muscles (Figure 11.4c). The first two affect the great toe and the third affects the fifth toe. The flexor hallucis brevis rests directly adjacent to the undersurface of the first metatarsal. It has multiple origins and divides and inserts into the medial and lateral aspects of the base of the first proximal phalanx. The adductor hallucis originates from two heads. The larger oblique head runs superficial to the peroneus longus. The transverse head joins the oblique head to insert into the lateral aspect of the base of the proximal phalanx of the great toe. The final muscle of the third layer is the flexor digiti minimi brevis. It arises from the base of the fifth metatarsal and inserts into the base of the fifth proximal phalanx running directly adjacent to the plantar surface of the fifth metatarsal bone.

The fourth layer includes the interossei seen within the intermetatarsal spaces (Figure 11.4c). Also included in this layer are the tendons of the tibialis posterior and peroneus longus, which were described earlier in the chapter.

Ligaments

The inferior tibiofibular joint is stabilized by three structures: anterior and posterior tibiofibular ligaments and the interosseous tibiofibular ligament. The anterior inferior tibiofibular ligament follows a slightly downward oblique course from the anterior margin of the fibular notch of the tibia to the distal aspect of the fibular shaft and proximal anterior lateral malleolus (Figure 11.5a). The posterior tibiofibular ligament is broader and thicker than its anterior counterpart. It travels from the posterior surface of the lateral malleolus and proximal aspect of the fibular malleolar fossa to the posterior aspect of the tibia, attaching as far medially as the medial malleolus. Between the anterior and posterior tibiofibular ligaments is the interosseous tibiofibular ligament, which is continuous with the more proximal crural interosseous membrane. It forms a strong attachment between the distal tibia and fibula, which prevents upward translation of the talus between the tibia and fibula.[12–15] The interosseous tibiofibular ligament extends from the mid aspect of the distal fibular shaft at the proximal border of the fibular malleolar facet to a roughened area on the lateral aspect of the distal tibia.

The ankle is stabilized medially by the deltoid ligament, which, as suggested by its name, is triangular, with the base forming the more distal component (Figure 11.5b). It originates proximal to the medial malleolus. Distal to this attachment, it is composed of deep and superficial layers with marked intermingling of the two layers. The superficial component is divided into three parts: the anterior tibionavicular, the intermediate tibiocalcaneal, and the posterior tibiotalar ligaments. The tibionavicular ligament attaches to the navicular tuberosity and to the medial edge of the spring ligament.[12,14] The tibiocalcaneal

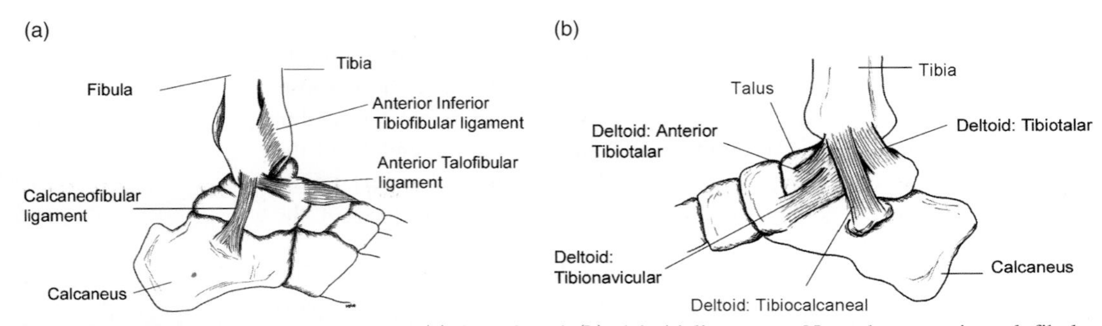

Figure 11.5. The ankle joint ligaments: (**a**) lateral and (**b**) deltoid ligaments. Note the posterior talofibular ligament is not seen due to its position in (**a**). The deltoid ligament is composed of superficial and deep layers.

ligament travels vertically downward to insert along the medial border of the sustentaculum tali. The posterior tibiotalar ligament runs in a posterolateral direction to insert at the medial talar tubercle and at the medial side of the talus. The deep layer of the deltoid ligament attaches distally to the medial border of the talar body. The deep layer is covered internally by synovium.

The lateral stabilizing ligaments of the ankle are considered to be one functional unit with three distinct components (Figure 11.5a).[12,15] The anterior talofibular ligament originates at the anterior border of the lateral malleolus. It follows an oblique anteromedial course to insert at the lateral surface of the talar neck. It is the weakest of the lateral three ligaments. The posterior talofibular ligament is the strongest of the three parts and is triangular in shape. It follows a posteromedial horizontal course from its origin in the posteromedial lateral malleolar fossa to insert into the lateral tubercle of the posterior process of the talus. From the posterior and superficial surface of the ligament, the intermalleolar ligament originates. This ligament extends across the posterior aspect of the ankle to insert on the posterior aspect of the tibia and medial malleolus. The third component of the lateral stabilizing ligament is the calcaneofibular ligament, which is the largest of the three. It runs deep to the peroneal tendons from the anteroinferior border of the lateral malleolus to insert on the superior aspect of the lateral portion of the calcaneus.

The remaining ligaments of the foot and ankle are not commonly evaluated with ultrasound; some of the more better known ligaments will be briefly reviewed. The superior talonavicular ligament is a broad, rectangular structure adding stability to the talonavicular joint. It travels from the dorsal aspect of the talar neck to the dorsal navicular bone. The inferior calcaneonavicular, or spring, ligament is a strong, thick ligament that attaches proximally to the anterior border of the sustentaculum tali and distally to the plantar aspect of the navicular bone. Medially it fuses with the distal aspect of the anterior deltoid ligament. Its importance includes stabilizing the head of the talus and thus maintaining, with the tibialis posterior and flexor hallucis longus tendons, the medial longitudinal arch of the foot.[12] The dorsal and plantar intermetatarsal ligaments pass between the bases of the metatarsal bones. The Lisfranc's ligament is a broad, strong ligament, deep in the sole of the foot. It attaches proximally to the distal plantar surface of the medial cuneiform and extends distally and laterally to the medial aspect of the base of the second metatarsal. It is partially contiguous with the capsules of the first and second tarsometatarsal joints.[12]

Retinaculae

The flexor retinaculum is an obliquely oriented thickening of the deep fascia running from the inferior border of the medial malleolus to the medial tubercle of the calcaneus and the medial aspect of the plantar aponeurosis (Figure 11.2b). It overlies the flexor tendons, the posterior tibial vessels, and the tibial nerve, thus forming the roof of the tarsal tunnel. From the undersurface of the retinaculum, several fine fibrous bands extend to the calcaneus, effectively dividing the tarsal tunnel into short ossofibrous canals.[13]

Along the extensor surface of the ankle, the deep fascia is focally thickened, forming the superior extensor retinaculum attaching to the anterior borders of the tibia and fibula. On the dorsum of the foot there is a Y-shaped thickening of the superficial fascia representing the inferior extensor retinaculum, which effectively prevents the extensor tendons from bowstringing as they pass the ankle joint (Figure 11.2a).[13] It arises from a common band at the anterolateral calcaneus with the inferior peroneal retinaculum. From this trunk, two medially coursing limbs arise. The upper limb attaches to the medial malleolus, and the lower limb coalesces with the plantar aponeurosis under the medial longitudinal arch of the foot. Most of the lower limb, however, traverses the extensor tendons, then slings under them to attach to the calcaneus. Only the superficial aspect of the retinaculum attaches to the medial aspect of the foot and ankle.

The posterolateral tendons are bound by two distinct retinaculae: the superior and inferior peroneal retinaculae. The superior peroneal retinaculum, at the level of the lateral malleolus, is defined by a band of deep fascia that extends from the posteroinferior aspect of the malleolus to the lateral surface of the calcaneus (Figure 11.2c). The inferior peroneal retinaculum is a band of fascia attached to the peroneal trochlea and to the calcaneus above and below the tendons, thus separating the tendons. Its more superior aspect is contiguous with the inferior extensor retinaculum.

Vessels and Nerves

The deep peroneal nerve courses lateral to the anterior tibial artery midway between the malleoli and deep to the tendons. It passes deep to the extensor digitorum brevis, after which it divides. The anterior tibial artery travels with a companion vein on either side. It changes its name to the dorsalis pedis as it crosses the anterior aspect of the tibiotalar joint just deep to the inferior extensor retinaculum. As it reaches the proximal aspect of the first intermetatarsal space, it dives deep through the first dorsal interosseous muscle to join the lateral plantar artery on the sole of the foot to complete the plantar arterial arch.

The posterior tibial nerve and artery travel between the flexor digitorum longus and flexor hallucis longus tendons deep to the flexor retinaculum where they end by dividing into medial and lateral plantar nerves and arteries (Chapter 12, Figure 12.20). The artery is accompanied by two venae comitantes, which often communicate with one another.

Technique

The patient lies supine on a couch with the lower limb exposed to the level of the knee, with the examiner sitting on the right side of the patient. Prior imaging and pertinent history should be reviewed prior to the study. The examination can then be tailored to the region of interest, or a full routine study, which will be described here, can be performed.[15] The study will be divided into the different anatomical zones: anterior, posteromedial, posterolateral, and posterior. Anatomy is assessed in orthogonal planes. Longitudinal and axial refer to the axis of the structure being imaged. Table 11.2 summarizes the ultrasound position for the different muscle compartments.

Insider Information 11.2

Knowledge of origin and insertion will allow correct transducer positioning in the identification of tendons and ligaments, particularly when there is significant local pathology present that may obscure normal anatomical relationships.

Table 11.2. Ultrasound Position in the Evaluation of Muscle Compartments.

Muscle	Position examined
Anterior compartment Tibialis anterior Extensor hallucis longus Extensor digitorum longus Peroneus tertius	Patient supine, knee flexed and plantar aspect of the foot flat on the table
Lateral compartment Peroneus longus	Patient supine, proximal: knee flexed and plantar aspect of the foot flat on the table and mild inversion
Peroneus brevis	Distal to cuboid groove: knee extended, toes pointing up Patient supine, knee flexed and plantar aspect of the foot flat on the table and mild inversion
Posterior compartment Achilles tendon (gastrocnemius, soleus) Plantaris	**Superficial group** Patient prone with the foot dorsiflexed, hanging over the table end
Posterior compartment Tibialis posterior Flexor digitorum longus Flexor hallucis longus	**Deep group** Patient supine, knee flexed and plantar aspect of the foot flat on the table for the distal component at the level of the ankle
Sole of the foot Flexor digitorum brevis Abductor hallucis Abductor digiti minimi	**First layer** Patient prone with the foot dorsiflexed, hanging over the table end
Flexor hallucis longus Flexor digitorum longus Flexor accesorius Lumbrical muscles	**Second layer** Patient prone with the foot dorsiflexed, hanging over the table end
Flexor hallucis brevis Adductor hallucis Flexor digiti minimi brevis	**Third layer** Patient prone with the foot dorsiflexed, hanging over the table end
Interossei Peroneus longus Tibialis posterior	**Fourth layer** Patient prone with the foot dorsiflexed, hanging over the table end

Anterior Ankle

The patient lies supine with the knee flexed to approximately 90° and the plantar aspect of the foot flat on the couch.

Tendons

The anterior compartment contains, from medial to lateral, the following tendons: tibialis anterior (TA), extensor hallucis longus (EHL), extensor digitorum longus (EDL), and the peroneus tertius (PT). The origin, insertion, and action of these muscles and their respective tendons are summarized in Table 11.1. The anterior compartment is initially evaluated in the transverse plane at the level of the ankle joint (Figure 11.6). The sagittal plane is then obtained by rotating the transducer 90°.

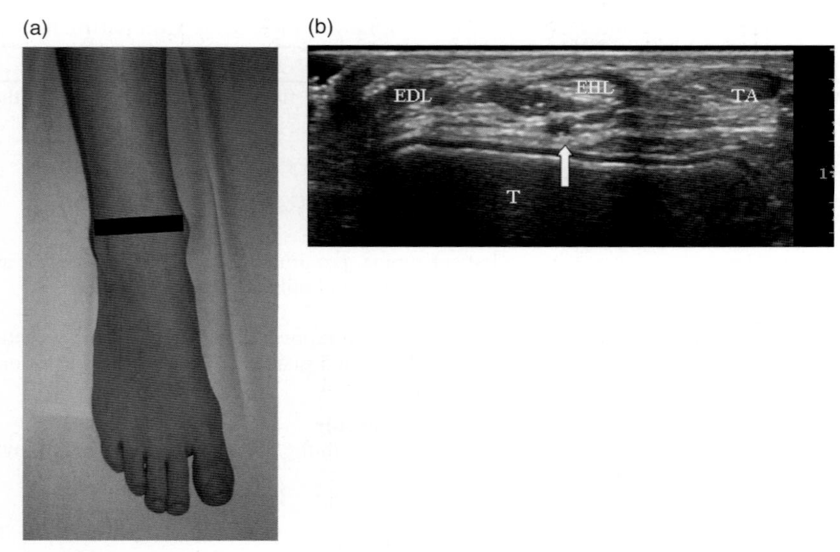

Figure 11.6. Anterior compartment: **(a)** transducer position and the corresponding **(b)** transverse ultrasound image at the level of the ankle joint. TA, tibialis anterior; EHL, extensor hallucis longus; EDL, extensor digitorum longus; T, tibia; arrow, dorsalis pedis artery and vein.

The TA is the most medial and largest of the tendons within the anterior compartment and inserts into the medial cuneiform and base of the first metatarsal (Figures 11.6 and 11.7a). The adjacent EHL lies lateral to the TA and can be differentiated by its smaller size, almost half that of the TA, and its insertion into the distal phalanx of the first toe (Figures 11.6 and 11.7b). Knowledge of origin and insertion allows correct identification of tendons, particularly when there is significant local pathology present, which may obscure normal anatomical relationships. The EDL musculotendinous junction may extend to or below the level of the ankle joint, as may the EHL (Figure 11.8). The four tendons of the EDL are hyperechoic and divide into three slips at the level of the proximal phalanx, with the central slip inserting into the base of the middle phalanx and the lateral slips reuniting to insert into the base of the distal phalanx. The PT is identified as a hyperechoic tendon lateral to the EDL. All tendons are evaluated from musculotendinous junction to point of insertion.

The synovial sheath of the Tibalis anterior (TA) is the only one to begin at, or just proximal to, the superior extensor retinaculum and normally contains no visible fluid. The remaining sheaths of the extensor tendons begin at the inferior retinaculum, with a common sheath for the EDL and PT. A small bursa lies between this tendon of the TA and the medial cuneiform, just at its point of insertion, which is not normally identified on ultrasound unless distended with fluid.

Insider Information 11.3

The tendons of the posteromedial and posterolateral compartments undergo significant change in angulation at the level of their respective malleoli. This requires the transducer to be continually adjusted to prevent anisotropy.

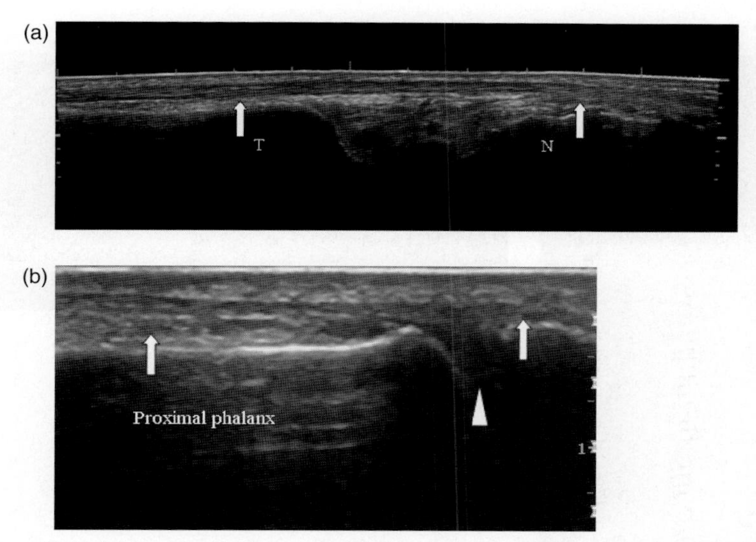

Figure 11.7. (**a**) Longitudinal extended field of view (EFOV) of the tibialis anterior (arrows). (**b**) Longitudinal ultrasound image of the insertion of the extensor hallucis longus (arrows). Arrowhead, first interphalangeal joint; T, tibia; N, navicular.

Retinaculum

The extensor retinaculum has two bands named according to their location with respect to the ankle joint: the superior and inferior. The superior extensor retinaculum (Figure 11.9) is identified by moving the probe in a transverse position, with respect to the extensor tendons as described previously, to just above the ankle joint. It is a thin, 1-mm, but strong hyperechoic band superficial to the tendons and attaching medially to the anterior distal shaft tibia and laterally to the fibula. The inferior extensor retinaculum (Figure 11.10) is Y-shaped with the stem on the lateral side. Once the lateral stem is identified, the medial end of the probe should be angled toward the medial malleolus where the upper slip inserts. The lower slip has a more horizontal course.

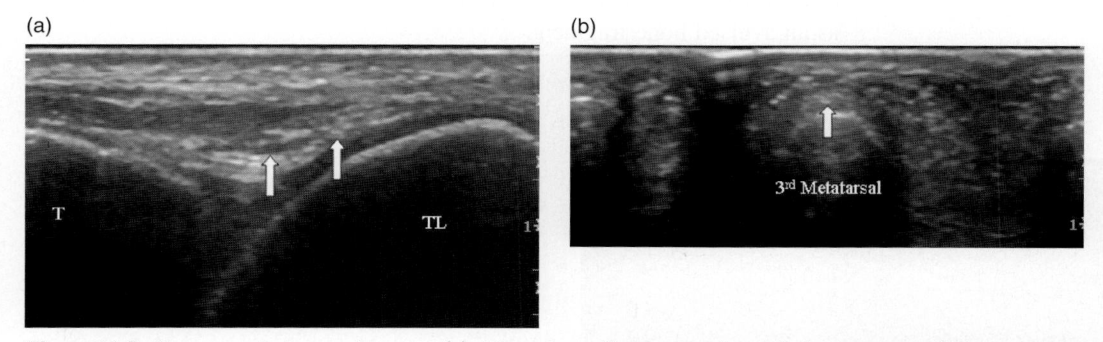

Figure 11.8. Extensor digitorum longus. (**a**) Musculotendinous junction of the extensor digitorum longus (arrows) at the level of the ankle joint, longitudinal view, and (**b**) transverse ultrasound image of the mid third metatarsal demonstrating hyperechoic tendon of the third extensor digitorum longus. T, tibia; TL, talus; AT, Achilles tendon.

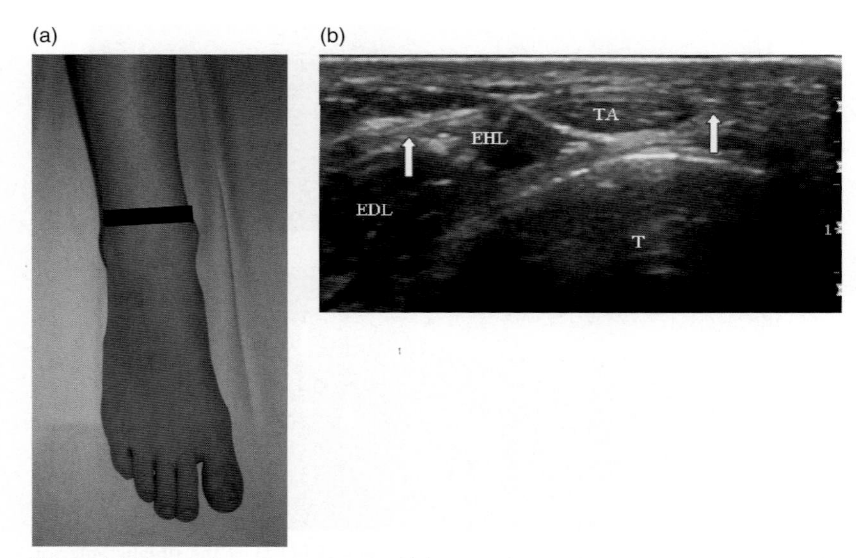

Figure 11.9. Anterior compartment: (**a**) transducer position and corresponding (**b**) transverse ultrasound image just proximal to the ankle joint. Arrows, superior retinaculum; TA, tibialis anterior; EHL, extensor hallucis longus; EDL, extensor digitorum longus; T, tibia.

Ankle Joint

The anterior recess is best studied in a longitudinal or sagittal plane (Figure 11.11). A small joint effusion may be present that normally measures less than 3 mm in depth. Remember that the joint capsule inserts onto the neck of the talus. The joint capsule is seen as a thin hyperechoic band. The articular cartilage is easily identified as a smooth hypoechoic covering, 2–4 mm in thickness. Cortical bone lies deep to the cartilage and on ultrasound appears as a smooth hyperechoic continuous line. The synovial membrane is attached to the articular margins of the joint and can be visualized deep to the medial, lateral, and posterior ligaments.

> **Insider Information 11.4**
> Occasionally, tendons may contain an internal ossicle or sesamoid, e.g., the peroneus longus or posterior tibialis; this should not be misidentified as an avulsed bone fragment.

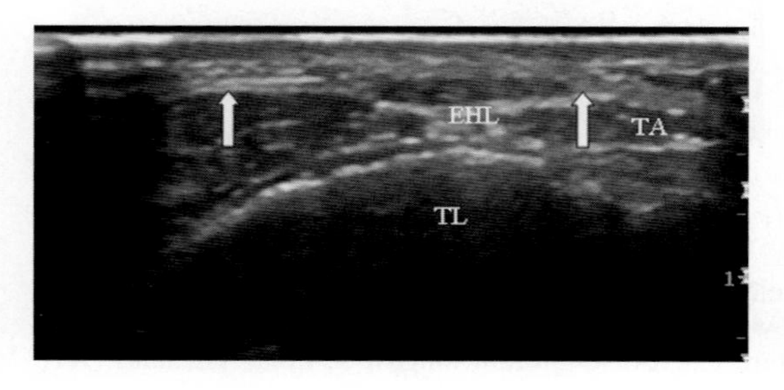

Figure 11.10. Inferior retinaculum (arrow) transverse ultrasound distal to the ankle joint

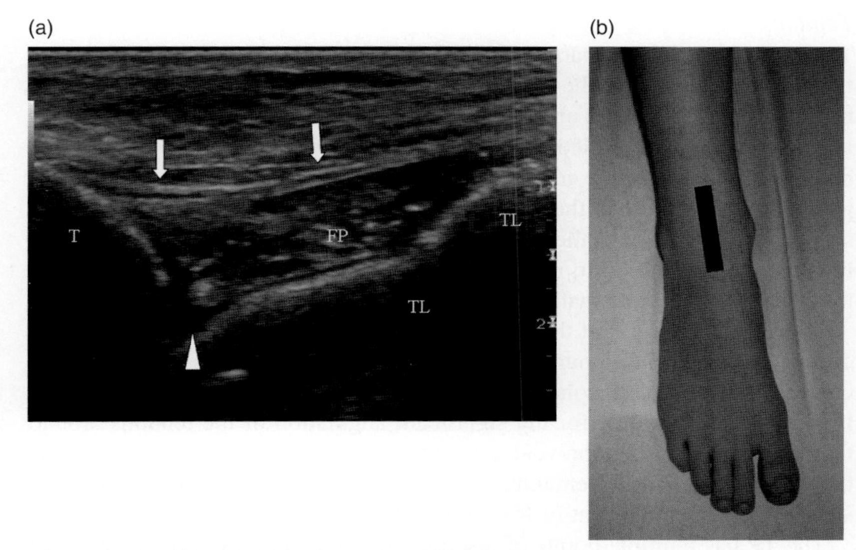

Figure 11.11. **(a)** Longitudinal ultrasound of the ankle joint demonstrating the thin linear hyperechoic capsule (arrows), deep to which is the anterior fat pad (FP) of the ankle joint. A minute amount of hypoechoic fluid is identified in the joint space between the talus (TL) and tibia (T) and corresponding transducer position **(b)**.

Posteromedial Ankle

The patient lies supine with the leg in a "frog-leg" position, hip abducted, knee flexed to 45°, and the foot resting on its lateral margin (Figure 11.12). If the patient finds this position uncomfortable, the medial compartment can be evaluated in the same position as the anterior study with abduction of the knee.

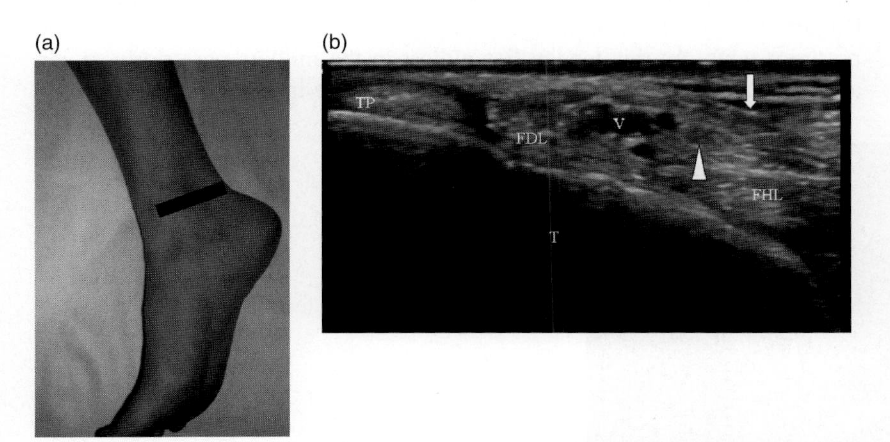

Figure 11.12. Posteromedial compartment: **(a)** patient and transducer position and **(b)** corresponding transverse ultrasound image of the tendons of the deep posterior compartment of the leg at the level of the medial malleolus. TP, tibialis posterior; FDL, flexor digitorum longus; arrow, flexor retinaculum; FHL, flexor hallucis longus; T, tibia; arrowhead, posterior tibial nerve; V, posterior tibial vessels.

Tendons

The posteromedial compartment tendons from anterior to posterior are the tibialis posterior (TP), the flexor digitorum longus (FDL), and the flexor hallucis longus (FHL) (Tom, Dick, and Harry). The examination is divided into supramalleolar, malleolar, and inframalleolar approaches. We normally begin at the level of the medial malleolus. Place the probe in a transverse position, with respect to the tendons, with the anterior margin on the medial surface of the medial malleolus (Figure 11.12). The transducer will have to be continually adjusted to remain in the transverse planes of the tendons as they course around the malleolus.

The TP is the largest of the tendons, measuring between 4 and 6 mm. It can contain a significant amount of fluid within its sheath, up to 4 mm, usually confined to its inframalleolar component.[16] In the inframalleolar examination, it is necessary to adjust for the significant angulation of the tendons around the medial malleolus to prevent anisotropy (Figure 11.13). The transducer is then moved superiorly, remaining in a transverse orientation, to evaluate the supramalleolar component of the tendons to the musculotendinous junctions.

The TP has multiple points of insertion as detailed in Table 11.1, the most prominent of which is the navicular tuberosity. Proximal to this insertion, the tendon fibers course obliquely and appear hypoechoic due to anisotropy (Figure 11.13). In addition, the tendon may contain an accessory ossicle, which appears hyperechoic with posterior shadowing. This should be recognized as such and not misinterpreted as an avulsed bone fragment.

The FDL tendon lies posterior to the TP and is normally half its size at the level of the malleolus (Figure 11.12). In its inframalleolar component, it travels forward and posteriorly into the sole of the foot, dividing into four tendons inserting onto the base of the distal phalanges (Figure 11.14). The evaluation of the distal component of the tendons requires repositioning the patient as described in the technique section on the sole of the foot. Due to its oblique orientation, it is usually easier to assess first in the longitudinal plane of the tendon.

The FHL tendon lies more posteriorly at the level of the malleolus (Figure 11.12), posterior to the neurovascular bundle, in a groove in the posterior talus. As this tendon lies almost in the midline posteriorly, it can also be evaluated from a posterior approach on the medial border of the AT.

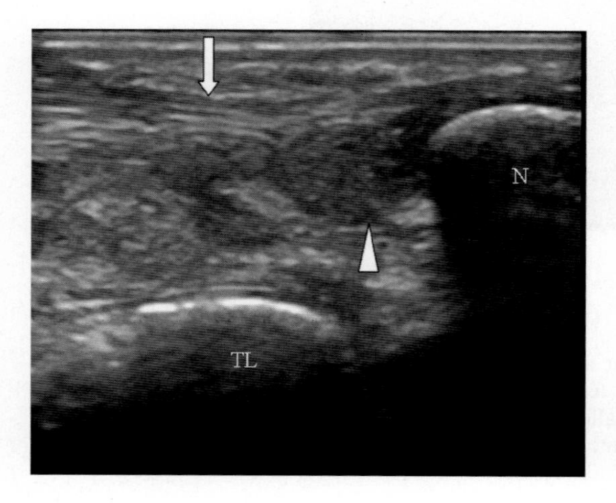

Figure 11.13. Anisotropy of the tibialis posterior (arrow) due to the obliquity of its fibers at insertion. N, navicular; TL, talus.

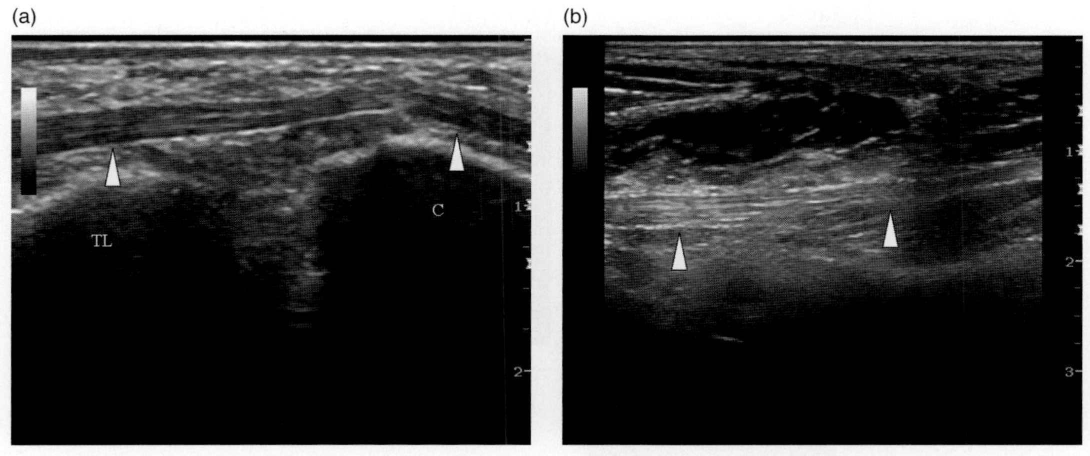

Figure 11.14. (**a**) Longitudinal ultrasound of the inframalleolar flexor digitorum longus (arrowheads). (**b**) Longitudinal ultrasound of the flexor digitorum longus (arrowheads) on the proximal sole of the foot. TL, talus; C, calcaneus.

The musculotendinous junction can be seen just proximal to the level of the ankle joint; its tendon sheath usually contains a small amount of fluid. The tendon passes distally into the sole of the foot on the undersurface of the sustentaculum tali, which can be used as a bony landmark (Figure 11.15), to its insertion at the base of the distal phalanx of the great toe. This is a useful starting point in its evaluation on the sole of the foot. Placing the transducer over the first metatarsal, its hyperechoic tendon is seen between the two hyperechoic sesamoids, within the flexor hallucis brevis tendons (Figure 11.16). The tendon can then be followed proximally and distally. This is easier to perform in the longitudinal plane initially. The same technique can be applied to the FDL tendons of the second to fifth metatarsals, noting that they are more obliquely oriented. All three tendon synovial sheaths begin proximal to and extend distal to the flexor retinaculum.

Accessory muscles at the level of the medial malleolus include the accessorius flexor digitorum, which runs within the tarsal tunnel, and the accessory FHL, which lies lateral to its parent tendon.

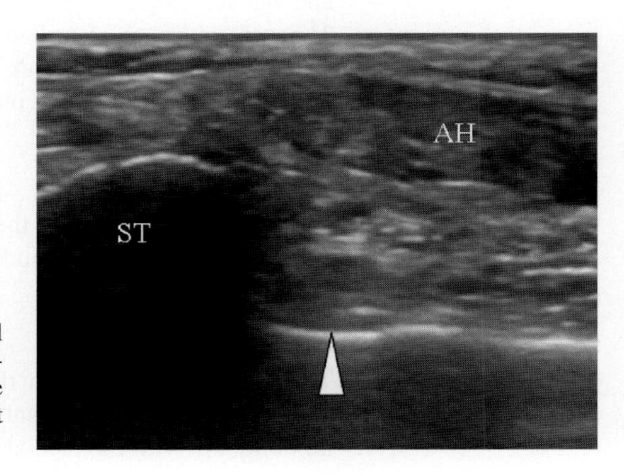

Figure 11.15. Transverse ultrasound image just distal to the medial malleolus at the level of the sustentaculum tali (ST) demonstrating the tendon of the flexor hallucis longus (arrowhead) and the adjacent abductor hallucis muscle (AH).

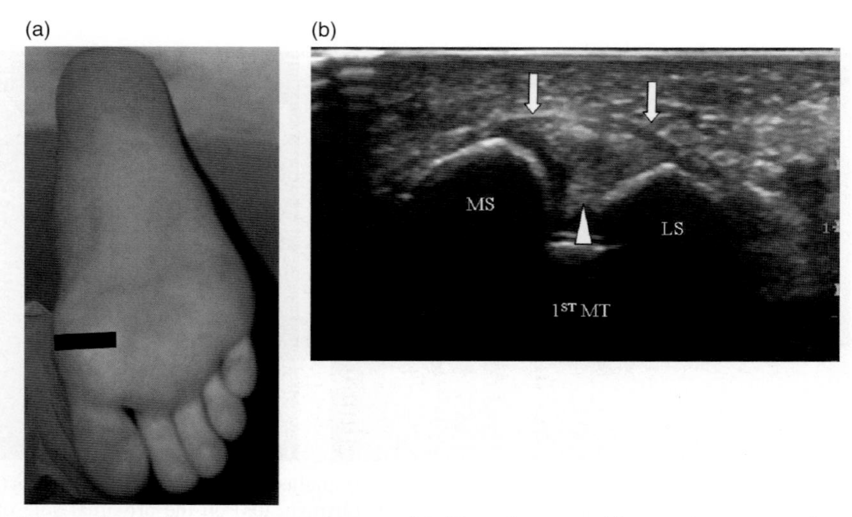

Figure 11.16. Flexor hallucis longus. (**a**) Transducer position and corresponding (**b**) transverse ultrasound image at the level of the first metatarsal head demonstrating the flexor hallucis longus tendon (arrowhead) between the medial and lateral sesamoids. Arrow, annular component of the fibrous flexor sheath; MS, medial sesamoid; LS, lateral sesamoid; 1st MT, first metatarsal.

Insider Information 11.5
The posterior tibialis tendon has multiple points of insertion. The distal tendon fibers fan out in multiple directions, causing anisotropy, which should not be mistaken for tendonosis.

Retinaculum

The medial flexor retinaculum or internal annular ligament forms the roof of the tarsal tunnel, attaching to the medial malleolus and to the calcaneus (Figure 11.12). Four individual tunnels are formed for the transmission of the TP, FDL, and FHL tendons and the neurovascular bundle. The patient remains in the same position as for examination of the posteromedial compartment, and the transducer is placed between the medial malleolus and calcaneus. The retinaculum is identified superficial to the tendons as a thin hyperechoic sheath, less than 2 mm thick. It blends superiorly with the deep fascia of the leg and inferiorly with the plantar fascia.

Posterior Ankle

Ultrasound evaluations of the AT and plantaris tendon, as well as the retrocalcaneal and retroachillean bursa, are detailed in Chapter 10.

Posterolateral Ankle

The patient lies supine in the same position as described for the anterior compartment with additional plantar inversion. Alternatively, the patient can lie obliquely with the medial aspect of the foot on the couch (Figure 11.17).

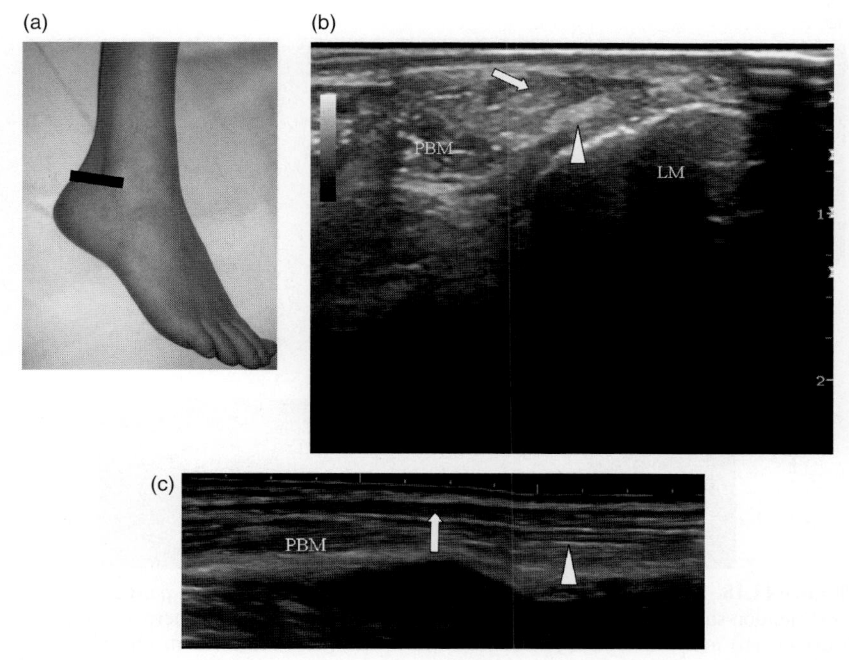

Figure 11.17. Posterolateral compartment: **(a)** transducer position for evaluation of the posterolateral compartment at the level of the lateral malleolus (LM) and **(b)** corresponding axial ultrasound image demonstrating the peroneus brevis muscle (PBM) and tendon (arrowhead) and the peroneus longus tendon (arrow). **(c)** Longitudinal supramalleolar ultrasound image of the peroneal tendons.

Tendons

The posterolateral compartment tendons include the peroneal longus (PL) and peroneal brevis (PB). At the level of the lateral malleolus, the PB lies anterior to the PL, and both are enclosed in a common synovial sheath. The relationship of the tendons may change in pathological states. The PL has a long tendon, as it name implies, whereas the PB tendon is shorter with its musculotendinous junction just proximal to the level of the ankle joint. Place the transducer on the anterior border of the lateral malleolus and orient to a transverse plane with respect to the tendons (Figure 11.17). The transducer will have to be continually adjusted to remain in the transverse planes of the tendons as they course around the malleolus. The tendons are identified, followed in their axial plane to their musculotendinous junctions, and then evaluated in their longitudinal plane. Inferior to the lateral malleolus, the tendons course anteroinferiorly. This significant change in angulation of the tendons requires careful transducer positioning to prevent anisotropy.

Distally they are separated by the peroneal tubercle or trochlea of the calcaneus, identified as a hyperechoic projection from the lateral margin of the calcaneus, with the PB lying on the superior aspect and the PL on the inferior aspect of this tubercle (Figure 11.18). The tendons now have two separate synovial sheaths. The PB then takes a horizontal course to insert onto the lateral margin base of the fifth metatarsal (Figure 11.18b).

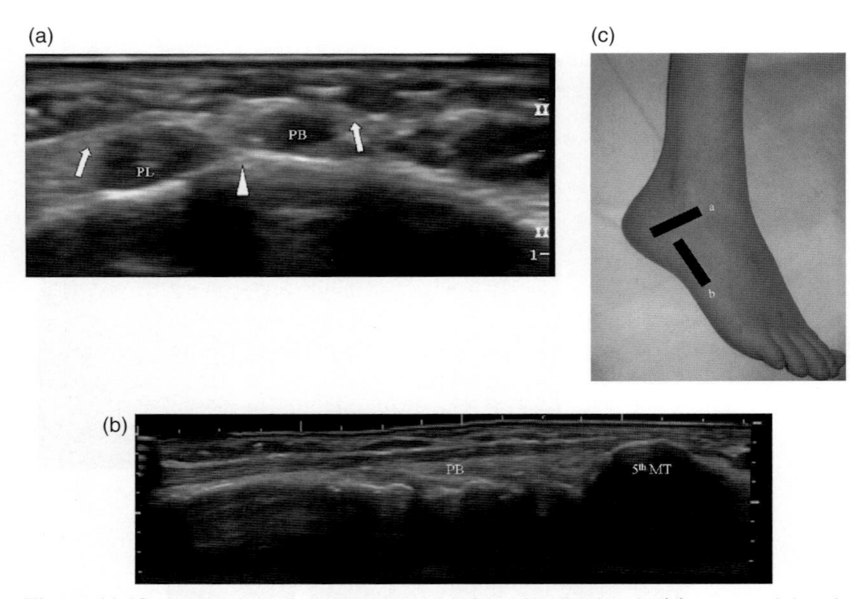

Figure 11.18. Posterolateral compartment, inframalleolar level: (**a**) peroneal brevis (PB) tendon superior and peroneus longus (PL) tendon inferior to the peroneal tubercle (arrowhead) and overlying hyperechoic inferior peroneal retinaculum (arrows). The tendons appear slightly hypoechoic due to anisotropy as it is difficult to achieve a normal hyperechoic appearance of the retinaculum and tendons on the one image. (**b**) EFOV ultrasound image of the PB insertion at the base of the fifth metatarsal (5th MT), and (**c**) corresponding transducer positions.

The PL runs in a groove on the cuboid bone (Figure 11.19) entering the plantar aspect of the foot and then inserting on the medial cuneiform and base of the first metatarsal. The os perineum, when present, is identified as a hyperechoic focus with posterior shadowing within the PL tendon at the level of the cuboid groove.

Dynamic evaluation at the level of the lateral malleolus to assess for subluxation is performed in the axial plane as described previously and by everting and dorsiflexing the foot. It is important not to apply pressure with the transducer, as excessive pressure may prevent subluxation. A common

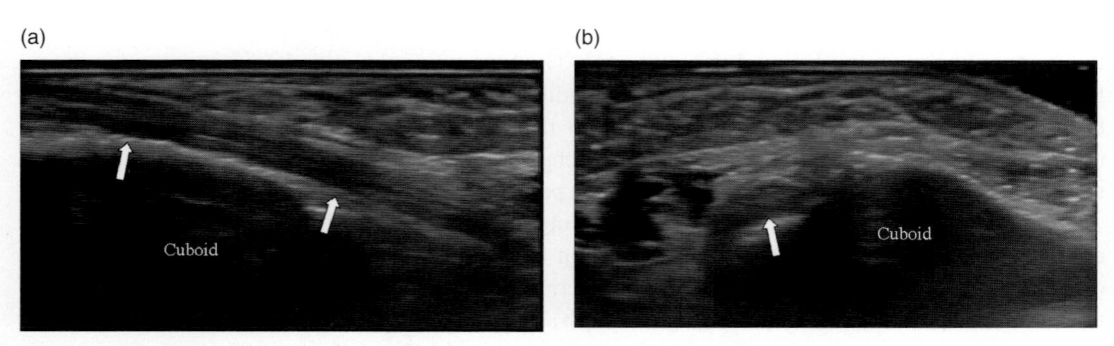

Figure 11.19. Peroneus longus (arrows): (**a**) longitudinal and (**b**) transverse ultrasound images at the level of the cuboid grove.

accessory tendon, the peroneus quadratus, may be present posteromedially at the level of the lateral malleolus, where it may present as a tendon or muscle. It is important to recognize this as a separate tendon rather than a split tear of the peroneal tendons.[9]

Retinaculum

Two retinaculae are present within the lateral compartment, the superior and inferior peroneal retinaculum. The retinaculae are best identified in their longitudinal planes by placing the transducer upon the anatomical plane of the retinaculae. The superior peroneal retinaculum extends from the tip of the lateral malleolus to the calcaneus, and the inferior peroneal retinaculum attaches to the calcaneus above and below the peroneal tubercle, as well as to the tubercle itself (Figure 11.18). The retinaculum, in both cases, is seen on ultrasound as a thin hyperechoic band (Figure 11.20).

Bursa

Subcutaneous bursae overlie the medial and lateral malleolus and are identifiable only when inflamed. The retrocalcaneal bursa lies anterior to the AT and may contain up to 3 mm of fluid. The walls are thin and hyperechoic. The retroachillean bursa or subcutaneous calcaneal bursa is seen only when inflamed posterior to the distal AT, close to its site of insertion, within the subcutaneous tissues.

Ligaments

The key to the assessment of ankle ligaments, listed in Table 11.3, is anatomy. Knowledge of the points of origin and insertion is essential for correct probe position and orientation. Placing the foot in different positions to stretch the ligament under evaluation is important.[4] The ligaments may be surrounded by fat, which appears hyperechoic. By gently angulating the probe, the ligaments will suffer from anisotropy and become hypoechoic, thus allowing visual differentiation from surrounding fat.

The anterior inferior tibiofibular ligament is oriented obliquely downward from the inferolateral margin of the tibia to the medial margin of the fibula. The transducer is placed in a transverse plane over the lateral margin of the distal tibia. A transversing thin hyperechoic band is seen, which is the distal component of the interosseous tibiofibular ligament (Figures 11.21a and b). Continue inferiorly, keeping the medial margin of the probe on the anterolateral tibial cortex; the anterior tibiofibular is identified as a thin band (Figure 11.21c). The posterior tibiofibular ligament is broader and thicker than its anterior counterpart, but is covered posteriorly by deep layers of soft tissues and is usually poorly visualized on ultrasound. The transducer should

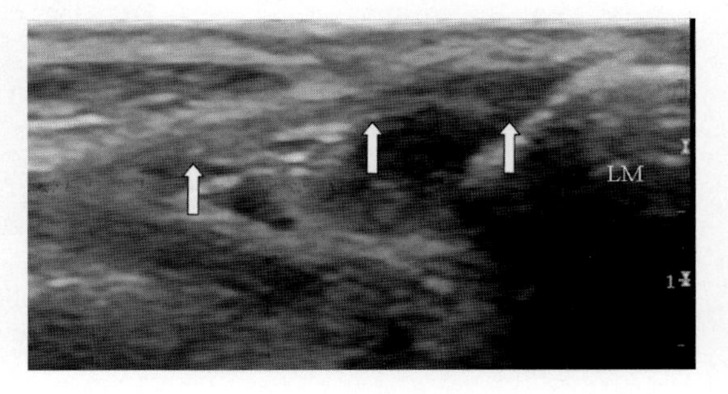

Figure 11.20. Superior peroneal retinaculum (arrows): transverse ultrasound image of the posterolateral compartment, demonstrating attachment to the lateral malleolar (LM).

Table 11.3. Ankle Ligaments.

Ankle Ligaments
Anterior
Anterior tibiofibular
Posterior tibiofibular
Interosseous tibiofibular
Medial-deltoid ligament (superficial layer and deep layers)
Anterior tibionavicular
Anterior tibiotalar
Deep tibiotalar
Tibiocalcaneal
Posterior tibiotalar
Lateral
Anterior talofibular
Calcaneofibular
Posterior talofibular

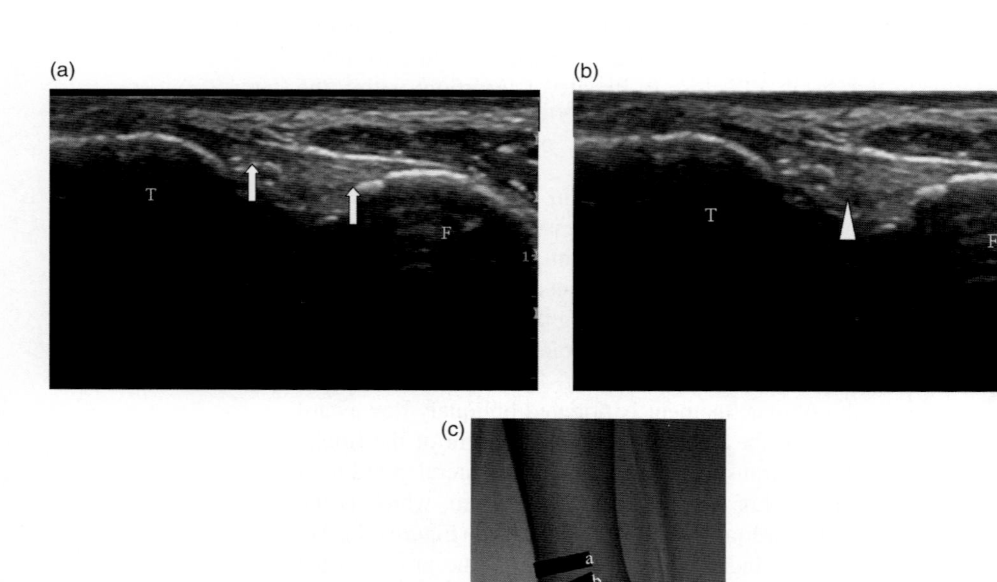

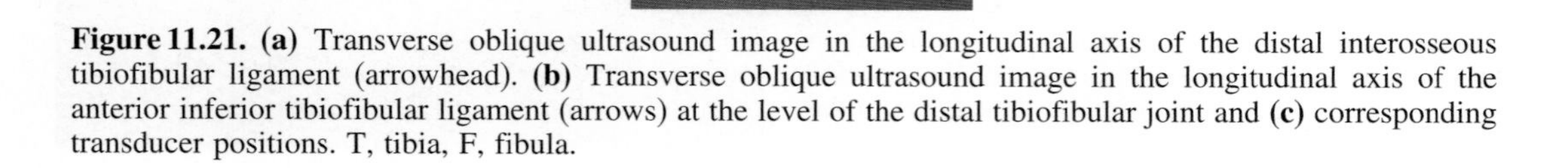

Figure 11.21. **(a)** Transverse oblique ultrasound image in the longitudinal axis of the distal interosseous tibiofibular ligament (arrowhead). **(b)** Transverse oblique ultrasound image in the longitudinal axis of the anterior inferior tibiofibular ligament (arrows) at the level of the distal tibiofibular joint and **(c)** corresponding transducer positions. T, tibia, F, fibula.

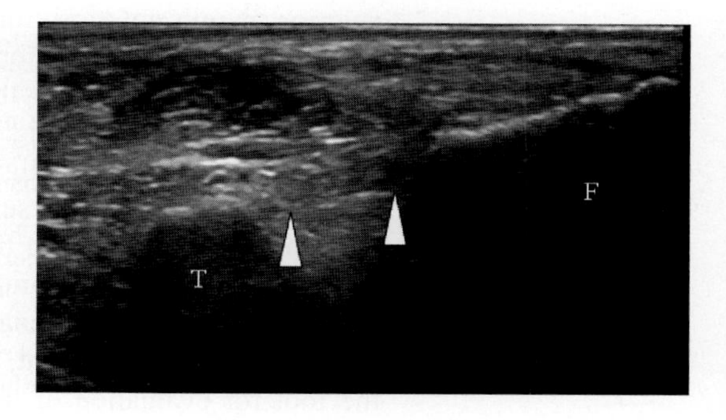

Figure 11.22. Transverse ultrasound of the distal tibiofibular joint in the longitudinal axis of the posterior tibiofibular ligament. T, tibia; F, fibula.

be placed in a horizontal orientation, with the anterior margin on the lateral malleolus and the posterior margin on the talus (Figure 11.22).

The lateral collateral ligament is composed of, from anterior to posterior, the following individual ligaments: anterior talofibular (ATF), calcaneofibular (CF), and posterior talofibular (PTF). It is examined in the same position as detailed in the evaluation of the lateral compartment. In addition, the ATF requires plantar flexion and the CF dorsal flexion in order to stretch their fibers. This action straightens the ligament, which normally measures less than 2 mm in thickness (Figure 11.23). The probe is placed in a horizontal oblique orientation with the posterior margin on the lateral malleolus and the

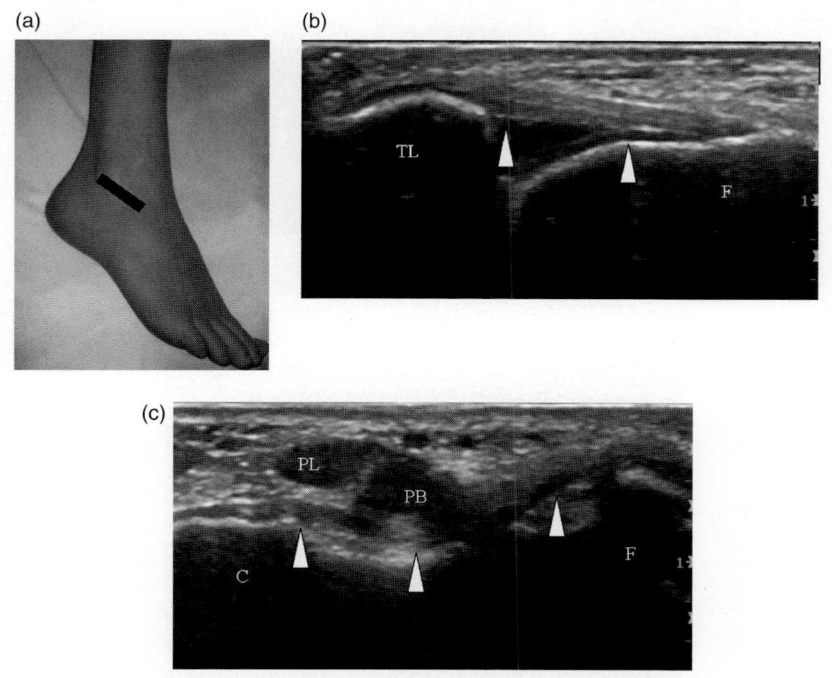

Figure 11.23. Anterior talofibular ligament: **(a)** transducer position and **(b)** corresponding ultrasound image in the longitudinal axis anterior to the talofibular ligament. **(c)** Longitudinal ultrasound of the calcaneofibular ligament (arrowheads). PL, peroneus longus; PB, peroneus brevis; C, calcaneus; F, fibula; TL, talus.

anterior margin anteriorly on the talus for the ATF. The transducer is then placed in a slightly posterior oblique orientation, in line with the orientation of the CF ligament, from the tip of the lateral malleolus to the calcaneus (Figure 11.23c). The CF ligament can be seen deep to the peroneal tendons.

The deltoid or medial ligament is composed of five parts that form two closely blended layers—a superficial and deep layer. It is triangular in shape with the apex attaching to the medial malleolus. From anterior to posterior it contains the anterior tibiotalar, tibionavicular, calcaneonavicular, tibiocalcaneal, and posterior tibiotalar. The patient is positioned as for the examination of the medial compartment, as described previously, with plantar flexion of the foot for evaluation of the anterior components and dorsiflexion for the posterior components. Inclusion of all components of the deltoid ligament can be challenging. The transducer is placed in an anteroinferior orientation with the posterior margin on the anterior margin of the medial malleolus. This will allow identification of the anterior tibiotalar ligament as a thin, less than 2-mm, hyperechoic fibrillar band (Figure 11.24). There is often a small amount of hypoechoic fluid identified deep to the ligament. This is the most important component to identify as it is often the first to rupture in trauma. Keeping the

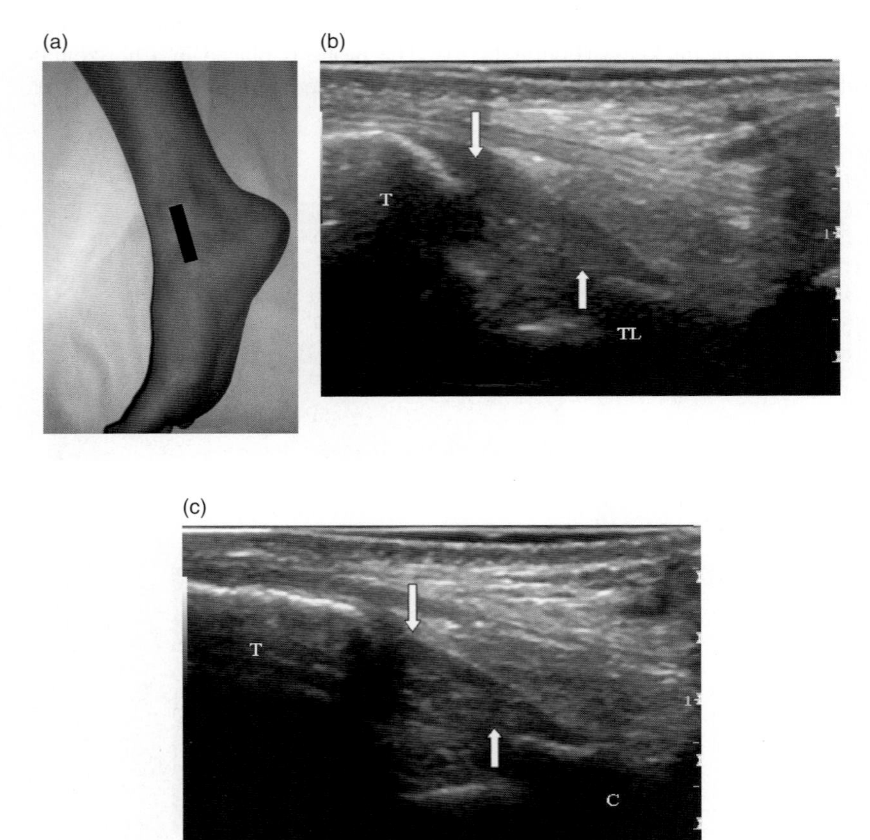

Figure 11.24. Deltoid ligament components: (**a**) transducer position for the anterior tibiotalar ligament and (**b**) corresponding ultrasound image in the longitudinal axis of the ligament. (**c**) Ultrasound image in the longitudinal axis of the tibiocalcaneal (deltoid) ligament. T, tibia; TL, talus; C, calcaneus.

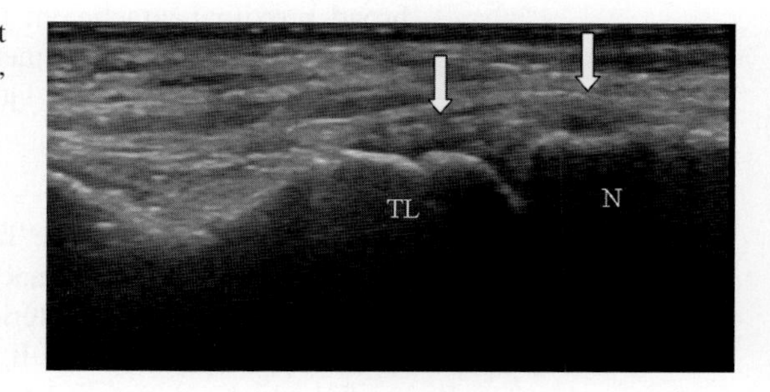

Figure 11.25. Superior talonavicular ligament (arrows), longitudinal ultrasound image. TL, talus; N, navicular.

posterior margin of the transducer on the medial malleolus and slowly rotating the anterior margin posteriorly for 180° will allow the remaining components of the deltoid complex to be visualized (Figure 11.24c). The deeper fibers of the deltoid ligament may appear hypoechoic due to anisotropy.

The remaining ligaments are rarely evaluated at our imaging center and are included for completeness. The superior talonavicular ligament, extending over the superior aspect of the talonavicular joint capsule, is a broad and thin ligament (Figure 11.25). It is identified by placing the transducer directly over the joint space in the longitudinal axis of the foot.

Insider Information 11.6
Ligaments should be stretched by manipulating the position of the ankle or foot. It is important to remain in the plane of the ligament to prevent anisotropy and a false diagnosis of pathology.

The inferior calcaneonavicular or spring ligament is a strong broad ligament running from the sustentaculum tali to the undersurface of the navicular (Figure 11.26). It is supported on its undersurface by the posterior tibial tendon. The sustentaculum tali is identified as a hyperechoic, medially projecting, bony prominence from the calcaneus deep to the inframalleolar component of the TP tendon. The transducer should be oriented in an anteroinferior oblique projection. The hyperechoic ligament is seen deep to the TP.

The intermetatarsal ligaments are seen as hyperechoic thin bands with the transducer axial to the bases of the metatarsals. Lisfranc's ligament is a strong and thick ligament, deeply situated in the sole of the foot. It has a relatively

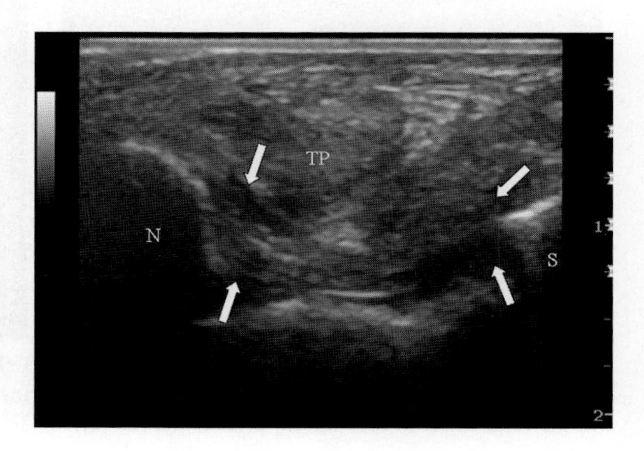

Figure 11.26. Ultrasound image in the longitudinal axis of the Spring ligament, inferior calcaneonavicular ligament (arrows). N, navicular; S, sustentaculum tali; TP, tibialis posterior.

broad proximal attachment to the plantar surface of the medial cuneiform adjacent to the first tarsometatarsal articulation.[4] From this attachment the ligament runs distally and laterally to attach to the medial aspect of the base of the second metatarsal.

Nerves

The posterior tibial nerve lies in a compartment within the tarsal tunnel formed by the medial retinaculum with the posterior tibial vessels, posterior to the FDL tendon and anterior to the FHL tendon, at the level of the medial malleolus (Figure 11.27). It divides into two terminal branches: the larger medial plantar nerve and the smaller lateral plantar nerve. The nerves are identified as a fascicular pattern of uninterrupted hypoechoic bands with intervening linear interrupted hyperechoic bands on longitudinal view and a mixture of hyperechoic and hypoechoic dots on axial view. Power Doppler is useful in separating the nerves from adjacent posterior tibial vessels. Digital branches of the medial or lateral plantar nerves are not normally identifiable. Evaluation for a Morton's neuroma is performed with the patient supine, or in a prone position, on the couch, and approaching the area between the metatarsal heads from a plantar approach (Figure 11.28). Gentle pressure from the dorsum of the foot can be applied over the intermetatarsal space being investigated. The dorsal approach can also be used in conjunction with the plantar approach if there are local artifacts from the thick plantar fascia. The dorsal approach requires additional plantar flexion of the toes. Chapter 12 describes in greater detail the assessment of nerves about the ankle and foot.

Sole of the Foot

Plantar Fascia

The plantar fascia or aponeurosis spans out, covering almost the whole of the sole of the foot, from its narrow attachment to the calcaneus to its distal division into five processes. It is composed of a thick central portion and thinner medial and lateral portions. The patient lies prone with the feet overhanging the bed (Figure 11.28). This is the usual position for evaluation

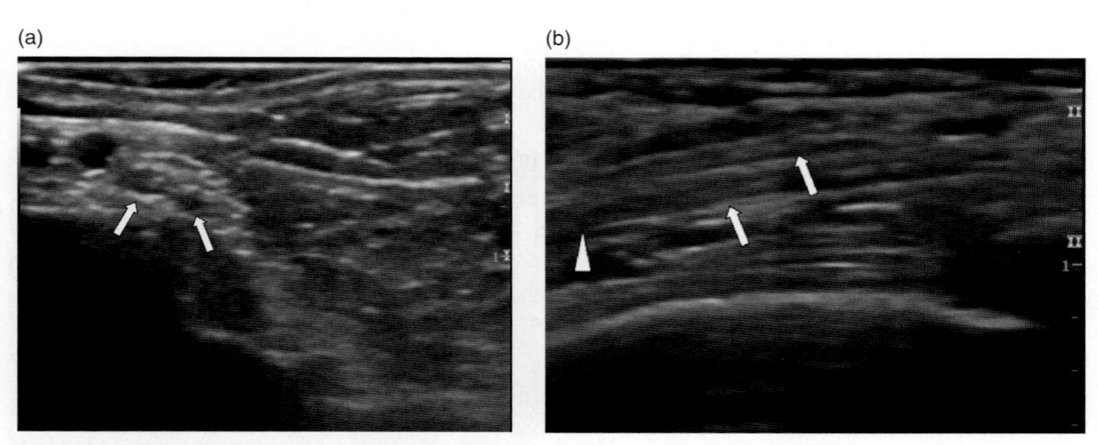

Figure 11.27. Posterior tibial nerve: **(a)** transverse and **(b)** longitudinal ultrasound images at the level of the tarsal tunnel, demonstrating the bifurcation of the posterior tibial nerve (arrowhead) into the medial plantar nerve and the larger and deeper lateral plantar nerves (arrows).

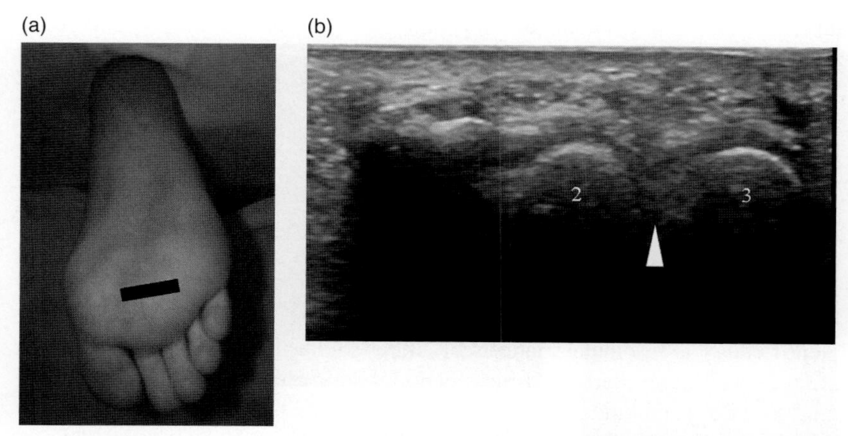

Figure 11.28. Morton's neuroma: **(a)** transducer position and **(b)** corresponding ultrasound image in the transverse plane at the level of the second (2) and third (3) metatarsal heads. Arrowhead, expected location of Morton's neuroma.

and allows for the AT to be evaluated at the same time, as pathologies in either the fascia or the tendon may present with heel pain. Alternatively, the patient can lie supine with the toes pointing up. The transducer is placed on the sole of the foot overlying the calcaneus and is slowly moved distally toward the metatarsals. The plantar fascia is seen as a superficial, relatively thick, less than 4-mm, hyperechoic band deep to the inhomogeneous heel fat pad (Figure 11.29). Examination should encompass the whole of the plantar fascia in the axial and longitudinal planes.

Muscles and Tendons

There are four layers of muscles as detailed in the anatomy section. Begin by locating the central origin of the plantar fascia with the transducer in the longitudinal axis of the foot (Figure 11.29). The hypoechoic muscle belly immediately deep to the plantar fascia is the flexor digitorum brevis in the first layer (Figure 11.29). By moving the probe in the same plane medially and laterally, the muscle bellies of the abductor hallucis and abductor digiti minimi are seen, respectively. The transverse plane allows identification of the proximal portion of all muscles and differentiation of the different layers (Figure 11.30). Deep to the abductor digiti minimi muscle, the peroneus longus tendon can be seen superficial to the hyperechoic cortex of the cuboid bone. Once the muscle belly is identified successfully, the musculotendinous junctions and tendons can be evaluated in orthogonal planes.

The transducer should be repositioned over the central portion of the plantar fascia. Deep to the fascia is the flexor digitorum brevis as previously described. Immediately deep to this is the hypoechoic muscle belly of the flexor accessories or quadratus plantae in the second layer (Figure 11.31). Initially, the transducer needs to be angled medially, then laterally, and moved toward the heel to access the two heads of origin of this muscle from the calcaneus. The lumbricals make up the second component of the second muscle layer. They are identified by first locating the tendon of the FDL on the sole of the foot (see the evaluation of the medial compartment of the ankle). The lumbricals originate from the four tendons of the FDL just

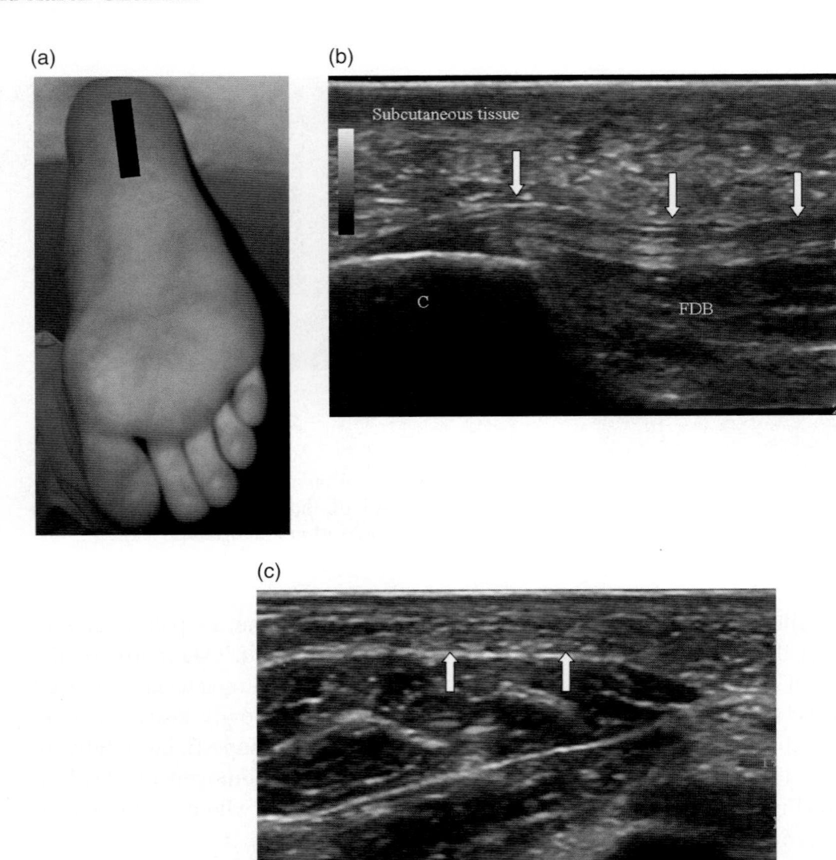

Figure 11.29. Plantar fascia: **(a)** transducer position and corresponding **(b)** longitudinal ultrasound image of the plantar fascia calcaneal origin. The hypoechoic muscle belly of the flexor digitorum brevis (FDB) is identified directly deep to the plantar fascia in the midline. **(c)** Transverse ultrasound image of the plantar fascia midfoot. C, calcaneus.

distal to their divergence. Each lumbrical has a thin hypoechoic muscle belly (Figure 11.32).

The third layer contains the flexor hallucis brevis (FHB), adductor (obliquus) hallucis (AH), adductor transverses hallucis (ATH), and flexor brevis digiti minimi (FDMB). The flexor hallucis brevis is evaluated first at the level of, and in the axial plane of, the first metacarpal head, where its two tendons contain hyperechoic sesamoid bones with posterior shadowing (Figure 11.33). The tendon of the FHL lies between the two heads of the FHB. The tendon heads of the FHB can then be traced proximally (Figure 11.34). The AH and ATH unite to form a common tendon of insertion. The AH lies directly on the lateral aspect of the lateral tendon of the FHB in an oblique plane to the bases of the second, third, and fourth metatarsals. Once visualized, turn the transducer into the axial plane, overlying the proximal

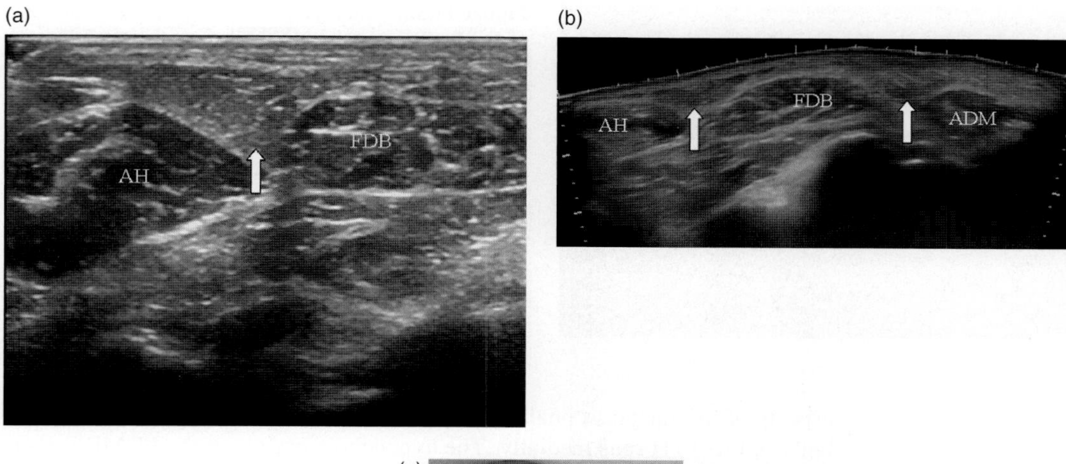

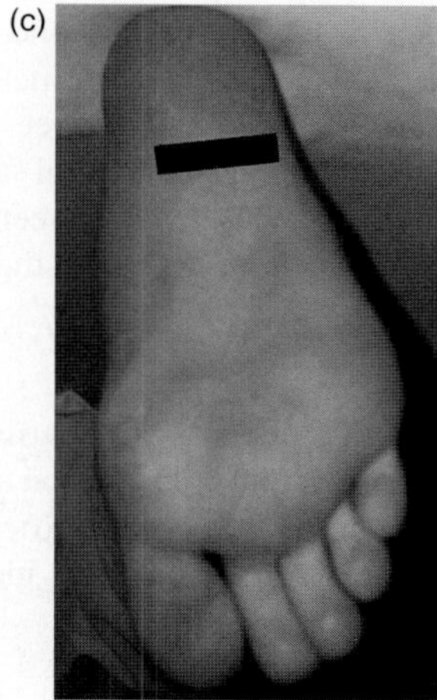

Figure 11.30. Sole of the foot: **(a)** transverse ultrasound image of the proximal and medial aspect of the sole of the foot demonstrating medial components of the first layer. **(b)** EFOV includes the lateral component and **(c)** corresponding transducer position. FDB, flexor digitorum brevis; AH, abductor hallucis; ADM, abductor digiti minimi; arrow, hyperechoic fat.

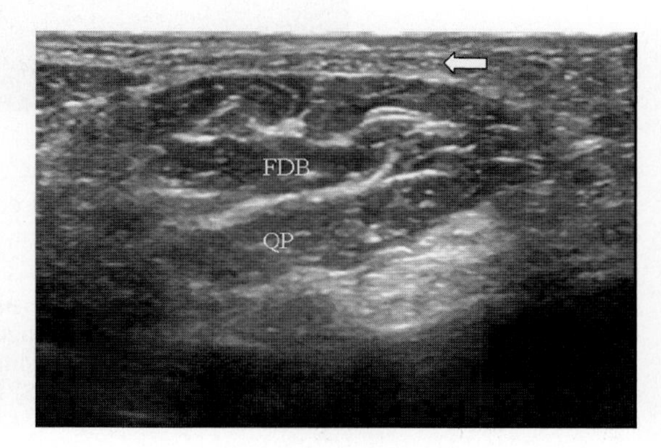

Figure 11.31. Transverse ultrasound of the proximal sole of the foot demonstrating the quadratus plantae (QP) deep to the flexor digitorum brevis (FDB) and plantar fascia (arrow).

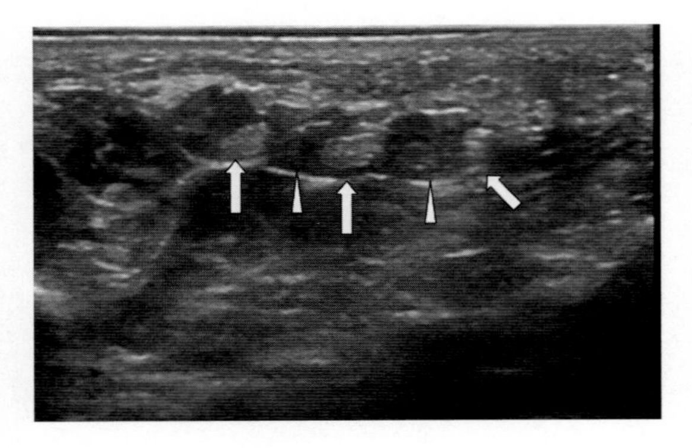

Figure 11.32. Transverse ultrasound of the mid sole of the foot demonstrating the hyperechoic tendons of the flexor digitorum longus (arrows) and the adjacent hypoechoic lumbrical muscle bellies (arrowheads).

aspects of the metatarsophalangeal joints, where the thin hypoechoic muscle belly of the ATH runs medially. The hypoechoic muscle of the FDMB lies on the lateral aspect of the sole deep to the hyperechoic tendon of the abductor digiti minimi at the level of the fifth metatarsal.

The fourth layer contains the three plantar and four dorsal interossei (Figure 11.35). The dorsal interossei are discussed in the evaluation of the dorsal compartment and lie between the metatarsal heads. The plantar interossei are on the plantar aspect of the third to fifth metatarsals.

Dorsum Foot

The tendons of the anterior compartment are followed from musculotendinous junctions to points of insertion as described previously. The extensor digitorum brevis muscle belly is identified on the dorsum of the foot, deep to the inferior extensor retinaculum. The identification of the latter is described

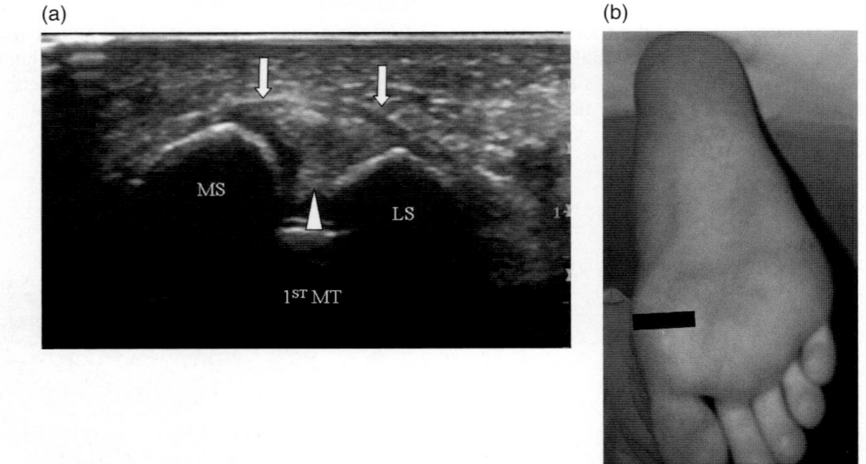

Figure 11.33. **(a)** Transverse ultrasound image of the first metatarsal head demonstrating the flexor hallucis longus tendon (arrowhead) between the medial and lateral sesamoids and **(b)** corresponding transducer position. Arrow, annular component of the fibrous flexor sheath; MS, medial sesamoid; LS, lateral sesamoid; 1st MT, first metatarsal.

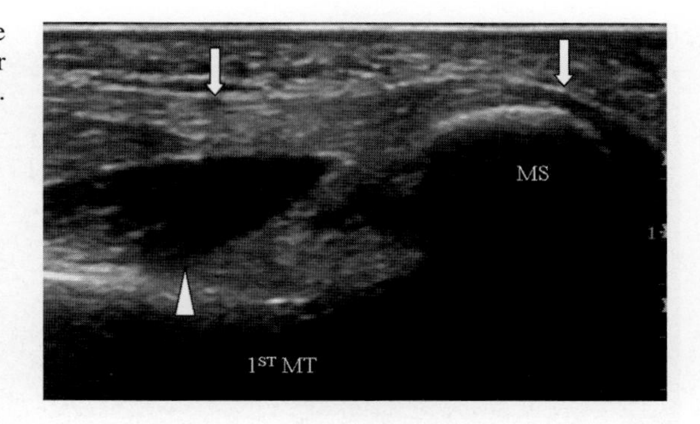

Figure 11.34. Longitudinal ultrasound image of the muscle (arrowhead) and tendon (arrows) of the flexor hallucis brevis in relationship to the medial sesamoid. 1st MT, first metatarsal; MS, medial sesamoid.

in the anterior evaluation of the ankle. Its muscle belly is hypoechoic when compared to the superficial surrounding anterior compartment tendons and the deep cuboid-navicular ligament (Figure 11.36). Placing the transducer upper margin at this level with the inferior margin pointing toward the first to fourth toes in sequence will allow identification of its four tendons, which arise just below the inferior retinaculum. The tendon slip extending to the great toe is considered separate, the extensor hallucis brevis, and inserts into the base of the proximal phalanx.

The four dorsal interossei muscles are initially evaluated in the axial plane by moving the transducer axial to and at the level of the metatarsals. The muscle belly is hypoechoic when compared to the hyperechoic metatarsal cortices. Their tendons can be followed to their insertion into the bases of the proximal phalanges.

Bones and Joints of the Foot

As in the study of all areas with complex anatomy, it is easiest to start in a region where one is confident of the anatomy and its appearance on ultrasound. The dorsal surface of the foot is a good starting point. The transducer should be placed in a longitudinal axis with respect to the foot at the level of the talar neck, with the plantar aspect of the foot flat on the table. This position was described in the section on the ankle joint. A hyperechoic line with posterior shadowing is identified deep to the joint space; this is the dorsal surface of the talus. Move the transducer slowly distally in the direction of the toes. The echogenic line of the talus ends at the talonavicular joint (Figure 11.37). It is

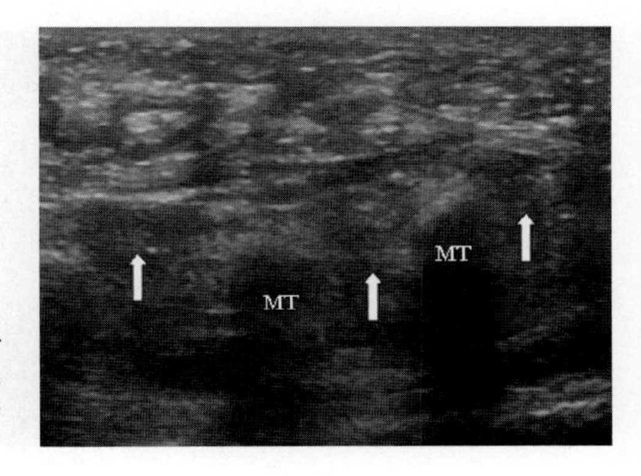

Figure 11.35. Transverse ultrasound image of the plantar surface of the foot demonstrating the metatarsal bones (MT), hyperechoic cortex and posterior shadowing, and the intervening hypoechoic plantar interossei muscles (arrows).

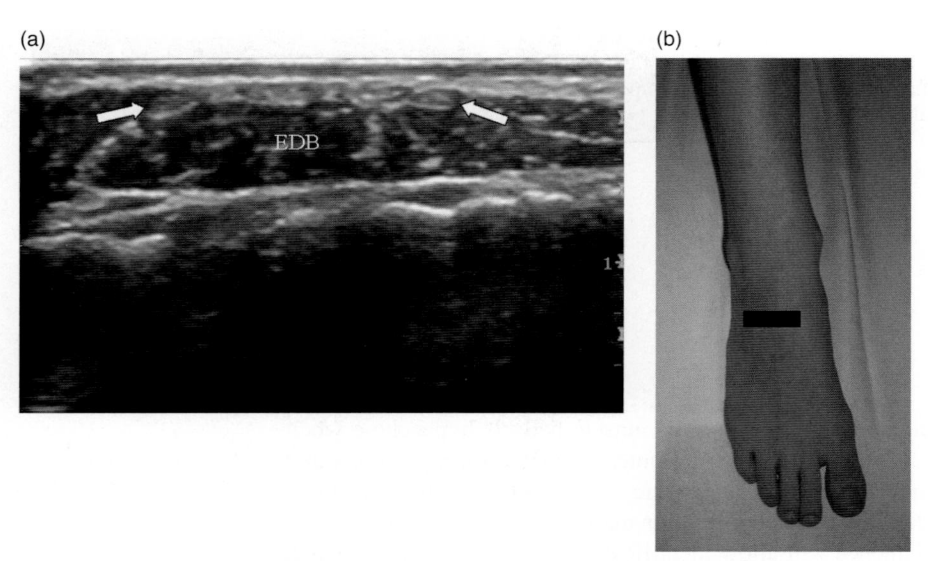

Figure 11.36. (**a**) Transverse ultrasound distal to the ankle joint demonstrating the hyperechoic tendons of the extensor digitorum longus (arrows) tendons superficial to the hypoechoic extensor digitorum brevis (EDB) muscle and (**b**) corresponding transducer position.

connected to the echogenic cortex of the navicular bone by the hyperechoic dorsal talonavicular ligament. Turn the transducer 90° and the navicular is seen medially and the cuboid bone laterally (Figure 11.37b). Return to the longitudinal plane of the foot with the distal end of the transducer pointing toward the first toe and slowly move the probe distally. The medial cuneiform articulates with the navicular proximally and the base of the first metatarsal (Figure 11.38). Turn the transducer 90° and the three cuneiforms—medial, intermediate, and lateral—can be identified on one image. Moving the probe

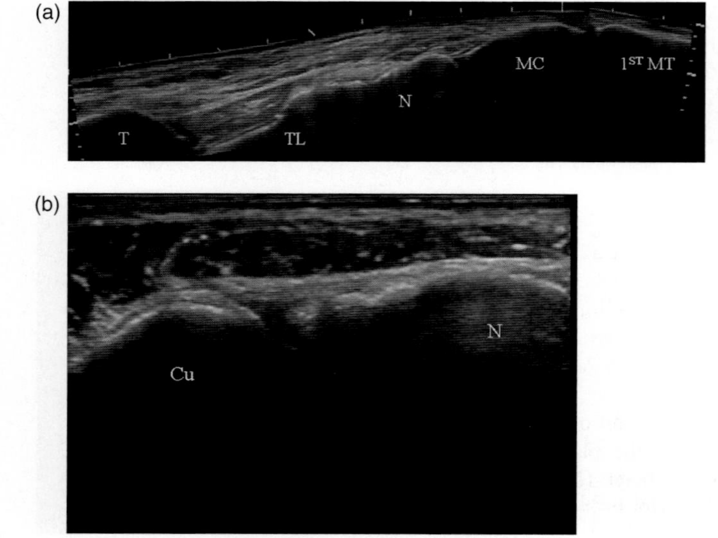

Figure 11.37. Articulations of the foot. (**a**) Longitudinal EFOV ultrasound image demonstrating the articulations of the foot. (**b**) Transverse ultrasound image of the navicular-cuboid joint. T, tibia; TL, talus; N, navicular; MC, medial cuneiform; 1st MT, first metatarsal; Cu, cuboid.

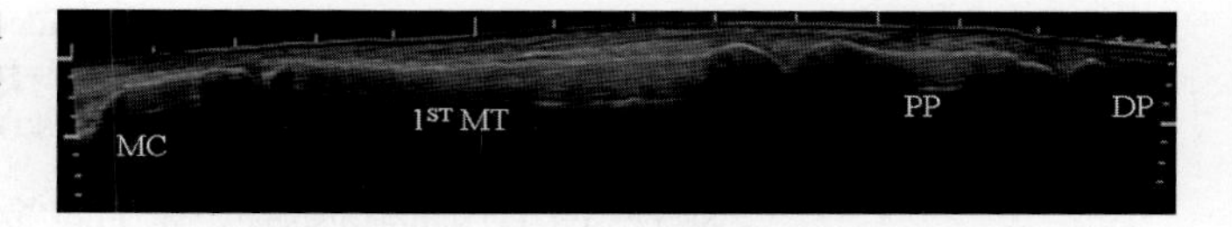

Figure 11.38. EFOV of the bones and articulations of the first toe. MC, medial cuneiform; 1st MT, first metatarsal; PP, proximal phalanx; DP, distal phalanx.

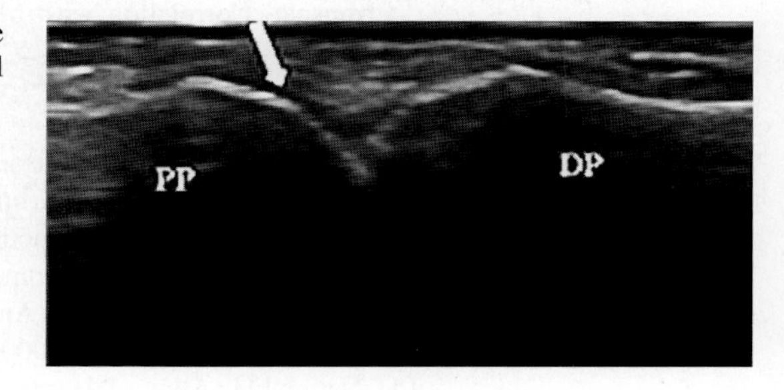

Figure 11.39. Longitudinal ultrasound image of the interphalangeal joint. PP, proximal phalanx; DP, distal phalanx; arrow, articular cartilage.

laterally, the cuboid bone can be identified. Return to the longitudinal plane at the level of the first tarsometatarsal joint. Move the probe distally in line with the long axis of the first metatarsal. Again the hyperechogenic cortex is smooth and continuous. The next joint space is the metatarsophalangeal joint, followed by the interphalangeal joint. This is the equivalent of the proximal interphalangeal joint in the second to fifth toes, which have in addition a distal interphalangeal joint. The joint spaces are similar, with the smooth cortical rounded surface covered by a thin hypoechoic rim of articular cartilage (Figure 11.39).

Imaging Protocol

The protocol adopted will depend on the referring clinical question and should be adaptable to any change in the patient's symptoms since referral. Development of good lines of communication with referring clinicians is essential; this ensures that the clinician understands the scope of ultrasound and requests a dedicated study to the region of concern. All anatomical structures within the symptomatic compartment are scrutinized. Rheumatological referrals are dedicated to specific joints as per request. An outline of the ankle imaging protocol at our imaging center is provided in the Appendix.

References

1. Fessell DP, Vanderschueren GM, Jacobson J et al. US of the ankle: Technique, anatomy and diagnosis of pathologic conditions. Radiographics 1998;18:325–340.
2. Shetty M, Fessell D, Femino et al. Sonography of ankle tendon impingement with surgical correlation. AJR 2002;179:945–953.
3. Fessell D, Jamadar D, Jacobson J. Sonography of dorsal ankle and foot abnormalities. AJR 2003;181:1573–1581.
4. Moran G, Busson J, Wybier M et al. Ultrasound of the ankle. Eur J Ultrasound 2001;14:73–82.
5. Magnano GM, Occhi M, Di Stadio M et al. High-resolution US of non-traumatic recurrent dislocation of the peroneal tendons: A case report. Pediatr Radiol 1998;28:476–477.

6. Sofka CM, Alder RS. Ultrasound-guided interventions in the foot and ankle. Semin Musculoskelet Radiol 2002;6(2):163–168.
7. Peetrons P, Creteur V, Bacq C. Sonography of ankle ligaments. J Clin Ultrasound 2004;32:491–499.
8. Fessell D, van Holsbeeck M. Foot and ankle sonography. RCNA 1999;37(4): 831–858.
9. Chepuri N, Jacobson J, Fessell D. Sonographic appearance of the peroneus quartus muscle: Correlation with MR imaging appearance in seven patients. Radiology 2001;218:415–419.
10. Quinn T, Jacobson J, Craig J. Sonography of Morton's neuromas. AJR 2000;174:1723–1728.
11. Oliver TB, Beggs I. Ultrasound in the assessment of metatarsalgia: A surgical and histological correlation. Clin Radiol 1998;53(4):287–289.
12. Primal Anatomy. Interactive foot and ankle: Sports Injuries Edition 2.0. http://www.anatomy.tv/home.
13. Sinnatamby CS. Last's Anatomy: Regional and Applied, 10th ed. St Louis: Churchill Livingstone, 2000.
14. Netter FH. Atlas of Human Anatomy, 5th ed. Ardsley, NY: Ciba-Geigy Corporation, 1996.
15. Bianchi S, Martinoli C, Gaignot C et al. Ultrasound of the ankle: Anatomy of the tendons, bursae, and ligaments. Semin Musculoskelet Radiol 2005;9(3):243–259.
16. Nazarian LN, Rawool NM, Martin CE et al. Synovial fluid in the hindfoot and ankle: Detection of amount and distribution with US. Radiology 1995;197: 275–278.

Section 4

The Peripheral Nerves

12

The Peripheral Nervous System

Srinivasan Harish

The advent of high-resolution ultrasound scanners has made possible the clear depiction of normal peripheral nerves. Ultrasound offers many advantages over magnetic resonance imaging (MRI) with respect to imaging of the peripheral nerves. It is faster, less expensive, and offers significantly higher spatial resolution. It also offers the ability to perform a dynamic study to assess the relationships of a nerve to surrounding structures, such as muscles, tendons, and ligaments. Comparison with the contralateral asymptomatic side is also a significant advantage in using ultrasound for the demonstration of peripheral nerves.

The choice of transducer for performing peripheral nerve ultrasound depends upon the regional anatomy of the nerve to be studied.[1] In general, for nerves that are literally superficial, such as the median nerve in the wrist, high-frequency transducers in the range of 12–15 MHz are appropriate. For nerves such as the sciatic nerve that have a deeper course, a 7.5-MHz transducer is more appropriate.

The regional anatomy, clinical indications for scanning, scanning technique, and normal appearance of the peripheral nerves that are commonly examined in clinical practice are described.

Normal Sonohistology of the Peripheral Nerves

The fundamental unit of the peripheral nerve is the nerve fiber, which is surrounded by the endoneurium (Figure 12.1).[2,3] The nerve fibers are made of axons, myelin sheaths, and Schwann cells. The combination of nerve fiber and its connective tissue covering, the endoneurium, together forms the nerve fascicles. The nerve fascicles are in turn surrounded by the capsular perineurium, which consists of connective tissue, vessels, and lymphatics. Multiple nerve fascicles are surrounded by a thick membrane called the epineurium. The epineurium has two parts: the superficial epineurium and the interfasicular epineurium. The superficial epineurium envelops the whole nerve trunk; the interfasicular epineurium is seen between the nerve fascicles. The epineurium consists of loose areolar tissue mixed with some elastic fibers and contains vessels. It is a relatively thicker membrane compared to the endoneurium and perineurium.

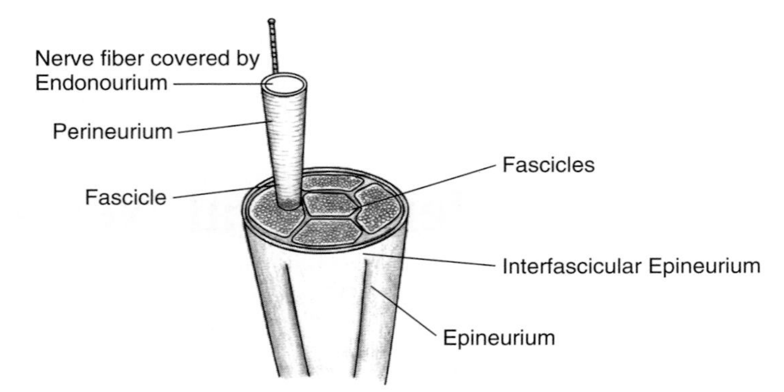

Figure 12.1. Cross section of the peripheral nerve demonstrating its internal structure.

The thin endoneurium is difficult to discern on ultrasound. The perineurium is seen as echogenic lines on ultrasound. The epineurium, being the thickest, reflects the ultrasound beam and hence appears as a thick echogenic line on ultrasound. The number of fascicles present in a given peripheral nerve depends upon factors such as the distance from its origin, type of nerve (motor, sensory, or mixed), and the amount of pressure that the nerve is subjected to in its compartment.[1]

Insider Information 12.1
The number of fascicles of a nerve seen on ultrasound depends not only on the type of nerve and its anatomical location, but also on the frequency of the transducer used. The number of individual nerve fascicles discerned in a given nerve decreases with the reduction in frequency of the transducer used.

On transverse sonography, the typical peripheral nerve demonstrates a reticular pattern with round hypoechoic areas surrounded by hyperechoic lines (Figure 12.2a). The hypoechoic dots correspond to the nerve fascicles, which are separated by a combination of echogenic perineurium and interfasicular

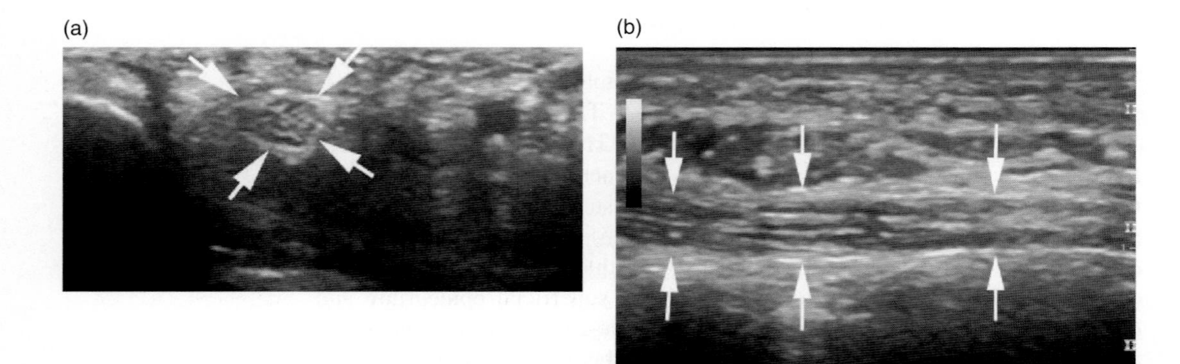

Figure 12.2. **(a)** A transverse ultrasound scan of the median nerve in the wrist shows a reticular pattern (arrows). **(b)** Ultrasound scan of a peripheral nerve shows parallel echogenic lines (arrows) in the longitudinal section.

epineurium.[2,3] The entire nerve trunk is surrounded by echogenic, thick, superficial epineurium. On longitudinal imaging, the typical peripheral nerve appears as multiple hypoechoic lines that are separated by echogenic bands (Figure 12.2b). The number of fascicles of a nerve seen on ultrasound depends not only on the type of nerve and its anatomical location, but also on the frequency of the transducer used. The number of individual nerve fascicles discerned in a given nerve decreases with the reduction in frequency of the transducer used.[1] The echotexture of a peripheral nerve is intermediate between that of skeletal muscle and tendon. The normal peripheral nerve can also demonstrate the anisotropic effect, but to a lesser extent compared to tendons.

Technique

The peripheral nerve should be examined in both the transverse and longitudinal planes. A copious amount of gel or a stand-off pad is necessary to improve the contact between the probe and the skin surface. The examination of the peripheral nerve is usually focused on the region in question, e.g., if there are clinical features suggestive of carpal tunnel syndrome, then the median nerve is examined in the wrist. As most compressive neuropathies occur in typical locations, the surface anatomy and bony landmarks should be utilized to identify the nerve on transverse images in a recognizable location in the first instance. The nerve can then be followed proximally and distally as required. In some patients, examination of the contralateral asymptomatic side may be needed to demonstrate any subtle changes in the dimension or echogenicity of the nerve. Since comprehensive sonographic examination of some of the peripheral nerves can be somewhat time consuming, it is important to rest the anatomical part being examined in a reasonably comfortable position for the patient, using a rolled towel or a pillow underneath the location to be examined. This also facilitates better examination of the nerve.

Anatomy of the Upper Limb Nerves

Nerves of the Arm (Figure 12.3)

Suprascapular Nerve

Regional Anatomy: The suprascapular nerve originates from the upper trunk of the brachial plexus with contributions from the fifth and sixth cervical roots (Chapter 13). It is a mixed nerve that carries pain sensation from both the glenohumeral and acromioclavicular joints and innervates the supraspinatus and infraspinatus muscles (Table 12.1). It has its origins in the posterior triangle of the neck. The suprascapular nerve runs outward, deep to the trapezius and parallel and deep to the omohyoid muscle, and enters the supraspinatus fossa through the suprascapular notch of the scapula, which is formed by the bridging transverse scapular ligament (Figure 12.4a). It winds around the lateral border of the spine of the scapula, passing through the spinoglenoid notch to reach the infraspinatus fossa. A branch to the supraspinatus muscle comes off just after it passes the suprascapular notch. After it enters the infraspinatus fossa, it supplies the infraspinatus.

> **Insider Information 12.2**
> An important problem to be recognized in imaging the spinoglenoid notch is that the prominent veins can mimic an enlarged nerve. However, these veins are relatively mobile and may change dimension and shape with movement of the shoulder.

Indications, Sonographic Anatomy, and Technique: One of the common indications for examining this nerve is to exclude ganglion and paralabral cysts compressing the nerve in the spinoglenoid notch. If the nerve is compressed around the scapular notch, then both the supraspinatus and the infraspinatus muscles are affected. When the compression is around the spinoglenoid

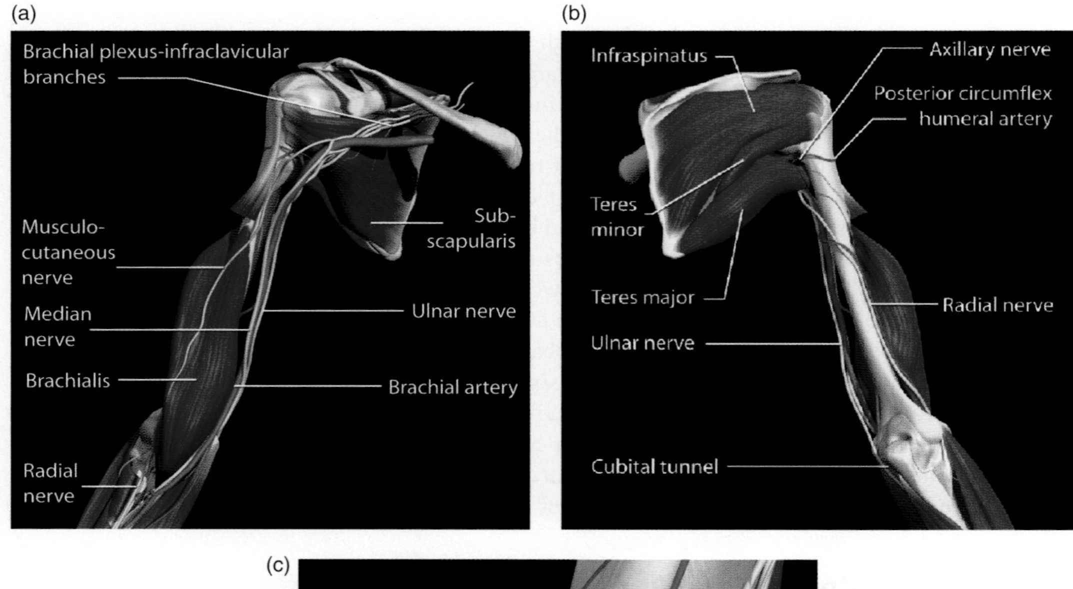

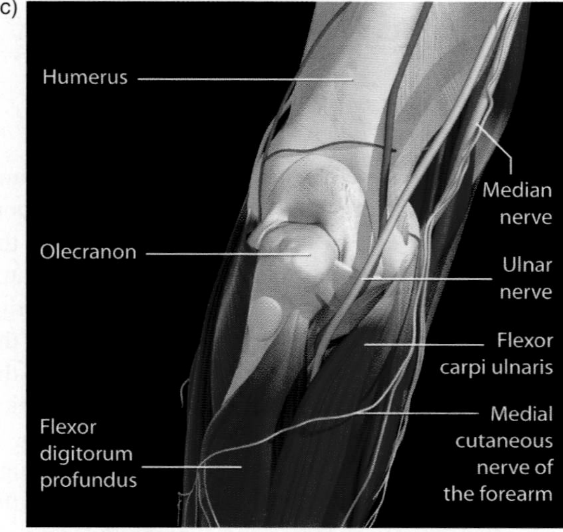

Figure 12.3. The major peripheral nerves of the arm: **(a)** anterior and **(b)** posterior views and **(c)** the ulnar nerve within the cubital tunnel.

Table 12.1. Major Nerves of the Upper and Lower Limb.

Nerve	Branches
Suprascapular nerve	Motor supply to supraspinatus and infraspinatus Pain fibers from the acromioclavicular joint and shoulder joint
Axillary nerve	Anterior branch—-supplies the deltoid and patch of skin over the deltoid Posterior branch—-teres minor and posterior aspect of the deltoid Upper lateral cutaneous nerve of the arm
Musculocutaneous nerve	Motor supply to biceps, brachialis and coracobrachialis muscles Lateral cutaneous nerve of the forearm Articular branch to the elbow joint
Median nerve	Palmar cutaneous branch proximal to the carpal tunnel Five branches in the hand—-radial motor branch and four sensory branches Anterior interosseous nerve—-flexor pollicis longus and radial parts of the flexor digitorum profundus
Radial nerve	Posterior cutaneous and inferior lateral cutaneous nerves of the forearm Muscular, deep, and superficial branches Posterior interosseous nerve (deep branch of the radial nerve) Superficial sensory branch
Ulnar nerve	Dorsal cutaneous branch—-before entering Guyon's canal Superficial sensory and deep motor nerves within the canal
Sciatic nerve	Common peroneal nerve Tibial nerve
Femoral nerve	Superficial sensory Deep motor Saphenous nerve
Common peroneal nerve	Superficial peroneal Deep peroneal
Tibial nerve	Sural nerve Medial plantar Lateral plantar Medial calcaneal

notch, only the infraspinatus is affected. To help visualize the nerve in the spinoglenoid notch, adduction of the shoulder with placement of the ipsilateral hand on the contralateral shoulder is useful; this brings the nerve slightly superficial to the plane of the scan (Figure 12.4b). To examine the suprascapular nerve at the level of the spinoglenoid notch, careful adjustment of the focal zones and magnification are necessary.[4] The normal nerve can be difficult to visualize, except in thin subjects, where it is seen as a low echogenicity structure located over the bony cortex of the spinoglenoid notch (Figure 12.4c). Doppler examination is of particular value in showing flow from the suprascapular artery; the nerve can then be identified adjacent to the artery. An important problem to be recognized in imaging the spinoglenoid notch is that the prominent veins can mimic an enlarged nerve.[4] However, these veins are relatively mobile and may change dimension and shape with movement of the shoulder.

Axillary Nerve

Regional Anatomy: The axillary nerve is a terminal branch of the posterior cord of the brachial plexus with contributions from the fifth and sixth cervical segments (Chapter 13). The nerve descends behind the axillary artery along

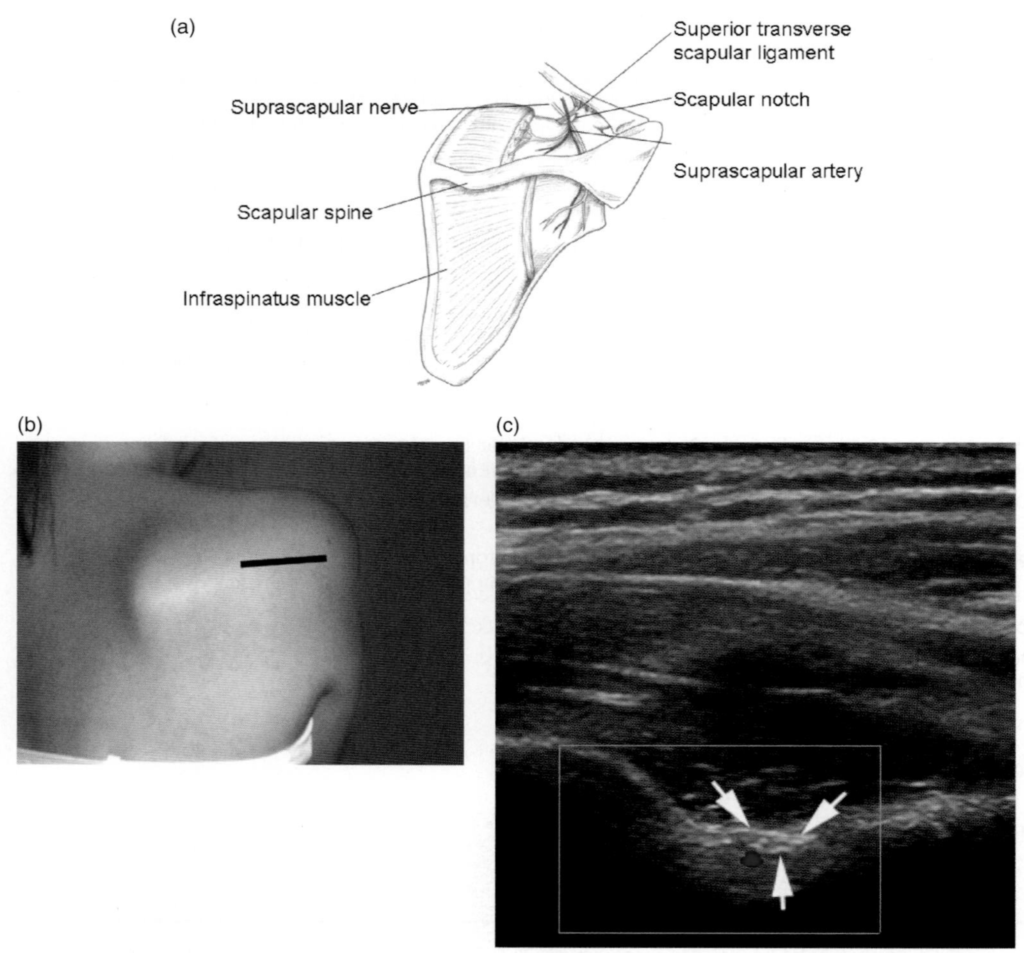

Figure 12.4. (**a**) The suprascapular nerve in the spinoglenoid notch. (**b**) The adducted arm position and probe position (black band) for examination of the suprascapular nerve in the spinoglenoid notch. (**c**) Ultrasound scan of the suprascapular nerve (arrows) in the spinoglenoid notch in the transverse section. Note the Doppler signal in the adjacent suprascapular vessels.

the lower lateral border of the subscapularis muscle, curves underneath the shoulder joint capsule, passes through the quadrilateral space along with the posterior circumflex humeral artery, and divides into two branches, anterior and posterior (Figure 12.3b). It has an anterior branch that winds around the posterior aspect of the surgical neck of the humerus, sending branches to the deltoid, and a patch of skin overlying the deltoid. The posterior branch of the axillary nerve supplies the teres minor muscle and also a small portion of the posterior aspect of the deltoid. As it descends around the posterior border of the deltoid, it forms the upper lateral cutaneous nerve of the arm, which supplies the skin over the lower deltoid and also along the lateral head of the triceps to the midpart of the arm. The quadrilateral space is bordered by the subscapularis muscle anteriorly, teres minor posteriorly, teres major inferiorly, long head of the triceps muscle medially, and the surgical neck of the humerus laterally.

Insider Information 12.3
Abduction/elevation of the arm coupled with the use of Doppler to identify the accompanying posterior circumflex humeral artery helps in identifying the axillary nerve near the posterior axillary fold.

Indications, Sonographic Anatomy, and Technique : The axillary nerve is typically compressed in the quadrilateral space syndrome, which involves compression of the nerve along with the posterior humeral circumflex artery. Demonstration of the normal axillary nerve is usually difficult due to its small dimension. The nerve can sometimes be located in the posterior aspect of the proximal arm at the level of the posterior axillary fold (Figure 12.5a). Maneuvers that help in demonstrating the nerve at this level include abduction/elevation of the arm coupled with the use of Doppler to identify the accompanying posterior circumflex humeral artery.[2] From the level of the posterior axillary fold, the nerve and the accompanying vessel can be traced across the posterior aspect of the shoulder in a more neutral position of the arm. The nerve is first located in transverse imaging; then it can be traced further with longitudinal imaging. The nerve is surrounded by the pectoralis major and latissimus dorsi muscles at this level (Figure 12.5b).

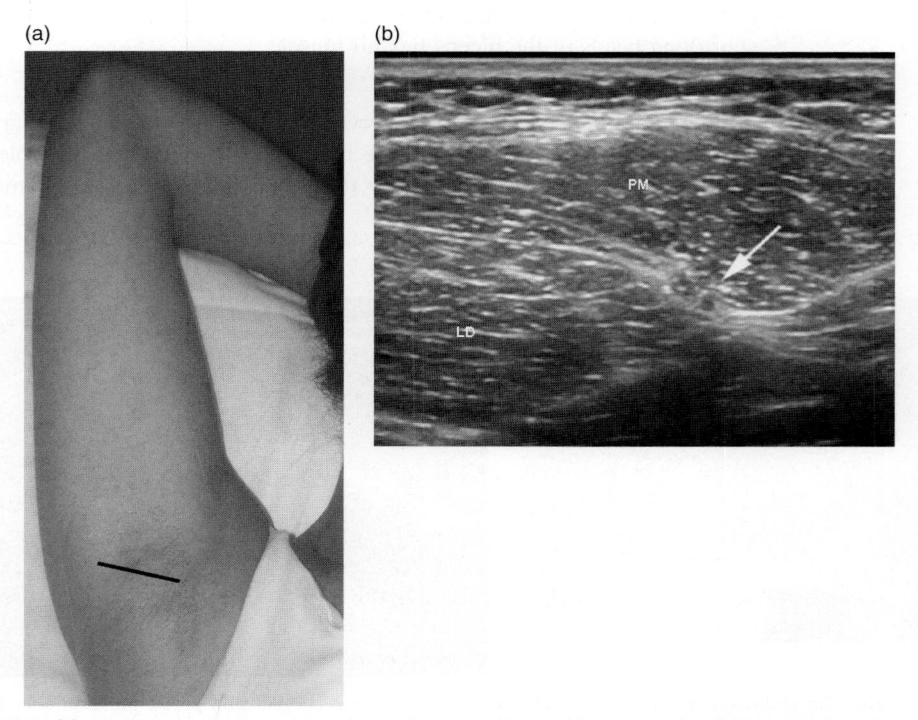

Figure 12.5. **(a)** The abducted arm position and probe position (black band) for examination of the axillary nerve near the posterior axillary fold. **(b)** The axillary nerve (arrow) is surrounded by the pectoralis major (PM) and latissimus dorsi (LD) muscles on transverse ultrasound section.

Musculocutaneous Nerve

Regional Anatomy: The musculocutaneous nerve is a mixed nerve with motor and sensory elements, which originates as a terminal branch of the lateral cord of the brachial plexus with contributions from the fifth to seventh cervical spinal segments. It courses along the medial border of the coracoid process, enters the coracobrachialis muscle, and continues downward and laterally between the biceps and brachialis muscles (Figure 12.3a). In its course, this nerve is usually covered by the short head of the biceps muscle. During its passage through the coracobrachialis, the nerve innervates the biceps, the brachialis, and the coracobrachialis muscles. At the level of the elbow, it pierces the deep fascia to continue as the lateral cutaneous nerve of the forearm. It gives an articular branch to the elbow joint.

Indications, Sonographic Anatomy, and Technique: There are no common compressive neuropathies involving the musculocutaneous nerve. It can sometimes be compressed by a humeral exostosis or be involved by tumor. The musculocutaneous nerve is a relatively small peripheral nerve. It can be demonstrated by transverse imaging medial to the coracoid process or between the biceps and the brachialis muscles.[2] The arm is usually kept in an abducted and supinated position with the hand on the occiput (Figure 12.6a). The ultrasound probe is placed transverse to the course of the axillary artery in the medial aspect of the proximal arm.[5] Since it is the only major nerve of the upper extremity embedded in a muscle, it can be easily demonstrated lateral to the axillary artery between the parts of the coracobrachialis muscle (Figure 12.6b). It can then be traced distally at the exit from the coracobrachialis, where the nerve lies between the coracobrachialis and the short/long heads of the biceps brachii muscle.

Median Nerve

Regional Anatomy: The median nerve is the largest nerve in the arm and arises from both the lateral and the medial cords of the brachial plexus at the distal end of the axillary artery (Chapter 13). It derives its name from

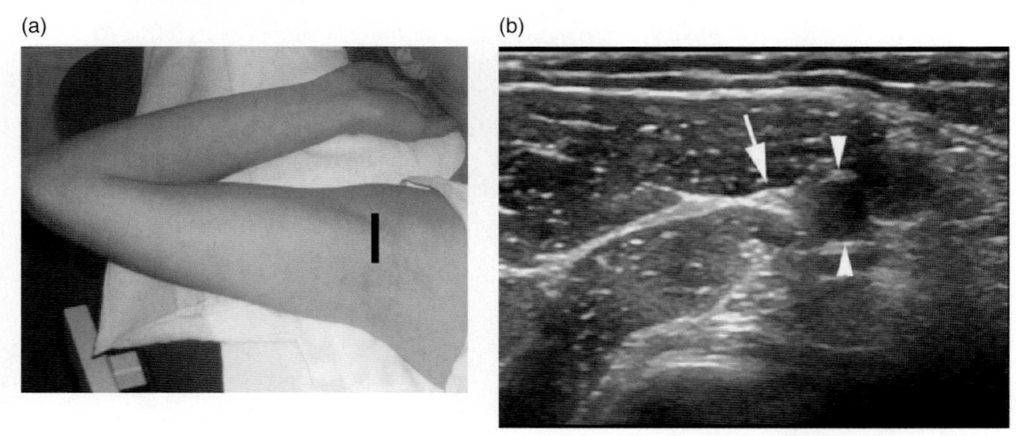

Figure 12.6. **(a)** The abducted arm position with the arm behind the occiput and probe position (black band) for examination of the musculocutaneous nerve in the medial proximal arm. **(b)** A transverse ultrasound scan shows the musculocutaneous nerve (arrow) between parts of the coracobrachialis muscle, lateral to the axillary vessels (arrowheads).

its position in the midarm between the ulnar and radial nerves. Proximally, the median nerve is located lateral to the brachial artery. It runs anterior to the brachial artery along the medial side of the bicipital groove, and distally it crosses to its medial border proximal to the elbow joint (Figures 12.3a and 12.7). There are variations in the course of the nerve near the pronator teres muscle. The median nerve descends distally toward the elbow to lie between the two heads of the pronator teres muscle in 95% of cases.[2] In a small proportion of patients, it can lie between the ulna and the ulnar head of the pronator teres. Sometimes it perforates the humeral head of the pronator teres muscle, which is supplied by the median nerve.

Indications, Sonographic Anatomy, and Technique: In the upper arm, the median nerve can be involved by tumors or posttraumatic hematoma. A potential site for compression of the median nerve in the upper arm is the ligament of Struthers, which connects the supracondylar process to the medial epicondyle. The supracondylar process, a beaklike bony projection that is usually an incidental finding in approximately 1% of the population, is located about 5 cm above the medial epicondyle.[6] For examination of the nerve, the patient is positioned supine with a pillow under the arm with the arm in mild external rotation to expose the medial aspect, or sitting on a chair with the elbow extended on the examining table. The nerve is first identified in the upper arm by transverse scanning. To begin, transverse scanning in the medial aspect of the upper/mid arm is performed to localize the brachial artery using Doppler examination. The nerve lies anterior to the brachial artery, medial to the bicipital groove (Figure 12.7).

Radial Nerve

Regional Anatomy: The radial nerve is a direct continuation of the posterior cord of the brachial plexus (C5 to C8) (Chapter 13). It gives rise to the posterior cutaneous and inferior lateral cutaneous nerves of the forearm and to muscular, deep, and superficial branches. It supplies the muscles of the extensor compartments. The nerve leaves the axilla, anterior to the origin of the latissimus dorsi muscle, winding around the posterolateral aspect of the humerus, also called the spiral groove of the humerus (Figure 12.3b). It reaches the proximal aspect of the groove of the radial nerve on the humerus between the medial and lateral heads of the triceps muscle. In its course, the

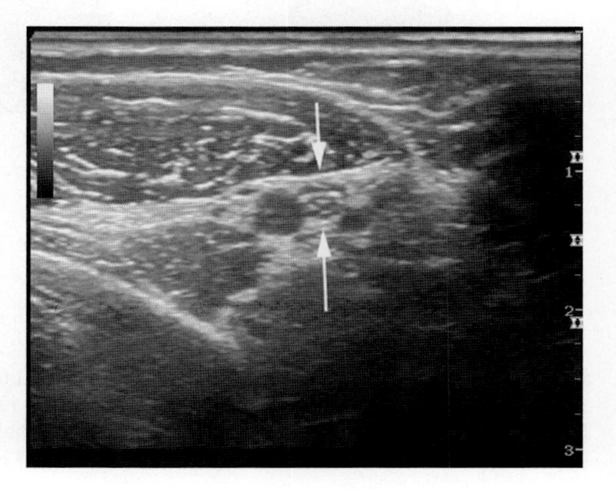

Figure 12.7. A transverse ultrasound section at the level of the medial aspect of the bicipital groove shows the median nerve (arrows) adjacent to the brachial artery.

nerve is accompanied by the deep brachial artery and vein. The nerve pierces the upper third of the lateral intermuscular septum, thus leaving the extensor compartment, and enters the cubital fossa; it finally lies on the anterior aspect of the elbow between the brachioradialis and brachialis muscle. It also supplies sensory branches to the posterior aspect of the arm.

Indications, Sonographic Anatomy, and Technique: The radial nerve can be entrapped in the spiral groove, particularly when people sleep with their upper arms in an improper posture. This leads to weakness of the triceps, brachioradialis, and extensor muscles of the hand and wrist. The nerve can be examined with the patients in a supine position, elbow flexed to 90° and positioned on a pillow to allow access to the posterolateral part of the arm (Figure 12.8a). The radial nerve is identified at the proximal part of the upper arm and is followed distally to the lateral epicondyle. It is identified at the posterolateral aspect of the humeral shaft, adjacent to the brachial artery, initially between the coracobrachialis and teres major and subsequently between the medial and lateral heads of the triceps. The nerve demonstrates a reticular appearance with an oval cross section and is seen between the heads of the triceps muscle (Figure 12.8b). The normal dimension of the nerve where it is closely applied to the humerus posteriorly is approximately 4.0 mm (mediolateral) and 2.3–3.5 mm (anteroposterior).[7]

Ulnar Nerve

Regional Anatomy: The ulnar nerve arises from the medial cord of the brachial plexus and receives fibers from the eighth cervical to first thoracic roots (Chapter 13). It descends on the medial aspect of the arm to the elbow, where

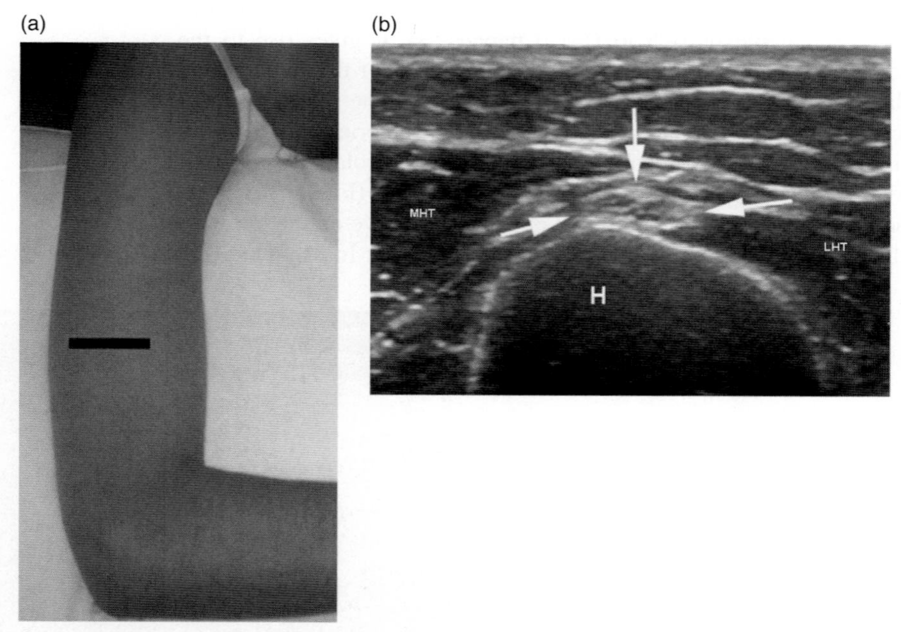

Figure 12.8. **(a)** The elbow flexed and positioned on a pillow to examine the posterolateral part of the arm and the probe position (black band) for examination of the radial nerve. **(b)** A transverse ultrasound section at the level of the posterolateral part of the arm shows the radial nerve (arrows) adjacent to the cortex of the humerus (H) between the medial (MHT) and lateral heads (LHT) of the triceps.

it lies in the cubital tunnel. The nerve descends in the upper arm along the medial aspect of the bicipital groove (Figure 12.3a and c). There are no motor or sensory branches coming off the nerve in the upper arm. At the medial elbow, the ulnar nerve courses in the groove behind the medial epicondyle in a space bordered by the olecranon and the medial epicondyle and bridged by the cubital tunnel retinaculum, also called Osborne's fascia. It then enters the cubital tunnel between the ulnar and humeral heads of the flexor carpi ulnaris muscle. The passage behind the medial epicondyle and the heads of the flexor carpi ulnaris are common sites of entrapment of the nerve. Loss of integrity of the Osborne's fascia can result in subluxation of the nerve out of the tunnel, with increasing flexion of the elbow. A normal variant at the cubital tunnel is the anconeus epitrochlearis muscle. It is present in 3–28% of cadaveric elbows.[8] It extends from the medial epicondyle to the medial aspect of the olecranon. The ulnar nerve may be subjected to static compression by the anconeus epitrochlearis muscle, of which the cubital tunnel retinaculum is thought to represent a remnant.[8] The location of the ulnar nerve within the cubital tunnel changes with different positioning of the elbow. As the elbow is flexed, the ulnar nerve can be entrapped between the retinaculum and the medial epicondyle of the humerus or it can sometimes be dislocated beyond the margin of the retinaculum.[9]

Insider Information 12.4
The location of the ulnar nerve within the cubital tunnel changes with different positioning of the elbow. As the elbow is flexed, the ulnar nerve can be trapped between the retinaculum and the medial epicondyle of the humerus or it can sometimes be dislocated beyond the margin of the retinaculum. Ulnar nerve dislocation can be seen in up to 20% of normal elbows.

Indications, Sonographic Anatomy, and Technique: Ulnar nerve entrapment at the elbow is the second most common entrapment neuropathy encountered in clinical practice. Ultrasound is usually requested to look for any nerve swelling, dislocation of the nerve out of the tunnel, or extrinsic compressive lesions. The nerve is best identified behind the medial epicondyle of the humerus in the elbow. The examination is performed initially with an extended elbow with slight external rotation of the shoulder (Figure 12.9a). The medial epicondyle and the olecranon process are palpated, and the probe is placed transversely between these two bony landmarks. The nerve can also be easily identified with the elbow in 90° of flexion with the palm of the hand resting on the table. Once again, the probe is placed between the bony landmarks of the olecranon and the medial epicondyle, with each end of the probe lying on these bony landmarks. The nerve is demonstrated as a fascicular structure behind the medial epicondyle (Figure 12.9b). Dynamic examination of the nerve is performed by active flexion of the elbow by keeping the probe stationary relative to the medial epicondyle. The nerve is examined as the elbow is flexed to look for any dislocation out of the cubital tunnel. However, it should be noted that ulnar nerve dislocation from the cubital tunnel can be seen in up to 20% of asymptomatic elbows. The nerve can then be followed more proximally into the arm from the level of the medial epicondyle. The nerve has a normal cross-sectional area of approximately 6.8 mm^2at the level

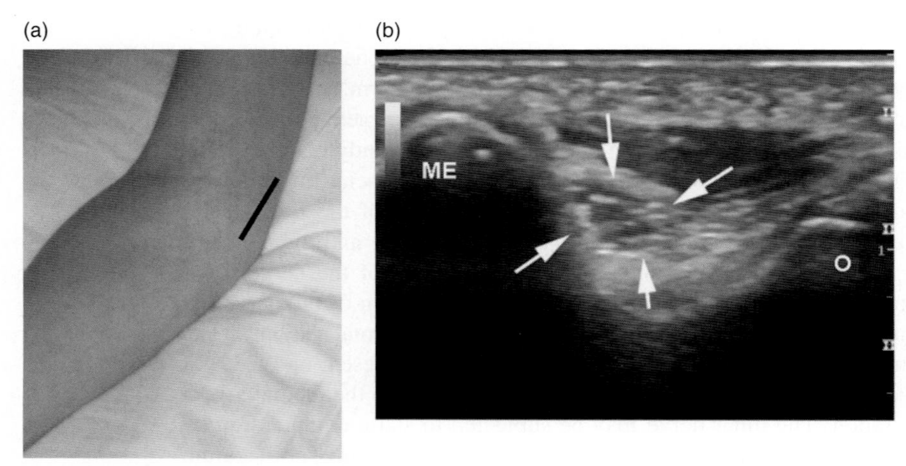

Figure 12.9. **(a)** The arm position and probe position (black band) for examination of the ulnar nerve behind the medial epicondyle of the humerus. **(b)** A transverse ultrasound section at the level of the medial epicondyle (ME) and the olecranon (O) shows the ulnar nerve (arrows).

of the medial epicondyle, 5.7 mm^2in the distal arm and approximately 6.2 mm^2in the proximal forearm.[4,10] After its exit from the ulnar groove, the nerve is identified between the humeral and ulnar heads of the flexor carpi ulnaris muscle in the proximal forearm.

Nerves of the Forearm and Wrist

Median Nerve

Regional Anatomy: At the level of the elbow, the median nerve passes deep to the bicipital aponeurosis superficial to the brachialis. It then courses between the humeral and ulnar heads of the pronator teres. This happens in approximately 80% of individuals, and the course of the median nerve with respect to the pronator teres can vary. It then passes beneath the edge of the fibrous arch of the flexor digitorum superficialis. It runs distally to the wrist between the superficial and deep flexor muscles of the hand (Figure 12.10a and Figure 12.10d and Figure 12.11a and Figure 12.11b). It innervates the flexor group of muscles in the forearm.

The anterior interosseous nerve is a motor nerve that is the largest branch of the median nerve. It originates on the lateral aspect of the median nerve approximately 5 cm distal to the medial humeral epicondyle. It courses through the pronator teres and then reaches the ventral aspect of the interosseous membrane along with the anterior interosseous artery. It supplies the flexor pollicis longus, the radial side of the flexor digitorum profundus, and the pronator quadratus muscles.

The carpal tunnel is bordered by the carpal bones and the flexor retinaculum, also called the transverse carpal ligament (Figure 12.10d). The tunnel is approximately 5 cm long, extending from the wrist to the mid-aspect of the palm. Apart from the median nerve, eight tendons of the flexor digitorum profundus, the flexor digitorum superficialis, and the flexor pollicis longus tendon pass through this fibroosseous tunnel. The flexor retinaculum is approximately 4 cm wide and 3 mm thick. It is attached to the tuberosity of the scaphoid and the trapezium on the lateral aspect and to the pisiform and the hook of hamate on the medial aspect. On its lateral aspect, the flexor retinaculum splits to enclose the flexor carpi radialis tendon. The median nerve passes superficial to the flexor digitorum superficialis proximal to the carpal tunnel and parallel to the flexor digitorum superficialis tendons to the second and third digits within the carpal tunnel. There are five branches given off by the median nerve in the palm. The radial branch innervates the thenar muscles and the four sensory branches innervate the medial three digits and the lateral half of the index finger. Approximately 5 cm proximal to the wrist crease, the palmar cutaneous branch supplying the proximal portion of the palm leaves the median nerve. This superficial branch runs between the palmaris longus and the flexor carpi radialis tendon, superficial to the flexor retinaculum.

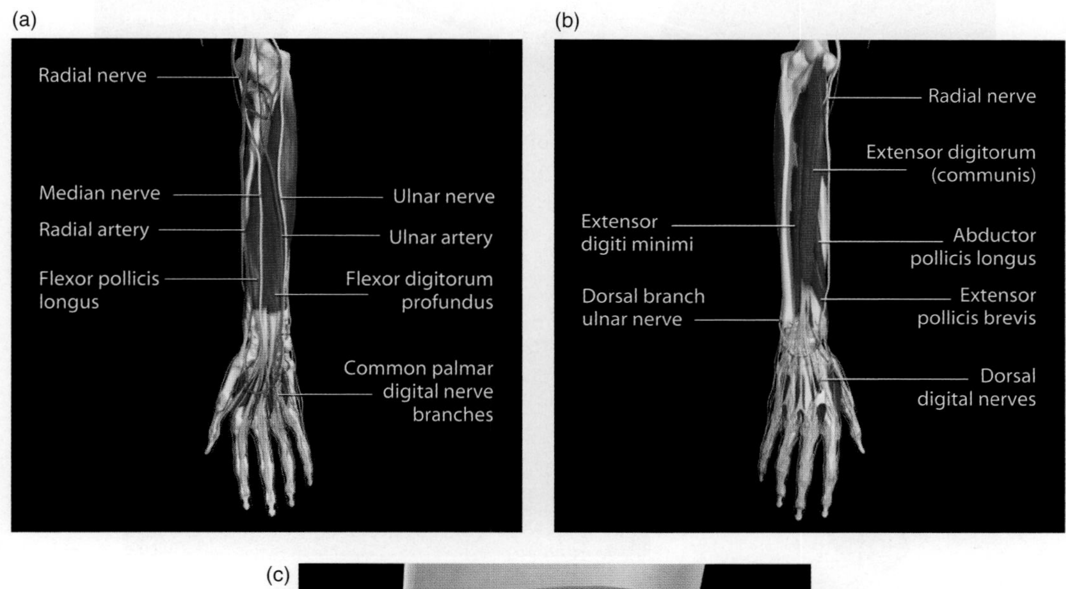

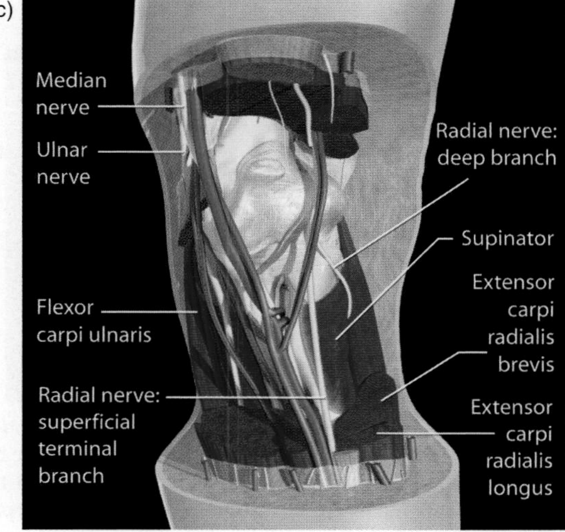

Figure 12.10. The major peripheral nerves of the forearm: **(a)** anterior, **(b)** posterior, **(c)** radial and median nerve of the anterior aspect of the elbow, and

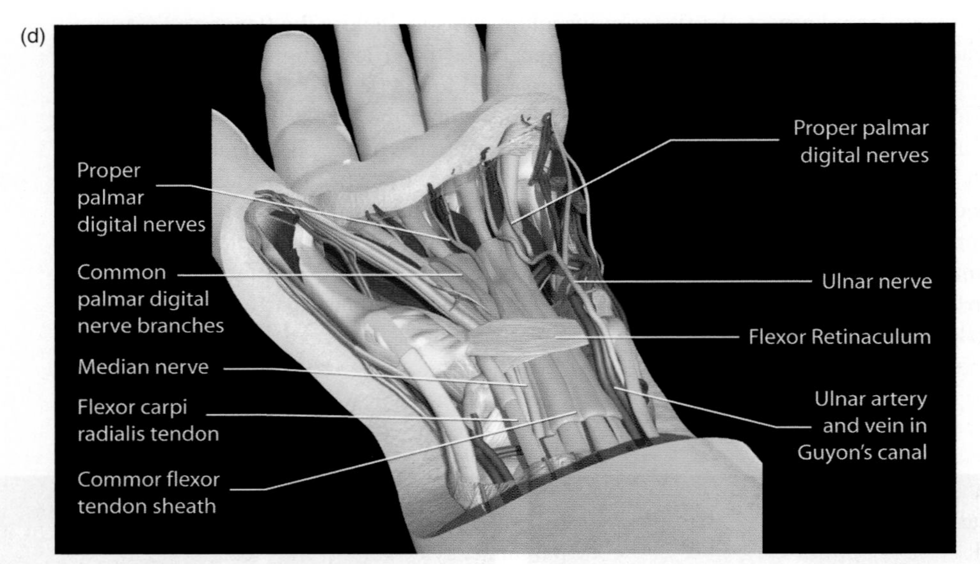

Figure 12.10. *(Continued)* The major peripheral nerves of the forearm: **(d)** the ulnar and median nerve on the volar aspect of the wrist.

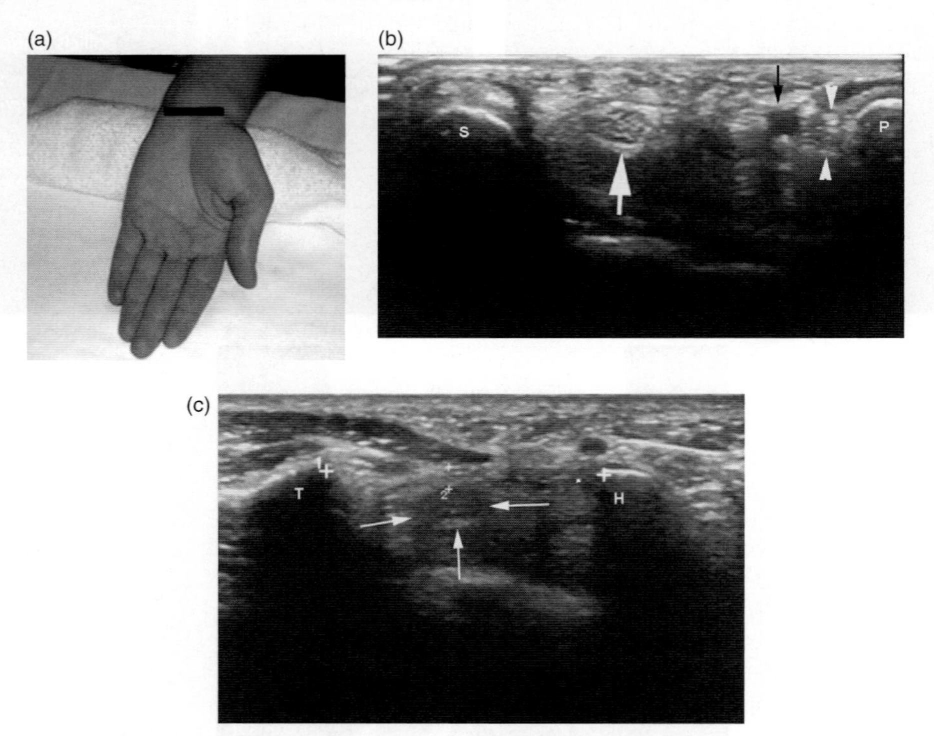

Figure 12.11. **(a)** The arm position and probe position (black band) for examination of the median nerve at the wrist. **(b)** A transverse ultrasound section in the carpal tunnel at the level of the scaphoid (S) and the pisiform (P) shows the median nerve (white arrow). The ulnar nerve (arrowheads) is seen at the level of Guyon's tunnel next to the ulnar artery (black arrow). **(c)** A transverse ultrasound section in the carpal tunnel at the level of the trapezium (T) and the hook of hamate (H) shows the median nerve (white arrows) and the method to measure the palmar bowing of the flexor retinaculum. Caliper 1 is the line connecting the hamate and the trapezium and Caliper 2 is the palmar bowing of the retinaculum.

Insider Information 12.5
The rounded appearance of the anterior pisiform is characteristic of the median nerve in the proximal carpal tunnel, and the hook of hamate is characteristic of the distal carpal tunnel.

Indications, Sonographic Anatomy, and Technique: In the region of the elbow, ultrasound is sometimes requested to exclude causes of the pronator syndrome such as a fibrous band of the bicipital aponeurosis or hypertrophied pronator teres muscle, the presence of an aberrant median artery, posttraumatic hematoma, or a soft tissue mass. Pronator syndrome is the most proximal entrapment neuropathy of the median nerve.

Entrapment neuropathy of the anterior interosseous nerve palsy is called Kiloh–Nevin syndrome. Ultrasound can be used to look for impingement on the nerve by fracture of the forearm bones or supracondylar fracture of the humerus, posttraumatic hematoma, soft tissue masses, or nerve swelling from any cause.

Median nerve compression at the wrist (carpal tunnel syndrome) is the most common peripheral nerve entrapment. This is the most commonly requested ultrasound examination of a peripheral nerve in routine clinical practice. The majority of cases of carpal tunnel syndrome are idiopathic. Secondary causes that can be identified with ultrasound include flexor tenosynovitis, ganglion, soft tissue mass, thrombosis of the median artery, and posttraumatic hematoma.

In the proximal forearm, identification of the median nerve on ultrasound can be slightly difficult due to the variability in the amount of surrounding connective tissue. However, it is easily identifiable at the wrist, from where it can be traced proximally. The patient is usually seated in a chair with the elbow flexed and the forearm extended (Figure 12.11a). The wrist is supported by a rolled towel placed dorsal to it. Transverse sonograms can be obtained proximal to the carpal tunnel at the level of the pronator quadratus muscle. The nerve can then be followed to the level of the proximal aspect of the carpal tunnel, and is identified by its fascicular appearance. The rounded appearance of the ventral aspect of the pisiform is characteristic of the median nerve in the proximal aspect of the carpal tunnel (Figure 12.11b). At this level, the flexor retinaculum appears as a thin echogenic band connecting the pisiform to the scaphoid. To avoid anisotropy, slight tilting of the transducer may be necessary to identify the nerve. The median nerve usually has an oval structure surrounded by the hyperechoic perineurium. At the distal aspect of the carpal tunnel, the palmar aspect of the hook of hamate serves as a bony landmark (Figure 12.11c). Once the nerve has been identified on transverse scanning, the probe can be turned to obtain longitudinal sonograms that demonstrate the characteristic appearance of the nerve as parallel hypoechoic bands separated by echogenic bands. In approximately 2–3% of normal subjects, the median nerve is bifid; this variation is usually seen at the proximal aspect of the carpal tunnel.[11,12] The normal value of the cross-sectional area of the median nerve in the region of the carpal tunnel is approximately 8–9 mm^2.[13]

To objectively measure the amount of palmar bowing of the flexor retinaculum, a straight line is drawn between the attachments of the flexor retinaculum to the trapezium tubercle and the hook of hamate. The distance between this line and the most palmar aspect of the flexor retinaculum is measured (Figure 12.11c). This is normally approximately 1.4 ± 0.5 mm.[14]

To objectively measure the amount of nerve flattening, the minor and major axes of the median nerve are measured on a transverse image at the level of the pisiform. The flattening ratio, which is the ratio of a nerve's major to minor axis, is normally approximately 2.07 ± 0.27.[14]

The anterior interosseous nerve can sometimes be demonstrated as a thin, hypoechoic, oval structure lying anterior to the interosseous membrane, deep to the median nerve, between the flexor digitorum profundus and the flexor pollicis longus muscle groups.

Ulnar Nerve

Regional Anatomy: The ulnar nerve leaves the elbow between the two heads of the flexor carpi ulnaris. In its course toward the wrist, it runs deep to the flexor carpi ulnaris, lying medial to the ulnar artery (Figure 12.10a and d). It innervates the flexor carpi ulnaris and the medial three parts of the flexor digitorum profundus muscle. In the distal forearm, it emerges from beneath the flexor carpi ulnaris tendon, which then lies on the medial and the ulnar artery at its lateral aspect.

The ulnar nerve runs superficial to the flexor retinaculum in the wrist and reaches the hand accompanied by the ulnar artery. At the wrist, the ulnar nerve passes through a fibroosseous tunnel called Guyon's canal. The tunnel extends from the palmar carpal ligament at the proximal aspect of the pisiform to the origin of the hypothenar muscles at the level of the hamulus. The floor of Guyon's canal is made of the pisiform, hamate, flexor retinaculum, and hypothenar muscle, and the roof is composed of the palmar carpal ligament, palmaris brevis muscle, and palmar fascia. The ulnar artery, veins, and ulnar nerve course through this space, which is surrounded by fat. The ulnar nerve enters Guyon's canal after giving off the dorsal cutaneous branch and divides into the superficial sensory and deep motor nerves within the canal. The deep motor branch innervates the palmaris brevis, hypothenar muscles, lateral lumbricals and interosseous muscles, adductor pollicis, and abductor digiti minimi muscles.

Insider Information 12.6

The accessory abductor digiti minimi lies in the superficial aspect of Guyon's canal as a hypoechoic structure, but does not have the fascicular appearance of the nerve. Doppler should be used to distinguish the artery from the ulnar nerve and ganglion in Guyon's canal.

Indications, Sonographic Anatomy, and Technique: Ultrasound can be requested to exclude causes of Guyon's canal syndrome such as ganglion, lipoma, trauma, and anatomic muscular variants, such as abductor digiti minimi coursing through this canal. Aneurysm and thrombosis of the ulnar artery due to repetitive trauma can result in hypothenar hammer syndrome.

The ulnar nerve is initially identified in the elbow and is then followed distally into the forearm. The patient lies in a sitting position with the forearm supinated. By transverse scanning, the nerve is identified behind the medial epicondyle and is followed distally deep to the flexor carpi ulnaris. More distally in the forearm, the nerve is identified between the ulnar artery and the flexor carpi ulnaris tendon.

The nerve is identified in Guyon's tunnel by transverse scanning (Figures 12.10d and 12.11). Images of the proximal aspect of Guyon's tunnel are obtained at the level of the pisiform, where the pulsatile nature of the ulnar artery can be demonstrated. Slight tilting of the transducer will enable clear demonstration of the ulnar nerve between the ulnar artery and the rounded ulnar aspect of the pisiform on the medial side. Scanning more distally in the transverse plane, the distal portion of Guyon's tunnel demonstrates the superficial branch of the ulnar artery and the superficial sensory branch of the ulnar nerve just overlying the hook of hamate. The abductor digiti minimi frequently has an accessory muscle inside Guyon's tunnel. This accessory muscle usually lies in the superficial aspect of the tunnel as a hypoechoic structure and does not have the fascicular appearance of the nerve. The normal anteroposterior diameter of the ulnar nerve in Guyon's canal is approximately 2.5 mm.[15] The mean transverse diameter of the nerve is approximately 3.7 mm.[15] The mean cross-sectional area of the nerve in Guyon's canal is 8.3–8.5 mm^2.[15] Doppler should be used to distinguish the artery from the nerve and any small ganglion in Guyon's tunnel.

Radial Nerve

Regional Anatomy: The radial nerve pierces the lateral intermuscular septum approximately 10 cm proximal to the lateral epicondyle of the humerus and enters the anterior aspect of the arm. Here it lies between the brachialis and the brachioradialis muscles. The nerve bifurcates into the superficial and deep branches just anterior to the level of the lateral epicondyle (Figures 12.3b and 12.10b and c).

The superficial branch of the radial nerve is a sensory nerve that runs distally along the medial aspect of the brachioradialis muscle, medial to the extensor carpi radialis longus/brevis muscles. The proximal aspect of the superficial branch runs anterior to the supinator muscle in the forearm. Distally, it runs in the dorsal subcutaneous region along with the distal part of the brachioradialis.

The deep branch of the radial nerve enters the radial tunnel. This tunnel is formed by a combination of muscles and aponeuroses. The radial tunnel is an anatomic space, approximately 5 cm long, extending from the capitellum to the distal aspect of the supinator muscle, through which the radial nerve courses. The tunnel is bounded posteriorly by the capitellum, anteromedially by the brachialis, and anterolaterally by the brachioradialis and extensor carpi radialis brevis muscles. The radial nerve divides into the superficial sensory branch and the deep motor branch, also called the posterior interosseous nerve, at a level between the lateral humeral epicondyle and superior aspect of the supinator muscle. The superficial branch passes superficial to the supinator muscle and continues to the radial aspect of the forearm, giving sensory supply to the posterolateral aspect of the hand. The posterior interosseous nerve passes in a plane between the superficial and deep heads of the supinator muscle. Here, the nerve can be compressed by the arcade of Frohse, which is a fibrous arch formed by the fibrous tissue between the brachialis and brachioradialis muscle anterior to the radial head. The posterior interosseous nerve travels deep along the extensor surface of the interosseous membrane, giving off the motor supply to the extensor muscles of the forearm.

(a)

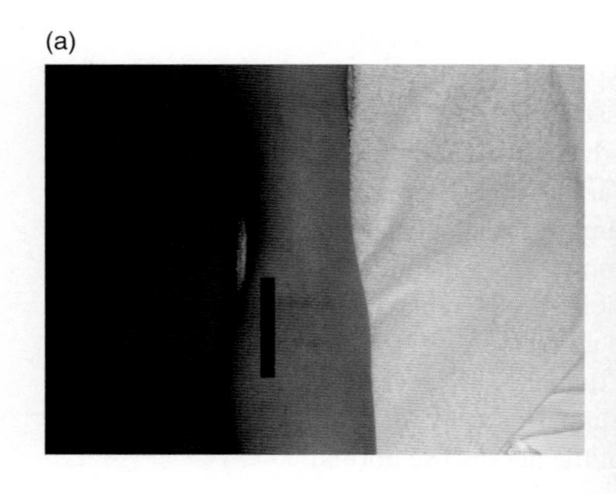

(b)

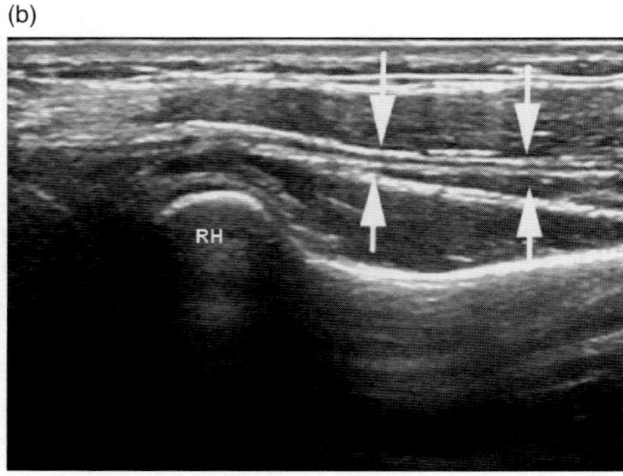

Figure 12.12. **(a)** The arm position and probe position (black band) for examination of the posterior interosseous nerve in the proximal forearm. **(b)** An ultrasound scan of the posterior interosseous nerve near the radial head (RH) between the supinator muscle shows parallel echogenic lines (arrows) in the longitudinal section.

Insider Information 12.7
It should be noted that in most asymptomatic people, the posterior interosseous nerve can show some change in diameter at the entry to the supinator muscle, which should not be mistaken as abnormal constriction.

Indications, Sonographic Anatomy, and Technique: Ultrasound can be requested to exclude nerve entrapment at the radial tunnel due to the ganglion, lipoma, vascular malformation, synovitis, bicipitoradial bursitis, posttraumatic hematoma, and radial head fractures or dislocation. Comparison with a contralateral asymptomatic side may be used to look for any abnormal fibrous bands and for swelling or flattening of the posterior interosseous nerve.

The radial nerve is best identified at the level of the midarm in the posterolateral aspect of the humerus by transverse scanning (Figure 12.8a). It is then followed distally to the level of the lateral epicondyle of the humerus. Following the radial nerve further distally by transverse scanning, the bifurcation of the radial nerve into the superficial and deep branches can be appreciated. For depiction of the posterior interosseous nerve, the elbow is positioned in semiflexion over the examination table with the forearm oriented transversely (Figure 12.12a). The posterior interosseous nerve can be depicted as hypoechoic fascicles embedded in the hyperechoic connective tissue plane between the superficial and deep portions of the supinator muscle (Figure 12.12b). It should be noted that in most asymptomatic people, the deep branch of the radial nerve shows some change in diameter at its entry into the supinator muscle.[2] The superficial branch of the radial nerve can be difficult to demonstrate with ultrasound due to its small diameter.

Anatomy of the Lower Limb Nerves

Nerves of the Groin

Sciatic Nerve

Regional Anatomy: The sciatic nerve is the largest peripheral nerve in the body. It has contributions from the L4 to S3 roots. The two main branches

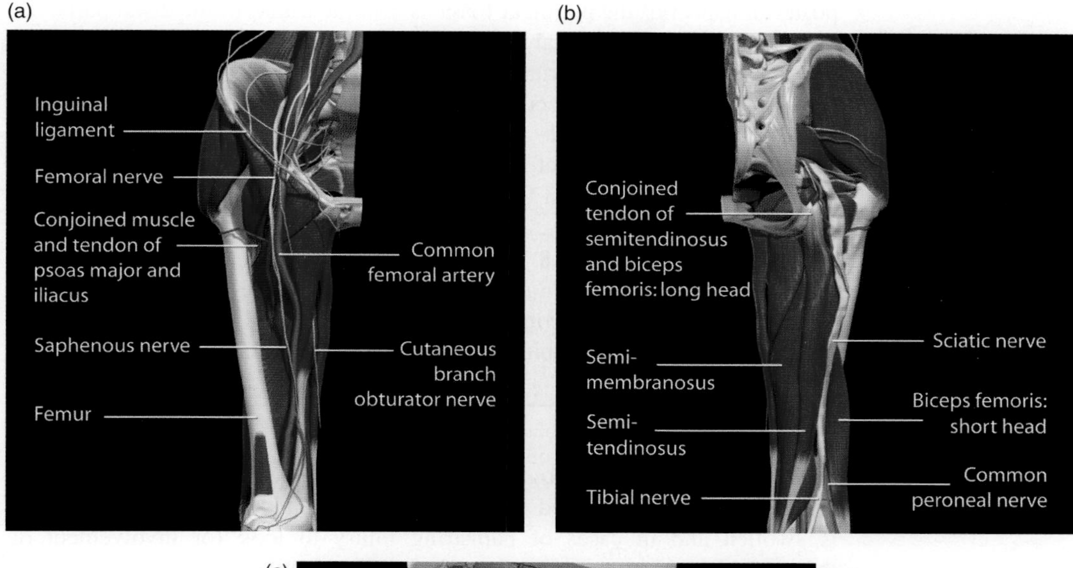

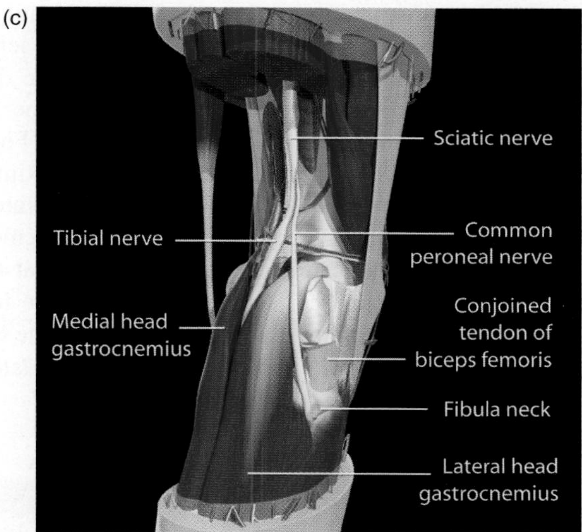

Figure 12.13. The exposed major peripheral nerves of the hip and thigh: **(a)** anterior, **(b)** posterior, and **(c)** popliteal fossa.

of the sciatic nerve are the common peroneal nerve and the tibial nerve (Figure 12.13b and c). In a majority of cases, the sciatic nerve passes along the ventral aspect of the piriformis, passing posteriorly along its inferior border, and exits the pelvis through the greater sciatic foramen along with the piriformis, accompanied by the superior and inferior gluteal neurovascular bundle. In some cases, a part of the sciatic nerve courses through the piriformis or above the muscle; in fewer cases, the entire sciatic nerve courses through the piriformis. After passing through the piriform fossa, the sciatic nerve lies between the greater trochanter and the ischial tuberosity. It passes deep to the gluteus maximus and takes a lateral course passing deep to the obturator internus and the gemelli muscles. After passing deep to the gluteal muscles, the sciatic nerve takes a more superficial course extending distally to the posterior aspect of the popliteal fossa as a single trunk. In the distal parts, the nerve divides into the tibial and common peroneal nerves; the level of this division shows a wide variation. At these levels, it lies between the biceps femoris on the lateral aspect and the semitendinosus and semimembranosus muscles on the medial side. The division of the sciatic nerve is sometimes seen as high as the level of the sacrosciatic foramen and sometimes as low as the level of the popliteal fossa.[16,17]

Insider Information 12.8
The division of the sciatic nerve can be as high as the level of the sacrosciatic foramen and sometimes as low as the level of the popliteal fossa. This should be borne in mind, particularly during ultrasound-guided nerve block procedures.

Indications, Sonographic Anatomy, and Technique: Sonography of the sciatic nerve is done in suspected piriformis syndrome to determine if the nerve is swollen and in cases of hamstring injury to look for involvement of the nerve by a hematoma or scar tissue. To identify the sciatic nerve, the patient is positioned prone (Figure 12.14a). The sciatic nerve can be seen in the gluteal region or the posterior aspect of the distal third of the thigh. It is best identified in the distal thigh between the biceps femoris and the semitendinosus/semimembranosus muscle groups (Figure 12.15b). The nerve is identified in axial imaging and can be traced proximally to the region of the buttock; it can also be traced distally to its division into the tibial and common peroneal nerves. Although the nerve can also be demonstrated at the level of the gluteal region by scanning in the axial plane at the level of the inferior gluteal fold, this technique is slightly difficult due to the increased bulk of the overlaying gluteal musculature at this point. The ischial tuberosity can be used as a bony landmark, and the nerve sits just lateral to it. Although the

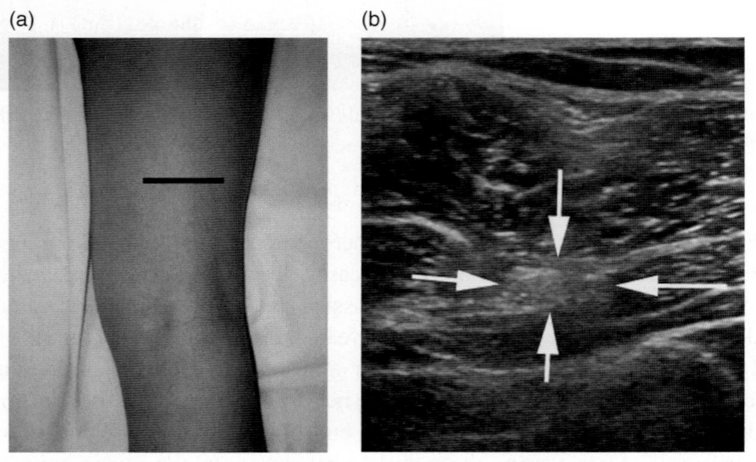

Figure 12.14. **(a)** The prone position and probe position (black band) for examination of the distal portion of the sciatic nerve in the thigh. **(b)** A transverse ultrasound section at the level of the distal thigh shows the sciatic nerve (arrows) between the medial and lateral hamstrings.

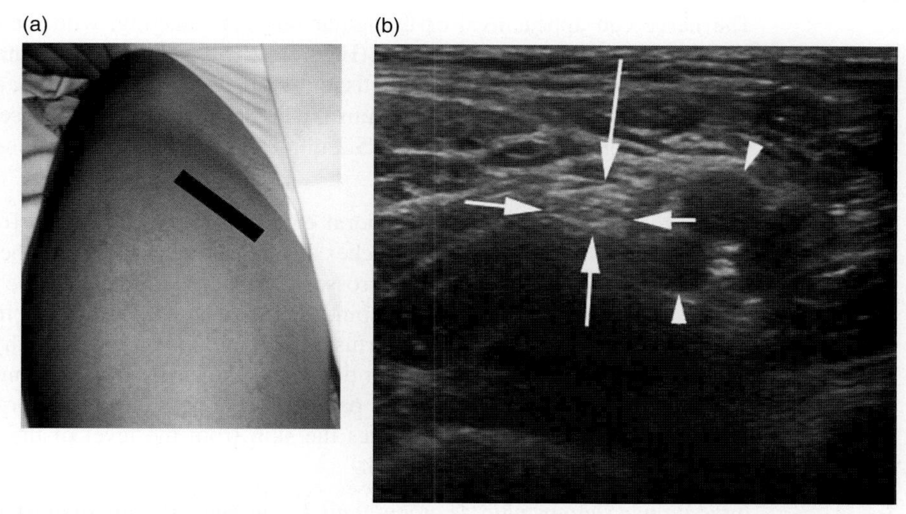

Figure 12.15. (**a**) The supine position and probe position (black band) in the groin for examination of the femoral nerve. (**b**) A transverse ultrasound section at the level of the groin shows the femoral nerve (arrows) lateral to the femoral vessels (arrowheads).

division of the sciatic nerve at the tibial and common peroneal nerve can be demonstrated consistently in all patients, the division is variable. This point should be considered when considering procedures such as ultrasound-guided nerve anesthetic block of the sciatic nerve.

Femoral Nerve

Regional Anatomy: The femoral nerve is a large peripheral nerve (Figure 12.13a). It is the largest branch of the lumbar plexus and has contributions from the L1 to L4 segments. It has motor supply to the quadriceps muscles and the sartorius. It supplies sensation to the skin of the anterior aspect of the thigh and from the medial aspect of the calf to the medial aspect of the ankle. The nerve follows the iliopsoas muscle toward the groin, lying between the iliac and psoas component of the iliopsoas. In the pelvis, the nerve is surrounded by loose areolar tissue. It leaves the region of the iliopsoas in the inguinal region at the medial aspect of the muscle; here the femoral artery lies medial to it (Figure 12.13a). The direction of the course of the femoral nerve in the thigh parallels that of the sartorius. The femoral nerve divides into the superficial sensory and deep motor branches. The saphenous nerve, which is the final branch of the femoral nerve, lies adjacent to the superficial femoral artery. It supplies the medial aspect of the knee and the lower leg, and runs quite close to the pes anserine tendons.

Indications, Sonographic Anatomy, and Technique: Ultrasound can be used to guide local anesthetic injections for femoral nerve blocks. It is also important to recognize the anatomical location of the nerve when performing ultrasound-guided femoral arterial or venous punctures. The femoral nerve is easily demonstrated on ultrasound. For sonographic demonstration of the femoral nerve, the patient is positioned supine. It is easily identified in the groin adjacent to the femoral vascular bundle by scanning in the axial plane (Figure 12.15a). Doppler can be used to identify the artery, and the nerve is seen just lateral to it. The iliopsoas lies lateral to the nerve in the groin.

The nerve can appear oval or triangular on axial imaging, with the typical reticulated hypoechoic dot pattern (Figure 12.15b). The normal anteroposterior diameter of the femoral nerve is approximately 3.1 ± 0.08 mm, and the mediolateral diameter is 9.8 ± 2.1 mm.[18] The normal average cross-sectional area of the femoral nerve is 21.7 ± 5.2 mm.[18]

Lateral Femoral Cutaneous Nerve

Regional Anatomy: The lateral femoral cutaneous nerve is formed from the lumbar plexus from the ventral branches of L2–L3. It emerges from the lateral border of the psoas major muscle, crosses the iliacus, and reaches the medial border of the anterosuperior iliac spine. It then passes deep to the inguinal ligament and superficial to the sartorius muscle into the proximal thigh, where it produces the anterior and posterior branches. The anterior branch innervates the skin of the anterior and lateral parts of the thigh. The posterior branch pierces the fascia lata and innervates the skin from the level of the greater trochanter to the middle of the thigh.

Indications, Sonographic Anatomy, and Technique: Meralgia paresthetica is a mononeuropathy of the lateral femoral cutaneous nerve characterized by pain, numbness, and tingling in the anterolateral aspect of the thigh. It can be idiopathic or secondary to trauma or surgical procedures that could injure the nerve. Injury to this nerve can be a complication during harvesting of bone grafts from the iliac bone.[19] Ultrasound is sometimes requested to exclude a significant swelling, hematoma, or neuroma in the nerve. An ultrasound-guided local anesthetic nerve block can result in temporary relief of symptoms. The normal nerve is difficult to visualize on ultrasound due to its relatively small size. It can be identified in some patients, in the supine position, where it enters the subcutaneous tissue between the sartorius and the tensor fascia lata muscle.

Nerves around the Knee

Common Peroneal Nerve

Regional Anatomy

The common peroneal nerve is the terminal branch of the sciatic nerve (Figure 12.13c). The division of the sciatic nerve to the tibial and common peroneal nerves can occur at a variable level in the distal thigh. From its division from the sciatic nerve in the distal aspect of the thigh, the common peroneal nerve courses anterolaterally along the biceps femoris tendon to the proximal fibula. In its course approaching the proximal fibula, the common peroneal nerve is located medial and slightly anterior to the biceps femoris tendon. It winds around the posterior and posterolateral aspect of the fibular neck (peroneal tunnel) and enters the musculature around the fibular aspect of the leg. At this point, the nerve divides into the deep and superficial peroneal nerves.

Indications, Sonographic Anatomy, and Technique

The common peroneal nerve is most often entrapped or compressed at the point at which it winds around the posterolateral aspect of the fibular neck, also called the peroneal tunnel. Nerve compression here causes pain along the dermatomal distribution of the common peroneal nerve, which can be mistaken for stress fractures, shin splits, or compartment syndrome. Fracture and hemorrhage around the proximal fibula, tight plaster casts around the knee, nerve sheath ganglion, ganglion arising from the proximal tibiofibular joint, and parameniscal cysts can also cause compression of the common peroneal nerve. The usual indication for sonographic examination of the common peroneal nerve is to demonstrate a local cause for foot drop. The examination of the common peroneal nerve is best performed with the patient in a prone position. Transverse scanning is performed at the level of the fibular neck, which can be palpated at the posterolateral aspect of the calf (Figure 12.16a). The slightly rounded landmark of the posterior cortex of the fibular neck is identified, and the nerve is identified lateral to it (Figure 12.16b). In the longitudinal section, the nerve can be identified medial and parallel to the course of the biceps femoris tendon, by having one end of the probe on the fibular head. The common peroneal nerve can also be visualized in the popliteal fossa by following the sciatic nerve to its division, and then following the course of the nerve to the region of the fibular neck. This division can be appreciated in transverse scanning between the biceps femoris on the lateral aspect and the semitendinosus/semimembranosus muscles on the medial aspect. The normal anteroposterior dimension of the common peroneal nerve is between 2.9 and 3.1 mm.[15] The mean transverse diameter of the nerve in men is 6.9–7.3 mm.[15] The mean cross-sectional area of the nerve is between 15.7 and 16.1 mm^2.[15]

Tibial Nerve

Regional Anatomy

The tibial nerve is a continuation of the sciatic nerve that is composed of the nerve fibers from the anterior branches of the sacral plexus. In the

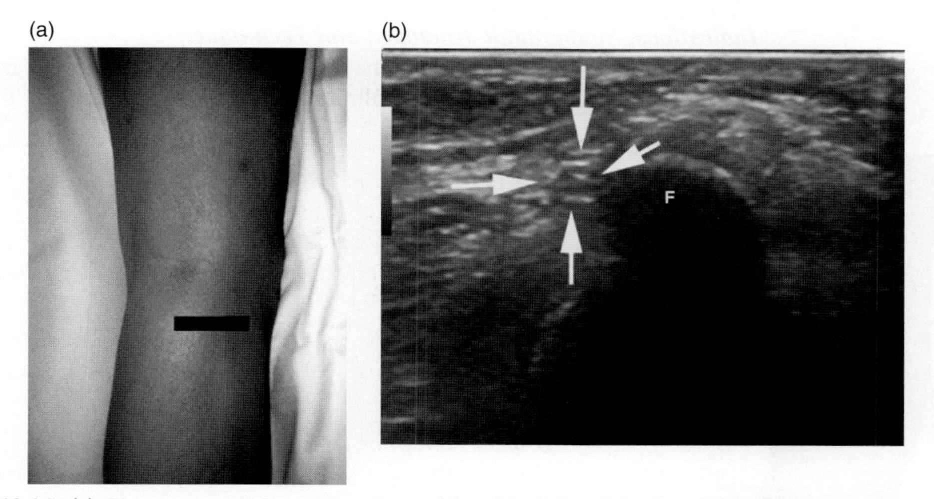

Figure 12.16. (**a**) The prone position and probe position (black band) in the posterolateral calf at the level of the neck of the fibula for examination of the common peroneal nerve. (**b**) A transverse ultrasound section at the level of the neck of the fibula (F) shows the common peroneal nerve (arrows).

popliteal fossa, the nerve lies superficially, lateral to the popliteal vessels (Figure 12.13c). It then crosses the vessels to their medial aspects and courses distally into the leg between and deep to the two heads of the gastrocnemius and the plantaris muscles. It passes over the popliteus muscle and deep to the tendinous arch of the soleus muscle on the medial aspect of the posterior tibial vessels. The tibial nerve enters the interface between the gastrocnemius and soleus muscles posteriorly, and enters the cranial aspect of the tibialis posterior. It supplies the muscles in the posterior aspect of the calf and sensory cutaneous supply to the posterior calf. The main cutaneous branch of the tibial nerve is the sural nerve, which accompanies the short saphenous vein to the lateral aspect of the ankle.

Indications, Sonographic Anatomy, and Technique

Entrapment or compression of the tibial nerve at the level of the popliteal fossa is not frequently encountered in routine clinical practice. It can involve tumors or be compressed by posttraumatic hematoma and large Baker's cysts. The patient is positioned prone for examination of the origin and proximal aspect of the tibial nerve (Figure 12.17). The sciatic nerve is identified between the biceps femoris and the semitendinosus/semimembranosus muscles. The sciatic nerve continues distally as the tibial nerve after it gives off the common peroneal nerve. In the region of the midcalf, the tibial nerve can be slightly difficult to visualize between the superficial and deep flexors of the foot.

Pudendal Nerve

Regional Anatomy

The pudendal nerve has contributions from the third and fourth sacral roots. The nerve is formed in the sacral plexus in the retroperitoneal space of the pelvis; it leaves the pelvis, along with the sciatic nerve, through the greater sciatic foramen to reach the deep gluteal compartment. It then winds around the sacrospinous ligament to reach the medial border of the ischial tuberosity and under the levator ani muscle in the fibroosseous tunnel called the pudendal canal or the canal of Alcock.

Indications, Sonographic Anatomy, and Technique

One application of ultrasound in the examination of the pudendal nerve is as guidance for local anesthetic infiltration of the pudendal nerve.[20] It is not

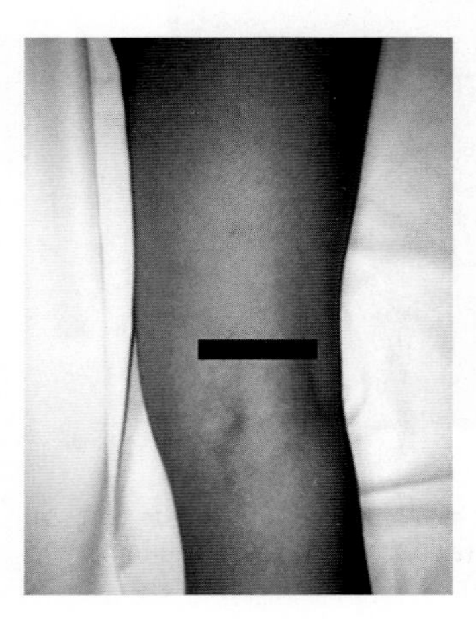

Figure 12.17. The prone position and probe position (black band) for examination of the proximal portion of the tibial nerve in the thigh.

always possible to visualize the normal nerve under ultrasound; however, in about half the cases, the nerve can be seen in the deep aspect of the gluteal compartment. For ultrasound guidance for pudendal nerve block, the patient is positioned prone. In transverse scanning, the sacrospinous ligament, pudendal artery, and accompanying nerve can be seen with ultrasound. Ultrasound can then be used to guide a needle medial to the artery for pudendal nerve block.

Nerves of the Calf and Ankle

Saphenous Nerve

Regional Anatomy

The saphenous nerve is a sensory nerve. It runs in the subcutaneous plane of the medial aspect of the ankle alongside the great saphenous vein. It is difficult to visualize the normal nerve on ultrasound given its relatively small size.[2]

Branches of the Common Peroneal Nerve

Regional Anatomy

As the common peroneal nerve winds around the posterolateral aspect of the neck of the fibula, it gives its terminal branches (Figure 12.18). These include the superficial and deep peroneal nerves. The deep peroneal nerve is positioned more posteriorly and enters the interface between the peroneus longus and peroneous brevis muscles along with the anterior tibial artery and veins. It supplies the peroneus longus/brevis muscles and the skin on the lateral aspect of the proximal calf.

The superficial peroneal nerve is located more anteriorly and enters the space between the peroneous brevis and the adjacent shaft of the fibula. It runs distally on the anterior aspect of the calf between the peroneal musculature and the extensor digitorum longus tendon. It then crosses the extensor muscles in the anterior compartment, coming to lie in the subcutaneous plane.

Sonographic Anatomy and Technique

It is difficult to visualize the normal superficial peroneal nerve on ultrasound.[2] The normal deep peroneal nerve can sometimes be visualized between the peroneous longus and brevis muscles in the prone position.

Tibial Nerve

Regional Anatomy

The tibial nerve, also called the posterior tibial nerve, runs in the calf between the two heads of the gastrocnemius muscles (Figures 12.17 and 12.18). It perforates the proximal aspect of the soleus muscle to enter the space between the deep and superficial muscles to the foot. It supplies branches to the soleus and gastrocnemius muscles and has sensory supply to the posterior calf. One of these branches, the sural nerve, runs distally along with the short saphenous venous vein to the posterolateral aspect of the ankle. The tibial nerve trifurcates into terminal branches of the medial calcaneal nerve, medial plantar nerve, and lateral plantar nerve (Figure 12.18c). The first branch is the medial calcaneal nerve, which demonstrates numerous anatomic variations.

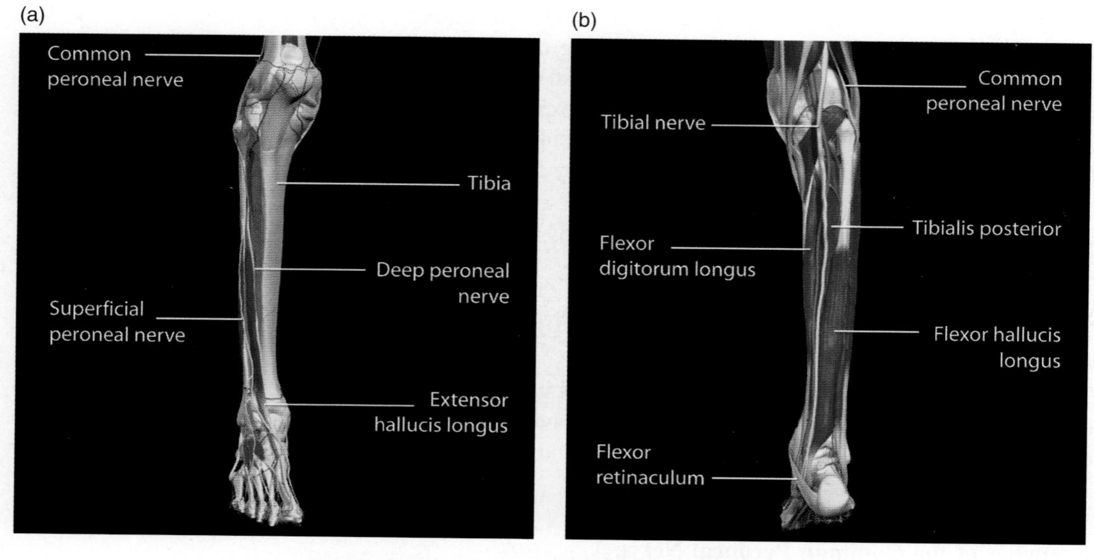

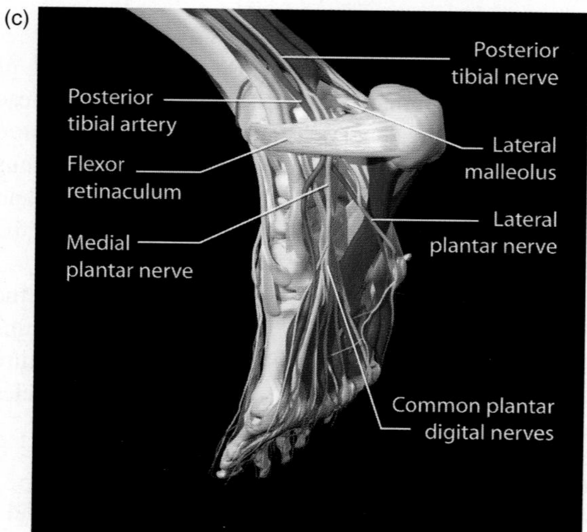

Figure 12.18. The major peripheral nerves of the leg: **(a)** anterior, **(b)** posterior, and **(c)** the posterior tibial nerve at the ankle.

The medial calcaneal branch originates proximal to the tarsal tunnel in 35–45% of cases, within the tunnel in 34% of cases, from the lateral plantar nerve in 16% of cases, and from multiple branches in 21% of cases.[21] The medial calcaneal branch provides sensory supply to the medial aspect of the heel and portion of the calcaneus. The tibial nerve continues through the tarsal tunnel and then divides into the medial and the lateral plantar nerves.

Indications, Sonographic Anatomy, and Technique

The tibial nerve is usually examined by ultrasound in cases of suspected tarsal tunnel syndrome, wherein a cause such as a ganglion compressing the nerve needs to be excluded. In tarsal tunnel syndrome, there is pain or other sensory disturbances from compression of the tibial nerve and its branches

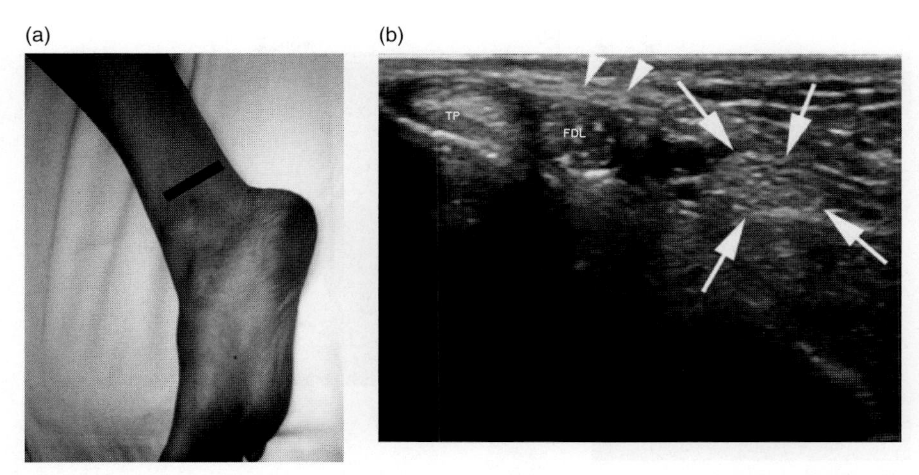

Figure 12.19. **(a)** The patient position and probe position (black band) in the posteromedial ankle for examination of the tibial nerve in the tarsal tunnel. **(b)** A transverse ultrasound section at the level of the tarsal tunnel shows the tibial nerve (arrows). The tibialis posterior (TP) tendon, flexor digitorum longus (FDL) tendon, and posterior tibial vessels are seen deep to the flexor retinaculum (arrowheads).

as they pass through the tarsal tunnel. The distribution of symptoms depends on whether the tibial nerve itself or one of the branches is compressed. The patient is positioned supine with the knee semiflexed and slightly externally rotated, with a pillow supporting the lateral aspect of the knee so that the medial aspect of the ankle is facing upward (Figure 12.19a). The patient can also be lying on the side to be examined so that the medial aspect of the ankle is facing upward. The nerve is identified in the tarsal tunnel, deep to the flexor retinaculum, by transverse scanning adjacent to the posterior tibial artery and vein (Figure 12.19b).

Nerves of the Foot

Branches of the Tibial Nerve

Regional Anatomy

Most of the motor and sensory supply is derived from the branches of the tibial nerve, mainly the medial and lateral plantar nerves (Figure 12.18c). The medial plantar nerve originates in the cutaneous branches innervating the medial two-thirds of the plantar aspect of the foot. The medial plantar nerve runs distally on the medial aspect along the flexor digitorum longus tendon. The lateral plantar nerve originates in the cutaneous branches innervating the lateral third of the plantar aspect of the foot. The tibial nerve essentially continues as the lateral plantar nerve. Trifurcation of the posterior tibial nerve occurs within the tarsal tunnel in 95% of cases, but in a very small percentage, it happens proximal to the tarsal tunnel.[22]

> **Insider Information 12.9**
> An intermetatarsal bursa of up to 3 mm in diameter is a normal finding (intermetatarsal bursa) that should not be mistaken for a Morton's neuroma or other pathology.

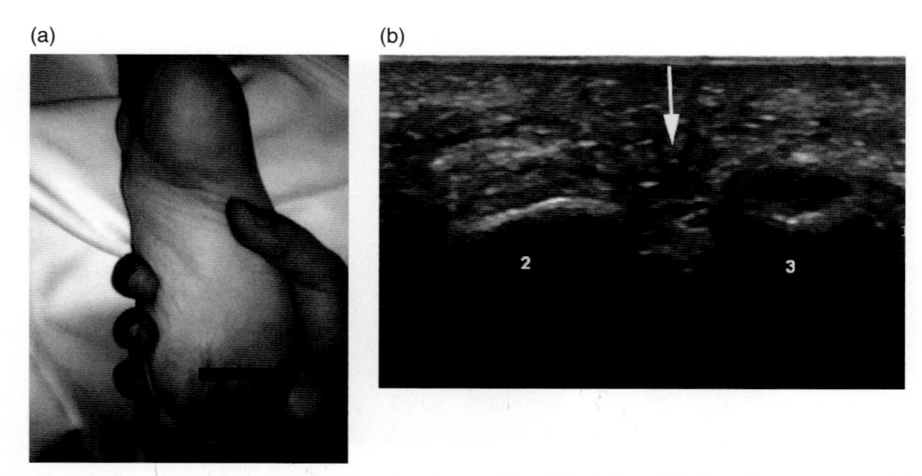

Figure 12.20. (**a**) The prone patient position and probe position (black band) in the plantar aspect of the foot for examination for the presence of Morton's neuroma. (**b**) Transverse ultrasound section at the level of the second (2) and third (3) metatarsal heads shows the position (arrow) where a Morton's neuroma would be expected to be seen (if present) with a metatarsal squeeze.

Indications, Sonographic Anatomy, and Technique

One indication for scanning the digital nerves is to look for entrapment near the transverse carpal ligament at the metatarsal head level. This gives rise to a nodular enlargement called a Morton's neuroma. Visualization of the normal medial and lateral plantar nerves of the foot is difficult due to its relatively small size.

To evaluate for Morton's neuroma, the patient is positioned prone; scanning is done from the plantar aspect of the foot (Figure 12.20a). Pressure is applied on the dorsal aspect of the foot with a finger or a gentle squeeze is applied to the metatarsal heads. This helps in viewing the intermetatarsal space by splaying the metatarsals (Figure 12.20b). The normal intermetatarsal space is echogenic due to the presence of fat and connective tissue. It should be noted that a small amount of fluid, up to 3 mm in diameter, is a normal finding (intermetatarsal bursa) that should not be mistaken for a neuroma or other pathology.[23]

References

1. Peer S. General considerations and technical concepts. In: Peer S, Bodner G (eds.). High Resolution Sonography of the Peripheral Nervous System, 1st ed., pp. 1–12. New York: Springer, 2003.
2. Gruber H, Kovacs P. Sonographic anatomy of the peripheral nervous system. In: Peer S, Bodner G (eds.). High Resolution Sonography of the Peripheral Nervous System, 1st ed., pp. 13–36. New York: Springer, 2003.
3. Chiou HJ, Chou YH, Chiou SY et al. Peripheral nerve lesions: Role of high-resolution US. Radiographics 2003;23(6):e15.
4. Martinoli C, Bianchi S, Pugliese F et al. Sonography of entrapment neuropathies in the upper limb (wrist excluded). J Clin Ultrasound 2004;32:438–450.
5. Schafhalter-Zoppoth I, Gray AT. The musculocutaneous nerve: Ultrasound appearance for peripheral nerve block. Reg Anesth Pain Med 2005;30:385–390.
6. Lordan J, Rauh P, Spinner RJ. The clinical anatomy of the supracondylar spur and the ligament of Struthers. Clin Anat 2005;18:548–551.

7. Bodner G, Buchberger W, Schocke M et al. Radial nerve palsy associated with humeral shaft fracture: Evaluation with US—-initial experience. Radiology 2001;219:811–816.
8. O'Driscoll SW, Horii E, Carmichael SW et al. The cubital tunnel and ulnar neuropathy. J Bone Joint Surg Br 1991;73:613–617.
9. Okamoto M, Abe M, Shirai H et al. Morphology and dynamics of the ulnar nerve in the cubital tunnel. Observation by ultrasonography. J Hand Surg [Br] 2000;25:85–89.
10. Okamoto M, Abe M, Shirai H et al. Diagnostic ultrasonography of the ulnar nerve in cubital tunnel syndrome. J Hand Surg [Br] 2000;25:499–502.
11. Iannicelli E, Chianta GA, Salvini V et al. Evaluation of bifid median nerve with sonography and MR imaging. J Ultrasound Med 2000;19:481–485.
12. Propeck T, Quinn TJ, Jacobson JA et al. Sonography and MR imaging of bifid median nerve with anatomic and histologic correlation. AJR 2000;175:1721–1725.
13. Keles I, Karagulle Kendi AT et al. Diagnostic precision of ultrasonography in patients with carpal tunnel syndrome. Am J Phys Med Rehabil 2005;84:443–450.
14. Altinok T, Baysal O, Karakas HM et al. Ultrasonographic assessment of mild and moderate idiopathic carpal tunnel syndrome. Clin Radiol 2004;59:916–925.
15. Peeters EY, Nieboer KH, Osteaux MM. Sonography of the normal ulnar nerve at Guyon's canal and of the common peroneal nerve dorsal to the fibular head. J Clin Ultrasound 2004;32:375–380.
16. Schwemmer U, Markus CK, Greim CA et al. Sonographic imaging of the sciatic nerve division in the popliteal fossa. Ultraschall Med 2005;26:496–500.
17. Schwemmer U, Markus CK, Greim CA et al. Sonographic imaging of the sciatic nerve and its division in the popliteal fossa in children. Paediatr Anaesth 2004;14:1005–1008.
18. Gruber H, Peer S, Kovacs P et al. The ultrasonographic appearance of the femoral nerve and cases of iatrogenic impairment. J Ultrasound Med 2003;22:163–172.
19. Mischkowski RA, Selbach I, Neugebauer J et al. Lateral femoral cutaneous nerve and iliac crest bone grafts—-anatomical and clinical considerations. Int J Oral Maxillofac Surg 2006;35:366–372.
20. Kovacs P, Gruber H, Piegger J et al. New, simple, ultrasound-guided infiltration of the pudendal nerve: Ultrasonographic technique. Dis Colon Rectum 2001;44:1381–1385.
21. Havel PE, Ebraheim NA, Clark SE et al. Tibial nerve branching in the tarsal tunnel. Foot Ankle 1998;9:117–119.
22. Lau JT, Daniels TR. Tarsal tunnel syndrome: A review of the literature. Foot Ankle Int 1999;20:201–209.
23. Zanetti M, Strehle JK, Zollinger H et al. Morton neuroma and fluid in the intermetatarsal bursae on MR images of 70 asymptomatic volunteers. Radiology 1997;203:516–520.

[illegible]

13

The Brachial Plexus

John O'Neill and Julian Dobranowski

The brachial plexus is one of the more challenging anatomical components of the peripheral nervous system to master, even before one picks up a transducer. The significant variation in the formation and arrangement of the plexus makes detailed anatomical knowledge essential to a complete ultrasound study. Ultrasound with its dynamic multiplanar high resolution capabilities allows the examiner to transform the acquired two-dimensional (2-D) anatomy into a more comprehensible three-dimensional (3-D) image.

Anesthesiologists have for many years successfully used ultrasound in the localization of the brachial plexus. Its use in this application dates back to 1978 when Doppler was used to assess the vasculature in supraclavicular nerve blocks.[1] It is only in recent years that radiology has begun to use ultrasound primarily for anatomical detail, achieving excellent resolution. Ultrasound has expanded its role to the assessment of plexopathies and may in the future be considered a primary imaging modality for this region.[2]

Clinical Indications

Ultrasound of the brachial plexus is commonly used in the localization of, and recently the real-time guidance of, the brachial plexus block in upper limb surgeries. Success is dependent upon correct placement of the anesthetic around the correct nerve.[3] There has been increasing interest in the radiological literature in the evaluation of brachial plexopathies by ultrasound.[2,4–9] Ultrasound offers high resolution, is dynamic, multiplanar, readily accessible, and well tolerated by patients. It clearly depicts the extraforaminal neural anatomy and the surrounding vascular structures. Ultrasound has been shown to be useful in assessing underlying etiologies, including posttraumatic pathology, primary and secondary tumors, and postradiation fibrosis.[2,10] It is also useful in guiding soft tissue biopsies. More studies are required to assess the diagnostic accuracy of ultrasound in brachial plexopathies. Magnetic resonance imaging (MRI) remains the gold standard for imaging

Technical Review

High-frequency linear array transducers of 12 to 15 MHz offer the best resolution. In patients of a larger habitus and in the infraclavicular region, transducers of 12 to 5 MHz may be required. Color or power Doppler will allow differentiation from the adjacent vasculature.

Anatomy

A plexus is a network of interlacing nerves. The brachial plexus allows multiple spinal segments to unite in a structured and efficient manner to supply the motor and sensory innervation to the upper limb. Each upper limb has its own plexus extending from the posterior triangle of the neck to the axilla, dividing into its main terminal branches at the level of the coracoid process. This somatic network of intersecting nerves supplies the innervation to the upper limb, excluding the levator scapula and trapezius muscles and the cutaneous innervation to the axilla, dorsal scapular region, and superior aspect of the shoulder (Table 13.1).[10]

Table 13.1. The Brachial Plexus and Major Branches.

Level	Origin	Anatomical location	Branches
Roots (5)	Anterior rami C5–T1 (prefixed C4–T1, postfixed C5–T2)	Lateral to neural foramina to interscalene level	Muscular branches—longus cervicis (C5–C6), scaleni (C5–C8), rhomboids (C5), serratus anterior via the long thoracic nerve (C5–C7) Communicating branch to phrenic nerve (C5)
Trunks (3)	Upper—C5–C6 roots Middle—C7 root Lower—C8–T1 roots	Interscalene to supraclavicular level	Subclavius (C5–C6) Suprascapular (C5–C6)
Divisions (6)	Formed from the anterior and posterior divisions of the three trunks	Posterior to clavicle	
Cords (3)	Lateral cord—anterior divisions upper and middle trunks	Infraclavicular and axillary levels	Lateral cord—musculocutaneous N (C5–C7), lateral root to median N (C6–C7), lateral pectoral N (C5–C7)
	Medial cord—anterior division lower trunk		Medial cord—ulnar N, medial root median N, medial pectoral N, medial cutaneous nerves arm and forearm (C8–T1)
	Posterior cord—all three posterior divisions		Posterior cord —radial nerve (C5–T1), axillary nerve (C5–C6), upper and lower subscapular N (C5–C6), thoracodorsal N (C6–C8)

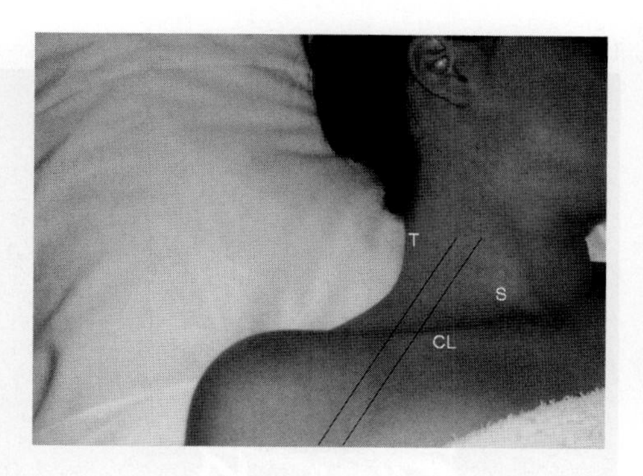

Figure 13.1. Surface anatomy of the brachial plexus, delineated by linear lines, within the posterior triangle of the neck. T, trapezius muscle; S, sternocleidomastoid muscle; CL, clavicle.

Surface Anatomy

The posterior triangle of the neck is defined by the posterior border of the sternocleidomastoid muscle anteriorly, the superior border of the clavicle inferiorly, and the anterior border of the trapezius posteriorly (Figure 13.1). The trunks of the plexus can be felt superficially, lateral to the lateral margin of the scalenus anterior. Within the supraclavicular region, the brachial plexus is deep to a line joining the midpoint of the sternocleidomastoid muscle and the midpoint of the clavicle.[4]

As the plexus descends under the clavicle, it passes just lateral to a midpoint between the center of the infraclavicular line between the jugular fossa and the anterior margin of the acromion.[11] The pulsating subclavian artery may be felt as it passes over the first rib in the inferior aspect of the supraclavicular fossa. The trunks of the brachial plexus may be felt as long bands running above and behind the artery. In the proximal infraclavicular region, the plexus is deep to the midpoint of the clavicle and distal within the axillary region. When the arm is abducted 90°, the plexus lays adjacent to the axillary artery, which can be felt high in the axilla.

Brachial Plexus

The plexus is divided anatomically into roots, trunks, divisions, and cords; the latter divides into branches—mainly the axillary, radial, median, and ulnar nerves (Figure 13.2). The plexus is derived from the ventral rami of the lower four cervical nerves, C5–C8, and the first thoracic nerve, T1. These ventral rami are of equal size, allowing for some variations outlined below, and are larger than their posterior counterparts and the preceding upper cervical roots.

> **Insider Information 13.1**
> The brachial plexus is anatomically divided into four components: roots, trunks, divisions, and cords.

There are many variations in the contributions to the plexus by C4 and T2, but the commonest are the prefixed and postfixed types. In the prefixed type, the C4 branch is prominent and the T2 contribution is frequently absent, with the T1 branch smaller than normal. The postfixed variation is the opposite

(a)

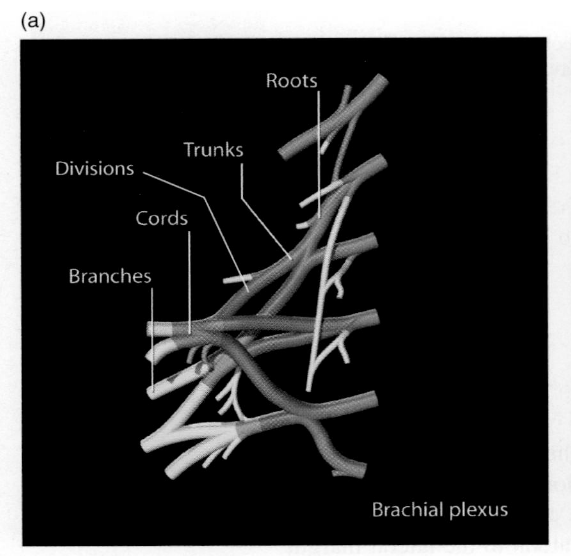

(b)

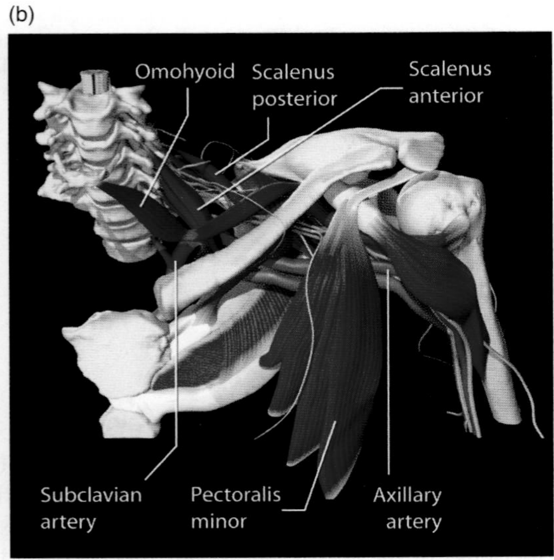

Figure 13.2. The brachial plexus: **(a)** overview of different components and **(b)** with related bony structures.

with the T2 branch always present, larger than a normal T1, with an absent or minimal contribution from C4 and a smaller than normal C5.[10] The plexus is symmetrical in approximately 60% of patients.

> **Insider Information 13.2**
> There are many anatomical variations to the plexus, the commonest being the prefixed and postfixed types. The prefixed type is commoner in the presence of a well-developed cervical rib. The brachial plexus is symmetrical in only 60% of patients.

The ventral rami form the roots of the brachial plexus, which in turn unite to form the trunks. This is also subject to variation. The commonest formation will be presented, with the upper trunk originating from the union of C5 and C6, the middle trunk from C7, and the lower trunk from C8 and T1. Each trunk then divides into anterior and posterior divisions. The anterior and posterior divisions essentially supply the flexor and extensor musculature of the upper limb, respectively.

The cords are formed by the union of the divisions and are named according to their relationship with the axillary artery; for example, the lateral cord lies lateral to the axillary artery. The lateral cord originates from the union of the anterior divisions of the upper and middle trunks, the medial cord from the anterior division of the lower trunk, and the posterior cord from the posterior divisions of all three trunks The posterior division of the lower trunk is significantly smaller and is composed primarily from the C8 root and frequently arises prior to formation of the lower trunk. The lateral and medial cords are also known as the outer and inner cords, respectively. Occasionally, only two cords will be formed.

Insider Information 13.3
The anterior and posterior divisions essentially supply the flexor and extensor musculature of the upper limb, respectively.

A neurovascular sheath composed of the prevertebral fascia and the fascia of the anterior and middle scaleni proximally, to the fascia of the brachialis and biceps distally, contains the brachial plexus and adjacent subclavian and axillary artery.

Branches

The branches of the brachial plexus are divided into two groups: supraclavicular (roots and trunks) and infraclavicular (cords) as detailed in Table 13.1. The major terminal branches arise from the cords in the following manner: the radial and axillary nerves from the posterior cord, the ulnar nerve from the medial cord, the median nerve from branches of the medial and lateral cord, and the musculotaneous nerve from the lateral cord. The anatomy and assessment of peripheral nerves are reviewed in Chapter 12.

Insider Information 13.4
The brachial plexus can be evaluated at five different levels: root, interscalene, supraclavicular, infraclavicular, and axillary.

Relations

The brachial plexus can be divided into five levels: root, interscalene, supraclavicular, infraclavicular, and axillary.

Root Level

There are eight cervical nerves and seven vertebrae; the C8 root exits at the C7/T1 neural foramen. The cervical spinal nerves of the brachial plexus exit obliquely downward and outward from the intervertebral foramina and enter the posterior triangle of the neck (Figure 13.3). They divide into an anterior and posterior ramus. The posterior ramus curves posteriorly around the superior articular process. The anterior ramus, which forms the root of the brachial plexus, lies upon a groove between the anterior and posterior tubercles of the transverse process.

The typical cervical vertebrae, C3–C6, have two transverse processes, one on either side, which are short and directed obliquely anterolaterally and are bifid at their tip (Figure 13.4).[10] The transverse processes are formed by two roots, anterior and posterior, and should not be confused with the neural ramus, ending in the anterior tubercle and the posterior tubercle. C7 is an exception with a large posterior tubercle and a vestigial anterior root (Figure 13.4). This anatomical variation allows for the identification of the C7 spinal nerve anterior ramus, which in turn allows for correct level identification of the remaining anterior rami.[8] The transverse process of T1 articulates with the head of the first rib and is directed posteriorly.

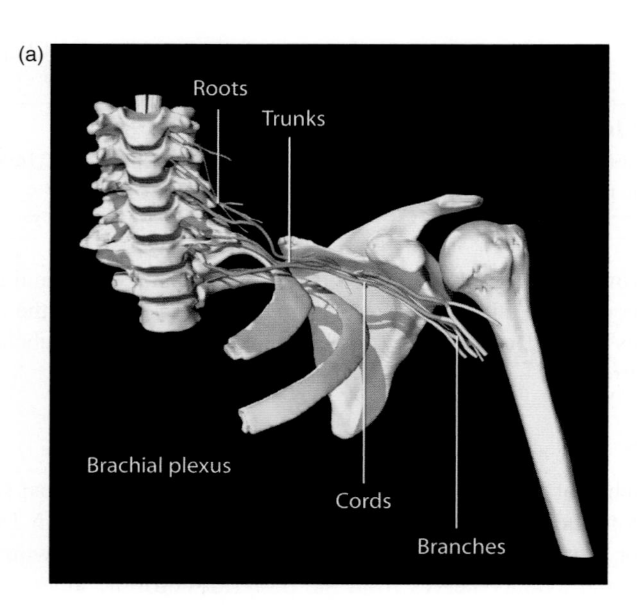

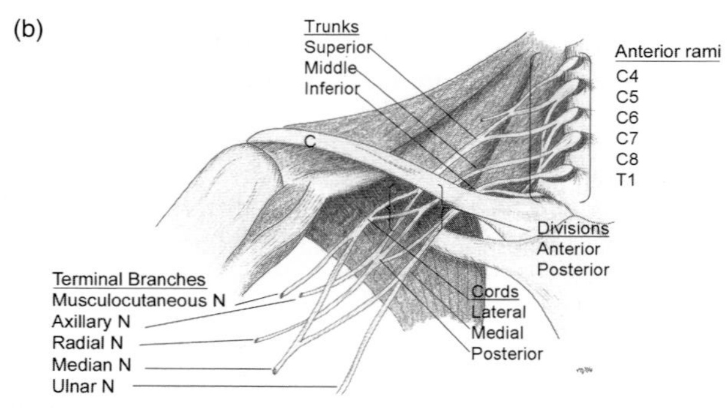

Figure 13.3. The brachial plexus: (**a**) supraclavicular and infraclavicular components of the brachial plexus *in situ* and (**b**) exposed brachial plexus.

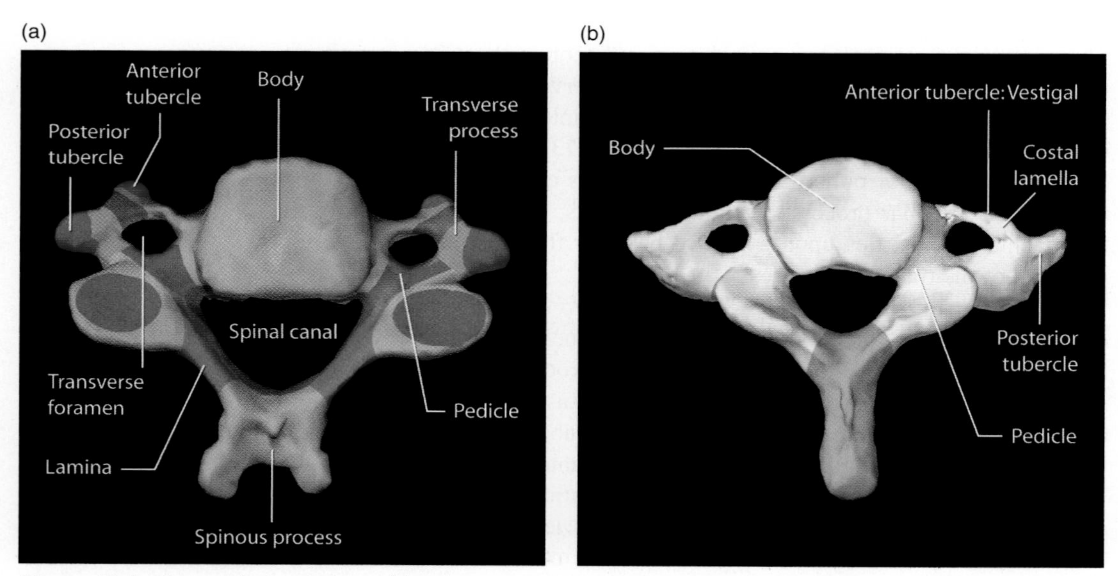

Figure 13.4. The cervical vertebrae: (**a**) C6 vertebra with normal anterior and posterior tubercles at the distal margin of the transverse process. (**b**) The C7 vertebra is identical except the anterior tubercle is vestigial.

Insider Information 13.5
The C7 vertebra is unique in that its transverse process has a large posterior tubercle with the anterior tubercle being vestigial. This anatomical variation allows for identification of the C7 vertebra on ultrasound.

Interscalene Level

The roots pass downward and outward on the groove between the anterior and posterior tubercles of the transverse processes and lie upon the scalenus medius muscle, posterior to the scalenus anterior muscle. The upper trunk unites early, and by the lateral margin of the scalenus anterior, all three trunks are usually formed. The anterior scalenus muscle is important in the anatomical landscape of the subclavian triangle. It arises from the transverse processes of C3–C6 and inserts on the anterior aspect of the first rib, Lisfranc's tubercle, and divides the subclavian artery into three parts. The subclavian vein is anterior to the muscle, separating it from the subclavian artery. The deep layer of the deep cervical fascia that covers the scalene muscles is reflected, forming a sleeve around the subclavian artery and brachial plexus.

Supraclavicular Level

The supraclavicular level of the brachial plexus occupies a space between the lateral margin of the scalenus anterior muscle and the superior border of the clavicle (Figure 13.3). The trunks divide into divisions at the lower aspect of this level and form cords below the level of the clavicle. The plexus is crossed by the transverse cervical artery, and more inferiorly by the inferior belly of the omohyoid muscle, at which point the plexus passes posterior to the clavicle and anterior to the first rib. The plexus lies in close relation to the subclavian artery, with the upper and middle trunks superolateral and the lower trunk lying posterior to the artery.

Infraclavicular and Axillary Levels

The plexus has now passed behind the clavicle, the subclavius muscle, and the suprascapular vessels and lies on the first serration of the serratus anterior and subscapularis muscles. Anteriorly from superficial to deep lie the pectoralis major and minor muscles. The nerves lie within the axillary sheath, a continuation of the deep layer of the deep cervical fascia. The axillary artery is divided into three parts by the pectoralis minor muscle: the first part medial, second part posterior, and the third part lateral to the muscle. The cords are named with respect to their relation to the second part of the axillary artery, e.g., the medial cord lies medial to the axillary artery. In the inferior aspect of the axilla, at the inferior margin of the pectoralis minor, the cords form peripheral nerves (Table 13.1).

Technique

The patient can either lie supine or seated with the examiner seated or standing to the side being examined. The ultrasound examination is divided into five levels: root, interscalene, supraclavicular, infraclavicular, and axillary. The brachial plexus can be examined in its entirety or dedicated to the area of clinical concern. Comparison with the contralateral side can be performed, but as noted previously there is often asymmetry to the plexus.

Root Level

The patient's head is in a neutral position or turned to the opposite side with the arm placed by the side of the body. Place the transducer axially at the level of the thyroid gland and move the probe laterally to the side being examined (Figure 13.5c). The carotid sheath—containing the common carotid artery, internal jugular vein, and the vagus nerve—is identified. The sympathetic trunk lies posteromedial and the phrenic nerve posterior to the carotid sheath.

Posterior to the carotid sheath is the longus colli muscle, behind which is a smooth, continuous, hyperechoic line representing the anterior cortex of the vertebral body (Figure 13.5a). This line has prominent posterior acoustic shadowing, secondary to a strong reflection of the ultrasound beam at the soft tissue–bone interface. As described in detail previously, in the case of the

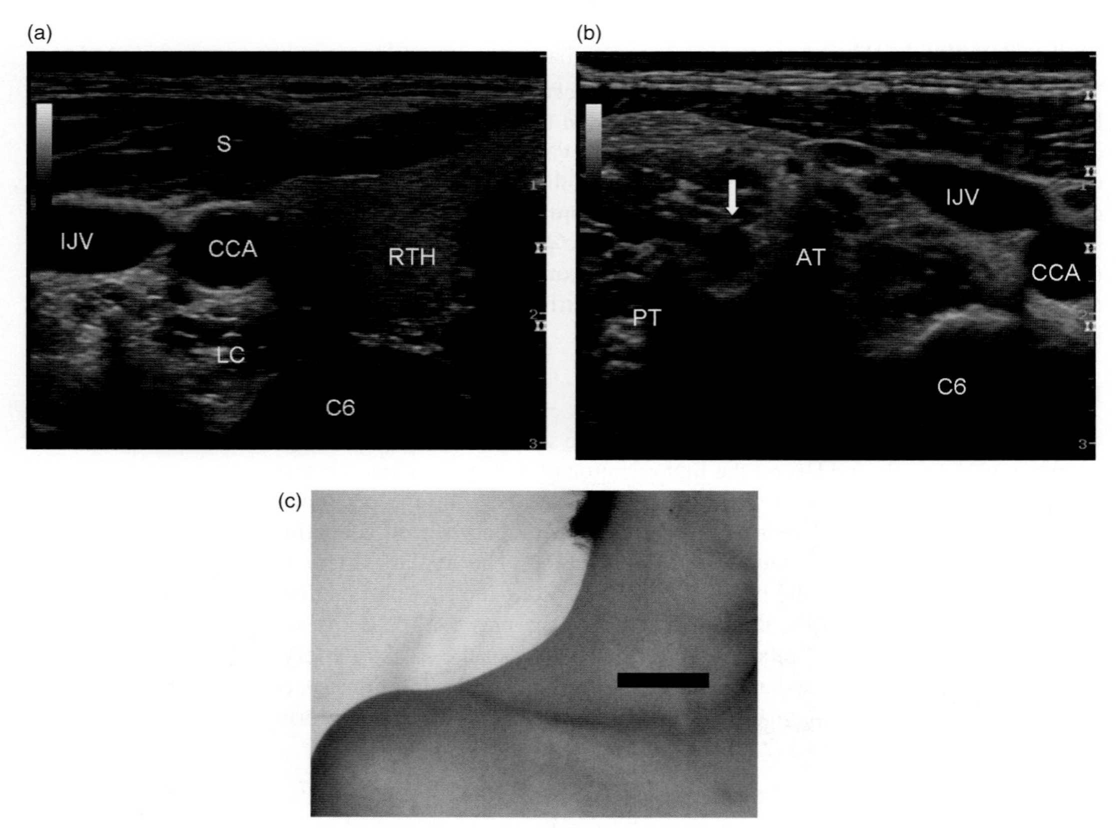

Figure 13.5. **(a)** Transverse ultrasound image of the lower right neck at the level of the thyroid gland and C6 vertebra. **(b)** Transverse ultrasound image of the lower right neck, lateral to **(a)**, demonstrating the anterior and posterior tubercles of the transverse process of C6, and **(c)** its corresponding transducer position. RTH, right lobe thyroid; CCA, common carotid artery; S, sternocleidomastoid muscle; IJV, internal jugular vein; LC, longus colli muscle; AT, anterior tubercle; PT, posterior tubercle of the transverse process; arrow, right C6 root.

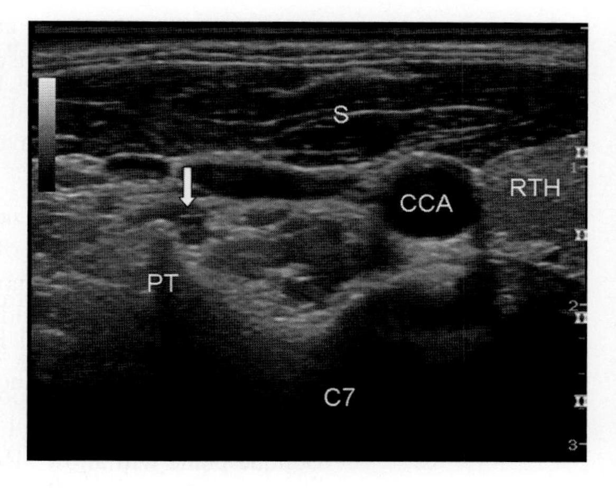

Figure 13.6. Transverse ultrasound image of the lower right neck at the level of the C7 vertebra with a vestigial anterior tubercle and a normal posterior tubercle. RTH, right lobe thyroid; CCA, common carotid artery; S, sternocleidomastoid muscle; PT, posterior tubercle of the transverse process; arrow, right C7 root.

C7 vertebra, the anterior tubercle is vestigial and a large posterior tubercle is present. This allows accurate identification of the C7 vertebra (Figure 13.6).[8]

The anterior ramus of the C7 spinal nerve lies upon the posterior root of the transverse process and is seen axially as a well-defined, hypoechoic, round or oval nodule (Figure 13.6). The hyperechoic fibrillar pattern secondary to the epineurium is poorly visualized proximally, but becomes more apparent as you travel distally along the plexus. Once the C7 anterior ramus is correctly identified, moving the probe in the same plane proximally or distally will allow visualization of the remainder of the brachial plexus, with the caveat that T1 is often difficult to examine as it lies caudal and deep.

By placing the probe in a coronal oblique plane, the longitudinal plane of the spinal nerve can be seen extending into the interscalene region (Figure 13.7). Color or power Doppler may be useful in separating the roots from adjacent vessels.

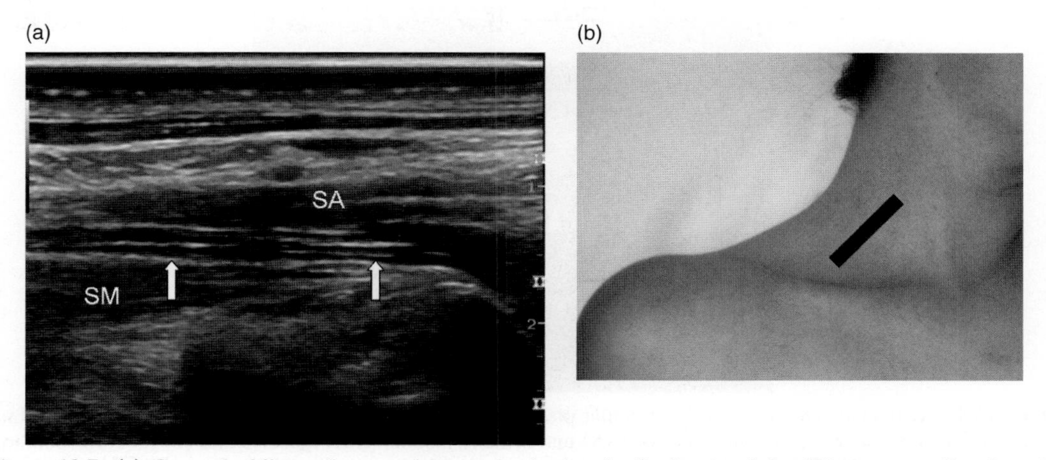

Figure 13.7. **(a)** Coronal oblique ultrasound image in the longitudinal axis of the C6 root extending into the interscalene space with the scalene anterior (SA) and scalene medius (SM) muscles as shown and **(b)** its corresponding transducer position.

> **Insider Information 13.6**
> The hyperechoic fibrillar pattern secondary to the epineurium is poorly visualized in the proximal component of the brachial plexus, but becomes more apparent as you travel distally along the plexus.

Interscalene

At the level of the cricoid cartilage, C6, the longitudinal plane of the roots of the brachial plexus are identified by following the nerve roots laterally in a coronal oblique plane. Turning the transducer 90°, several hypoechoic nodules representing the roots can be seen to converge to form the trunks of the brachial plexus (Figure 13.8a). Moving distally and returning to the coronal oblique plane will allow visualization of the relatively homogeneous, hypoechoic, tubular trunks (Figure 13.8c).[1,5–7,12] Identifying the individual trunks and distal branches may be difficult due to the inherent variation in anatomy.

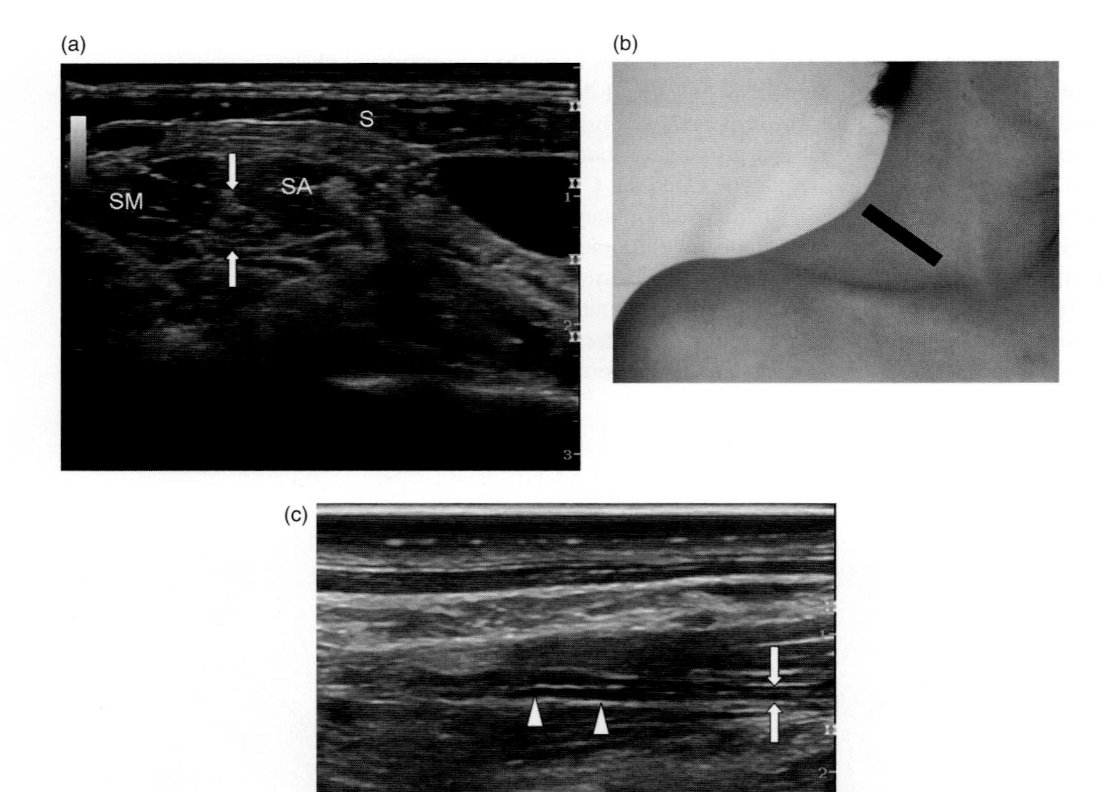

Figure 13.8. **(a)** Interscalene level of the brachial plexus. Transverse oblique ultrasound image of the brachial plexus (arrows) between the scalene anterior (SA) and scalene medius (SM) muscles and **(b)** its corresponding transducer position. **(c)** Coronal oblique ultrasound image in the longitudinal axis roots. The roots can be seen to unite distally and become thicker, thus forming the trunks (arrowheads) of the brachial plexus. S, sternocleidomastoid muscle.

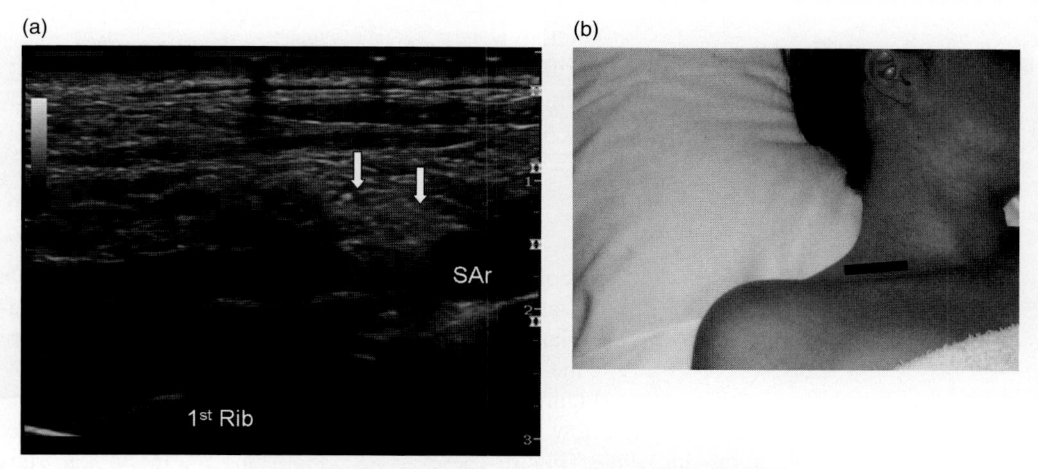

Figure 13.9. Brachial plexus, supraclavicular level. **(a)** Transverse ultrasound image mid-supraclavicular level demonstrating the relationship of the brachial plexus (arrows) to the subclavian artery (SAr) and **(b)** its corresponding transducer position.

Supraclavicular

The probe is again placed in an axial oblique plane directly above the midpoint of the clavicle. The first rib is identified as a smooth, hyperechoic line with the subclavian artery lying superiorly. The plexus lies in close relation to the artery, as detailed previously, and is seen as multiple hypoechoic nodules (Figure 13.9). The transverse cervical artery can be seen passing in front of or through the brachial plexus (Figure 13.10). Turning the probe into the longitudinal axis of the nerves will identify the trunks as hypoechoic tubular structures dividing into their divisions before delving posterior to the clavicle (Figure 13.10c).[1,5–7,12]

Infraclavicular

The probe is placed 2 cm medial to the coracoid process in a parasagittal plane. The plexus lies deep to the pectoralis major and minor muscles. The cords have formed by this time and as per their name lie medial, lateral, and posterior to the axillary artery. Turing the probe in the orthogonal plane allows assessment in their axial plane (Figure 13.11).[1,5,7,12]

Axillary

The ipsilateral arm is abducted and the elbow flexed to 90°. The cords of the plexus maintain their relation to the axillary artery as in the infraclavicular region (Figures 13.11 and 13.12). The short head of the biceps and coracobrachialis lie laterally. The main terminal branches of the plexus can be seen in the inferior aspect of the axilla.[1,7,9,12] For a more detailed review of these terminal branches, please refer to Chapter 12.

Imaging Protocols

The ultrasound imaging protocol will depend upon the clinical question. In the case of brachial plexus block, this is usually selected by the anesthetist,

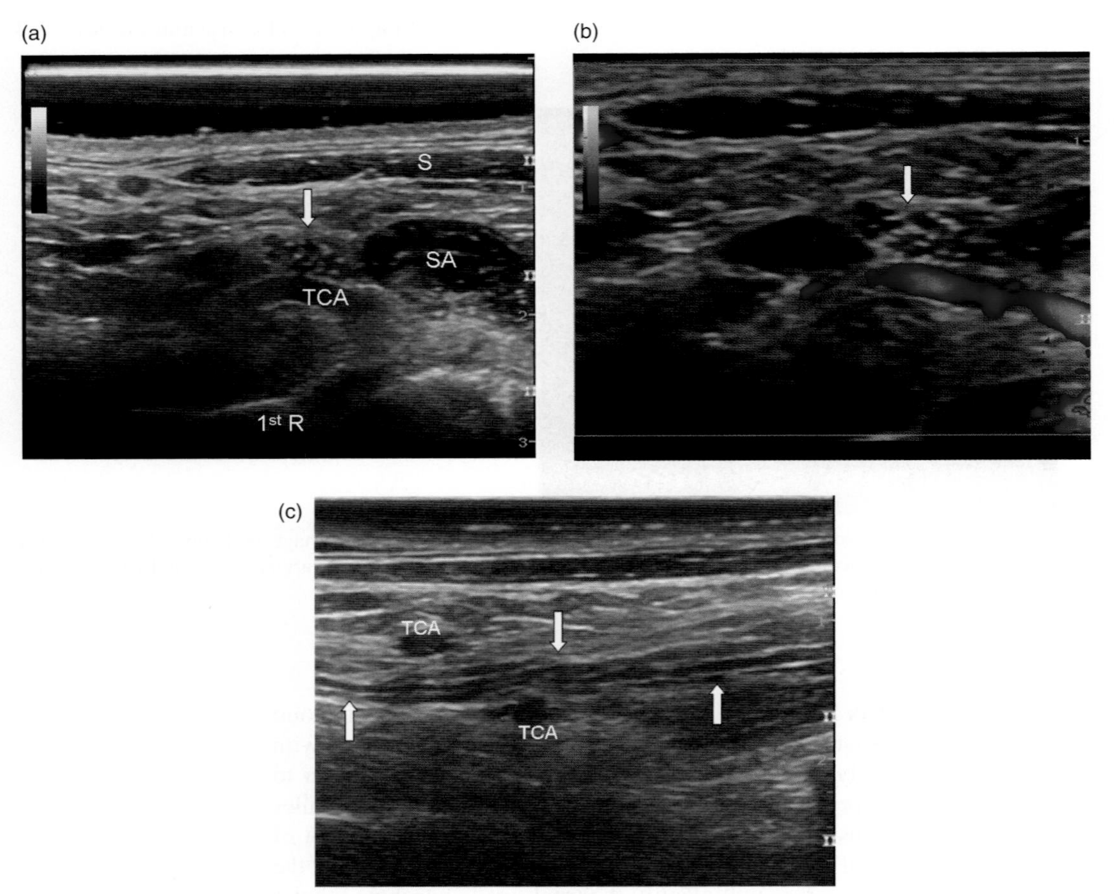

Figure 13.10. Brachial plexus, supraclavicular level. **(a)** Transverse ultrasound image of the proximal supraclavicular level demonstrating the relationship to the transverse cervical artery (TCA), which often passes through or in front of the divisions of the brachial plexus, **(b)** with color Doppler and **(c)** orthogonal longitudinal image. SA, scalene anterior muscle; S, sternocleidomastoid muscle.

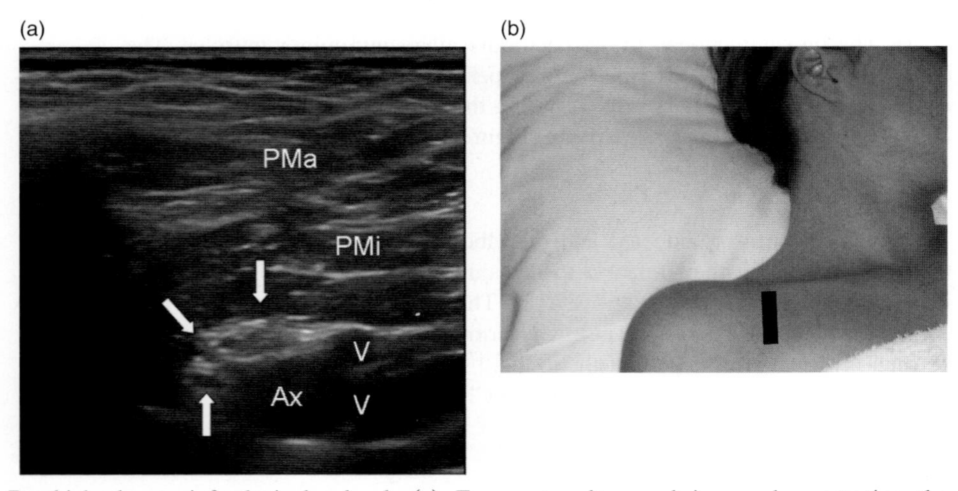

Figure 13.11. Brachial plexus, infraclavicular level. **(a)** Transverse ultrasound image demonstrating the relationship to the axillary artery (Ax) and veins (V) with overlying pectoralis major (PMa) and pectoralis minor (PMi) muscles and **(b)** its corresponding transducer position.

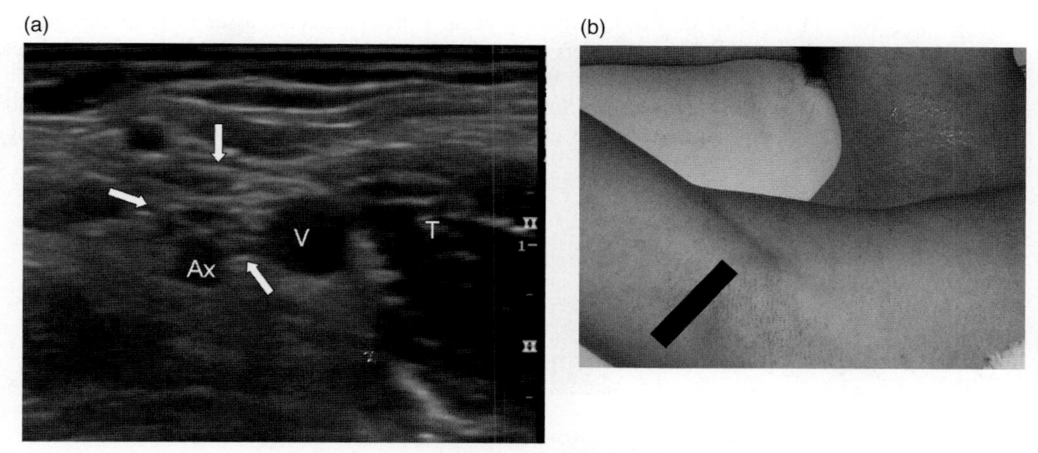

Figure 13.12. Brachial plexus, axillary level. **(a)** Transverse ultrasound image demonstrating the relationship to the axillary artery (Ax) and veins (V) with the adjacent triceps muscle (T) and **(b)** its corresponding transducer position.

and several levels, from interscalene to axillary, may be employed. In the case of trauma, primary or secondary tumors, radiation fibrosis, as well as other etiologies of brachial plexopathies, it is usually clinically apparent if the involved region is supraclavicular or infraclavicular and the examination can be tailored appropriately.

References

1. La Grange P, Foster P, Pretorius L. Application of the Doppler ultrasound bloodflow detector in supraclavicular brachial plexus block. Br J Anaesth 1978;50(9):965–967.
2. Graif M, Martinoli C, Rochkind S et al. Sonographic evaluation of brachial plexus pathology. Eur Radiol 2004;14(2):193–200.
3. De Andres J, Sala-Blanch X. Ultrasound in the practice of brachial plexus anesthesia. Reg Anesth Pain Med 2002;27:77–89.
4. Apan A, Baydar P, Yylmaz S et al. Surface landmarks of brachial plexus: Ultrasound and magnetic resonance imaging for supraclavicular approach with anatomical correlation. Eur J Ultrasound 2001;13(3):191–196.
5. Sheppard D, Iyer R, Fenstermacher R et al. Brachial plexus: Demonstration at US. Radiology 1998;208:402–406.
6. Yang W, Chui P, Metreweli C. Anatomy of the normal brachial plexus revealed by sonography and the role of sonographic guidance in anesthesia of the brachial plexus. AJR 1998;171:1631–1636.
7. Demondion X, Herbinet P, Boutry N et al. Sonographic mapping of the normal brachial plexus. Am J Neuroradiol 2003;24:1303–1309.
8. Martinoli C, Bianchi S, Santacroce E et al. Brachial plexus sonography: A technique for assessing the root level. AJR 2002;179:699–702.
9. Retzl G, Kapral S, Greher M et al. Ultrasonographic findings of the axillary part of the brachial plexus. Anesth Analg 2001;92:1271–1275.
10. Gray H. Brachial plexus. In: The Complete Gray's Anatomy, 16th ed., pp. 897–909. London: Longman, Green, and Co., 1905.

11. Greher M, Retzl G, Niel P et al. Ultrasonographic assessment of topographic anatomy in volunteers suggests a modification of the infraclavicular vertical brachial plexus block. Br J Anaesth 2002;88:632–636.
12. Perlas A, Chan V, Simons M. Brachial plexus examination and localization using ultrasound and electrical stimulation: A volunteer study. Anesthesiology 2003;99(2):426–435.

Appendix

Musculoskeletal Ultrasound Imaging Protocols

Shoulder

Date: ____________
History: ____

Biceps—long head ________________________________
Subscapularis ____________________________________
Infraspinatus ____________________________________
Supraspinatus ____________________________________

Posterior Labrum _________________________________
Spinoglenoid Notch _______________________________
ACL Joint & Acromion _____________________________
Fluid: SASD[1]
Joint ________________________
Bicipital Sheath ________________
Other ________________________
Cortical Margin[2] ______________________________________

Impingement: Supraspinatus ________________________
Subcoracoid ________________________
Other:

____

Additional comments:
____
____

Sonographer ____________________

Note: Tendon tears should be measured in orthogonal planes, distance from key landmarks, e.g., rotator cuff interval for supraspinatus tears, involvement of musculotendinous junction, muscle belly atrophy/fat infiltration, description tear, e.g., partial, delaminating, etc.

[1]Subacromial-subdeltoid bursa.
[2]Greater and lesser tuberosities.

Elbow

Date: ___________
History: ____

Joints Space:

Effusion___________

Synovial Proliferation___________

Cartilage___________

Cortex___________

Coronoid fossa______ Radial fossa______ Radial neck recess[1]______
Olecranon fossa ______

Anterior

Biceps Tendon___________

Brachialis___________

Median Nerve___________

Radial Nerve___________

Medial

Common Flexor Tendon___________

Ulnar Collateral Ligament___________

Medial Epicondyle___________

Lateral

Common Extensor Tendon___________

Radial Collateral Ligament___________

Lateral Epicondyle___________

Posterior

Triceps Tendon___________

Olecranon/Fossa___________

Ulnar Nerve___________

Additional comments:
____
____

Sonographer

Note: Usually a dedicated study performed as per clinical request and/or symptoms.

[1]Includes the proximal radioulnar joint.

Wrist

Date: ____________
History:____

Wrist Volar

Flexor Tendons:
FDS/FDP/FPL____________
FCR/FCU____________
Flexor Retinaculum____________

Nerves: Median N____________
Ulnar N____________

Dorsal

Compartments:

1 ________________________ 2 ________________________
3 ________________________ 4 ________________________
5 ________________________ 6 ________________________

Scapholunate Ligament ____________
Lunotriquetral Ligament____________

Triangular Fibrocartilage Complex

TFC____________
Ulnar Collateral Ligament____________
Tendon Sheath Extensor Carpi Ulnaris____________

Joint

Effusion____________
Synovial Proliferation____________
Cartilage____________
Cortex____________
DRUJ____________ Radiocarpal joint____________
Additional comments:
____
____

Sonographer

Note: Usually a dedicated study performed as per clinical request and/or symptoms.

Hip

Date: ____________
History: ____

Joint:

Effusion____________
Synovial Proliferation____________
Cartilage____________
Cortex____________
Anterior Labrum____________

Anterior

Femoral Triangle____________
Iliopsoas Tendon and Bursa____________
Sartorius____________
Rectus Femoris____________

Medial

Pectineus____________Adductor Longus____________
Adductor Brevis____________Adductor Magnus____________
Gracilis____________

Lateral

Bursae around the Greater Trochanter____________
Gluteus Maximus____________Gluteus Medius____________
Gluteus Minimus____________
Tensor Fascia Lata____________Iliotibial Band____________

Posterior

Gluteus Maximus____________Gluteus Medius____________
Gluteus Minimus____________________________________
Hamstrings: Semimembranosus________________________
Conjoint Tendon Semitendinosus/Biceps Femoris____________
Sciatic Nerve ____________
Additional comments:
____
____

Sonographer

Note: Usually a dedicated study performed as per clinical request and/or symptoms.

Knee

Date: ____________
History: ____

Anterior

Quadriceps Tendon____________
Patellar Tendon____________
Patella ____________
Patellar Retinaculum____________
ACL[1]____________
Superior Joint Recess____________
Bursae____________

Medial

Semitendinous________________________ Gracilis________________________
Sartorius________________________
Medial Collateral Ligament__________________
Medial Meniscus (Anterior Horn and Body)__________________

Lateral

Iliotibial Band_____ Fibular Collateral Ligament_____Biceps Femoris_____
Lateral Meniscus (Anterior Horn and Body)____________
Common Peroneal Nerve____________

Posterior

Semimembranosus____________
Gastrocnemius: Medial Head ____________Lateral Head____________
PCL__________ACL____________
Bursae____
Posterior Horns Menisci: Medial____________Lateral____________
Popliteal Fossa Vessels ____________
Tibial Nerve________

Joint:

Effusion____________
Synovial Proliferation____________
Cartilage____________
Cortex____________

Additional comments:
____
____

Sonographer

Note: Usually a dedicated study performed as per clinical request and/or symptoms.

[1] ACL: may not be identifiable in all patients.

Ankle and Foot

Date: ____________

History: ____

Joint:

Effusion____________

Synovial Proliferation____________

Cartilage____________

Cortex____________

Anterior

Tibialis Anterior____________Extensor Hallucis Longus____________

Extensor Digitorum Longus ____________Peroneus Tertius____________

Posteromedial

Tibialis Posterior____________Flexor Digitorum Longus____________

Flexor Hallucis Longus____________

Flexor Retinaculum____________

Posterolateral

Peroneus Brevis ____________ Peroneus Longus____________

Extensor Retinaculum____________

Posterior

Achilles____________________________________

Retrocalcaneal Bursa__________________________

Retroachillean Bursa__________________________

Kagar's Fat Pad ____________

Ligaments

Anterior Tibiofibular________Distal Interosseous Membrane____________

Lateral: Anterior Talofibular______

Calcaneofibular____________

Posterior Talofibular[1]____________

Medial: Deltoid________

Additional comments:

____

____

Sonographer

Note: Usually a dedicated study performed as per clinical request and/or symptoms.

[1]May not be identifiable in all patients.

Soft Tissue Mass: Upper/Lower Limb

Date: ________
History: ____

Site[1] ________

Overlying Skin________

Size AP_____Longitudinal_____Transverse

Shape_____Contour[2] ______

Internal Echotexture[3] ________

Compressible[4] ________

Posterior Acoustic Enhancement________

Doppler________

Extension[5] ________

Surrounding Fluid________

Surrounding Tissues (Displacement/Invasion)________

Examine adjacent joint if in close proximity

Additional comments:
____
____

Sonographer

Notes

1. Plane, e.g., subcutaneous, intramuscular, intermuscular.
2. Contour, e.g., smooth, lobulated, ill-defined, etc.
3. In/homogeneous, hyper/hypo/anechoic, calcification, air, vascularity.
4. Compressibility: also assess with Doppler.
5. Extension, e.g., along nerve or fascial plane.

Synovitis Protocol: Wrist and Hand

Date: ________
History: ____

Distal Radioulnar Joint.____________________________________

	1	2	3	4	5
MCPJ					
PIPJ					
DIPJ					

Radiocarpal Joint
Space____________________

Midcarpal Joint
Space____________________

Carpometacarpal
Joints____________________

Additional comments:
____
____

Sonographer

Notes

1. Usually a dedicated examination limited to the symptomatic joints is performed and agreed upon with referring clinicians.
2. Assess joints in longitudinal and transverse planes, volar and dorsal aspects, and, where accessible, the lateral joint recesses.
3. Assess the following: (a) fluid and synovium: compressibility and displacement, power Doppler; (b) articular cartilage; (c) cortex: smooth/irregular/erosions.
4. Overlying tendons and sheaths.

Synovitis Protocol: Ankle and Foot

Date:________
History: ____

Ankle Joint____________________________________
Intermetatarsal Joint Spaces__________________________

	1	2	3	4	5
MTPJ					
PIPJ					
DIPJ					

Tarsometatarsal Joint Spaces_____________________________
Additional comments:
____
____

Sonographer

Notes:

1. Usually a dedicated examination limited to the symptomatic joints is performed and agreed upon with referring clinicians.
2. Assess joints in longitudinal and transverse planes, volar and dorsal aspects, and, where accessible, the lateral joint recesses.
3. Assess the following: (a) fluid and synovium: compressibility and displacement, power Doppler; (b) articular cartilage; (c) cortex: smooth/irregular/erosions.
4. Overlying tendons and sheaths.

Index

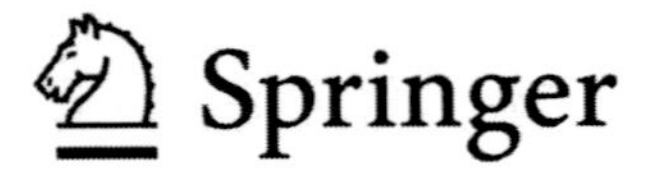